ISSUES IN BIOMEDICAL ETHICS

Reproductive Health and Human R

The concept of reproductive health promises to pl
women's health and rights around the world. It was ....
United Nations conference in 1994, but remains controversial because of the challenge
it presents to conservative agencies: it challenges policies of suppressing public discussion on human sexuality and regulating its private expressions. *Reproductive Health
and Human Rights* is designed to equip health care providers and administrators to
integrate ethical, legal, and human rights principles in protection and promotion of
reproductive health, and to inform lawyers and women's health advocates about
aspects of medicine and health care systems that affect reproduction.

Rebecca Cook, Bernard Dickens, and Mahmoud Fathalla, leading international
authorities on reproductive medicine, human rights, medical law, and bioethics, integrate their disciplines to provide an accessible but comprehensive introduction to
reproductive and sexual health. They analyse fifteen case studies of recurrent problems,
focusing particularly on resource-poor settings. Approaches to resolution are considered at clinical and health system levels. They also consider kinds of social change
that would relieve the underlying conditions of reproductive health dilemmas. Supporting the explanatory chapters and case studies are extensive resources of epidemiological
data, human rights documents, and research materials and websites on reproductive
and sexual health.

In explaining ethics, law, and human rights to health care providers and administrators, and reproductive health to lawyers and women's health advocates, the authors
explore and illustrate limitations and dysfunctions of prevailing health systems and
their legal regulation, but also propose opportunities for reform. They draw on the values and principles of ethics and human rights recognized in national and international
legal systems, to guide health care providers and administrators, lawyers, governments,
and national and international agencies and legal tribunals.

Reproductive Health and Human Rights will be an invaluable resource for all those
working to improve services and legal protection for women around the world.

ISSUES IN BIOMEDICAL ETHICS

General Editors
John Harris and Søren Holm

Consulting Editors
Raanan Gillon and Bonnie Steinbock

The late twentieth century witnessed dramatic technological developments in biomedical science and in the delivery of health care, and these developments have brought with them important social changes. All too often ethical analysis has lagged behind these changes. The purpose of this series is to provide lively, up-to-date, and authoritative studies for the increasingly large and diverse readership concerned with issues in biomedical ethics—not just health care trainees and professionals, but also philosophers, social scientists, lawyers, social workers, and legislators. The series will feature both single-author and multi-author books, short and accessible enough to be widely read, each of them focused on an issue of outstanding current importance and interest. Philosophers, doctors, and lawyers from a number of countries feature among the authors lined up for the series.

Reproductive Health and Human Rights

Integrating Medicine, Ethics, and Law

REBECCA J. COOK,

BERNARD M. DICKENS,

and

MAHMOUD F. FATHALLA

CLARENDON PRESS · OXFORD

OXFORD

UNIVERSITY PRESS

Great Clarendon Street, Oxford OX2 6DP

Oxford University Press is a department of the University of Oxford.
It furthers the University's objective of excellence in research, scholarship,
and education by publishing worldwide in

Oxford New York

Auckland Bangkok Buenos Aires Cape Town Chennai
Dar es Salaam Delhi Hong Kong Istanbul Karachi Kolkata
Kuala Lumpur Madrid Melbourne Mexico City Mumbai Nairobi
São Paulo Shanghai Taipei Tokyo Toronto

Oxford is a registered trade mark of Oxford University Press
in the UK and in certain other countries

Published in the United States
by Oxford University Press Inc., New York

British Library Cataloguing in Publication Data

Data available

Library of Congress Cataloging in Publication Data

Data available

ISBN 0-19-924132-5
ISBN 0-19-924133-3 (pbk.)

10 9 8 7 6 5 4 3 2 1

Typeset by Graphicraft Limited, Hong Kong
Printed in Great Britain
on acid-free paper by Biddles Ltd., Guildford & King's Lynn

Foreword

The concept of reproductive health is one of the landmarks of twentieth-century social history. Developed as the result of experience in the 1970s and the 1980s, the consensus at the 1994 International Conference on Population and Development gave it universal validity. The greatest single difference between women in rich countries and women in poor ones is in their reproductive health status. Reproductive health—an important component of the 'state of physical, mental and social well-being' that defines health—is in jeopardy when women lack the power to realize their reproductive and other goals in life. As Chapter 2 of this book rightly concludes, the 'powerlessness of women is a serious health hazard'.

The danger to women's reproductive health comes from multiple oppressions and denials of opportunities and choice in their families, communities, cultures, and national political systems. Relieving this burden has become a human rights commitment for legal systems and practical systems of ethics alike.

This book, the work of three of the leading experts in the medical, legal, and ethical advancement of the human right to health care in general and to women's reproductive health in particular, sets out the elements of the medical health care system, and the ethical, legal, and human rights dimensions of reproductive and sexual health. It goes on to analyse fifteen representative case studies drawn from different regions of the world and experiences such as women frequently face in real life. The emphasis is on resource-poor settings in which service providers have little support.

The authors examine the medical background and the ethical, legal, and human rights aspects of each case, indicating options for response at the levels of clinical care and health system development. In addition they suggest ways for health service providers, working together as professionals and in collaboration with others in their communities, to address the social factors that create disadvantage and distress. The authors take care not to be definitive, but rather invite readers to understand their reasoning and to become engaged themselves in determining how to analyse medical, ethical, legal, and human rights issues.

The book is both an academic text and a training tool designed to equip health care providers to uphold and advance the human rights principles on which reproductive and sexual health depends. It will also help lawyers, ethical analysts, health policy administrators, and legislative aides to understand how laws appropriate for earlier times can create ethical and practical difficulties today. Such laws often fail to promote women's reproductive health. They fail to protect families, which can flourish only when mothers, wives, and women care-givers enjoy health, self-esteem, and the power of reproductive choice.

The book will also be a resource for those who wish to undertake further research. It includes charts of reproductive health statistics, countries' human rights treaty commitments, and the texts and summaries of key international documents and guidelines, including a table of annotated legal cases, a select chapter-specific bibliography, and an annotated list of relevant websites.

I believe that the book will inspire its readers, and I hope that it will become a springboard for some of them to plunge into the promotion of women's rights in general and reproductive rights in particular.

Dr Nafis Sadik

Special Adviser on Gender Issues to the United Nations Secretary-General, and former Executive Director of the United Nations Population Fund

September 2002

Acknowledgements

The authors are grateful to many people for providing invaluable explanations of different dimensions of reproductive and sexual health, reviewing particular sections of previous drafts and providing data for Part III, laws, policies, and court decisions, and often their translations. They include Dina Bogecho, Anne Carbert, Beatriz Galli, Noah Gitterman, Jaya Sagade, Julie Stanchieri, Kibrom Teklehaimanot, all of our students at the Faculty of Law of the University of Toronto during the last five years, and Marylin Raisch, the International and Comparative Law Librarian of our Law Library. The Dean of the Law Faculty, Ron Daniels, facilitated this project in endless ways, not the least of which was providing release time from teaching for two of its authors. Our colleagues at the Center for Reproductive Law and Policy in New York, including Anika Rahman, Kathy Hall Martinez, Luisa Cabal, Monica Roa, and Julia Zajkowski, provided invaluable assistance in finding laws and providing explanations of how they are implemented in particular national contexts. We thank our colleagues at IPAS, including Charlotte Hord, Liz MacGuire, and Barbara Crane, for holding our feet to the fire to ensure that the case studies might make a difference in practice.

Our colleagues in Colombia at Profamilia and their Legal Services for Women, Maria Isabel Plata and Maria Christina Calderon, were tireless in their support of this project, and overcame our inability to read Spanish, as did our colleague, Pedro Morales, in Mexico. Charles Ngwena in South Africa provided insights and scholarship that proved invaluable, and Ken Wafula in Kenya provided information that gave us insight into the lives of adolescent girls facing female genital cutting. One of the authors remains grateful to the ReproCen project of the University of the Philippines for inviting her to give a series of lectures based on a previous draft of the book in their Law School and Medical School.

We are all grateful to the Committee on Women's Sexual and Reproductive Rights of the International Federation of Gynecology and Obstetrics for being able to test the ideas and insights reflected in the book at meetings of the Committee. We thank our colleagues at the World Health Organization, Paul Van Look, Iqbal Shah, and Jane Cottingham, who perceptively reviewed drafts, and Jelka Zupan and Carla Maklouf Obermeyer, who provided information and insights, as did Wariara Mbugua and Wilma Doedens of the United Nations Population Fund. Vasantha Kandiah of the United Nations Population Division was overly generous with her time and explanations of

UN data that helped us to prepare the chart of country data on reproductive indicators in Part III.

Tracey Pegg, the coordinator of the Law Faculty's International Reproductive and Sexual Health Law Programme, was steady and constant in her management of the project throughout its years of development, making the task of preparation of the text not only possible, but enjoyable. Jeanette Williams responded readily to our untimely calls for help in typing and retyping manuscripts. Peter Momtchiloff, our editor at Oxford University Press (OUP), proved insightful with his suggestions for the book, and John Harris of Manchester University, the overall co-editor of the series in which this book appears, was endlessly patient. We benefited from and are grateful to the anonymous reviewers, to whom OUP submitted the text, for their observations and recommendations.

Two of the authors were able to work on the book for a month at Rockefeller Foundation's Bellagio Study and Conference Center in Italy, and will always be grateful for the serenity and inspiration that they derived from their time in residence and the gracious hospitality. The three authors are indebted to our funders, Ford Foundation, Hewlett Foundation, and UNFPA. They provided us with the means, but even more importantly the understanding, to undertake the research and writing of the text and for the three of us to meet in person at least three times a year for four years to discuss drafts, design case studies, and plan future drafts.

Earlier versions of sections of chapters in Part I have appeared in previous publications, and have been revised for Chapters 2, 3, 5 and 7. Earlier versions of sections of Chapters 2 and 3 appeared in M. F. Fathalla, *From Obstetrics and Gynecology to Women's Health: The Road Ahead* (New York and London: Parthenon, 1997). Earlier versions of sections of Chapters 5 and 7 appeared in R. J. Cook and B. M. Dickens, *Considerations for Formulating Reproductive Health Laws* (Geneva: World Health Organization, 2000) and earlier versions of parts of Chapter 6 appeared in R. J. Cook and B. M. Dickens, *Advancing Safe Motherhood through Human Rights* (Geneva: World Health Organization, 2001).

Summary Table of Contents

Detailed Table of Contents

Part II. From Principle to Practice

List of Tables

Abbreviations

ACOG	American College of Obstetricians and Gynecologists
ADR	alternative dispute resolution
AGI	Alan Guttmacher Institute
AIDS	Acquired Immune Deficiency Syndrome
CAT	Committee against Torture
CATWAP	Coalition against Trafficking in Women—Asia Pacific
CEDAW	Committee on the Elimination of Discrimination against Women
CERD	Committee on the Elimination of Racial Discrimination
CESCR	Committee on Economic, Social and Cultural Rights
CIOMS	Council for International Organizations of Medical Sciences
CLADEM	Comité de América Latina y el Caribe para la Defensa de los Derechos de la Mujer
ComMAT	Commonwealth Medical Association Trust
CRC	Committee on the Rights of the Child
CRLP	Center for Reproductive Law and Policy
CRO	contract research organization
DALY	disability-adjusted life year
DHS	Demographic and Health Survey
EC	emergency contraception
FGC	female genital cutting
FCI	Family Care International
FGM	female genital mutilation
FHI	Family Health International
FIGO	International Federation of Gynecology and Obstetrics
HIV	human immunodeficiency virus
HRC	Human Rights Committee
ICASO	International Council of AIDS Services Organizations
ICPD	International Conference on Population and Development
ICSI	intra-cytoplasmic sperm injection
ICTR	International Criminal Tribunal for Rwanda
ICTY	International Criminal Tribunal for the Former Yugoslavia
ILO	International Labour Organization
INVIMA	Instituto Nacional de Vigilancia de Medicamentos y Alimentos
IPPF	International Planned Parenthood Federation
IRB	Institutional Review Board
IVF	*in vitro* fertilization

IWRAW	International Women's Rights Action Watch
MAR	medically assisted reproduction
MCH	maternal and child health
MMR	maternal mortality ratio
ODA	official development assistance
PAHO	Pan American Health Organization
PATH	Program for Appropriate Technology in Health
PGD	pre-implantation genetic diagnosis
PHR	Partners for Health Reform
PHMWG	Population and Health Materials Working Group
RHR	Reproductive Health and Research
RTI	reproductive tract infection
RVF	recto-vaginal fistula
RVVF	recto-vesico-vaginal fistula
STD	sexually transmitted disease
STI	sexually transmitted infection
UNDP	United Nations Development Programme
UNFPA	United Nations Population Fund
UNHCHR	United Nations High Commissioner for Human Rights
UNICEF	United Nations Children's Emergency Fund
URD	Unité de Recherche Démographique
VVF	vesico-vaginal fistula
WHO	World Health Organization
WHRR	Women's Human Rights Resources
WMA	World Medical Association

Biographical Notes

REBECCA J. COOK AB (Barnard), MA (Tufts), MPA (Harvard), JD (Georgetown), LL M (Columbia), JSD (Columbia), called to the Bar of Washington, DC, holds the Faculty of Law Chair in International Human Rights and is a Professor in the Faculty of Law, the Faculty of Medicine, and the Joint Centre for Bioethics at the University of Toronto; Co-Director, International Programme on Reproductive and Sexual Health Law, University of Toronto. She is ethical and legal issues co-editor of the *International Journal of Gynecology and Obstetrics*, and serves on the editorial advisory boards of *Human Rights Quarterly* and *Reproductive Health Matters*. Her publications include over 150 books, articles, and reports in the areas of international human rights, the law relating to women's health, and feminist ethics. She is the recipient of the Certificate of Recognition for Outstanding Contribution to Women's Health by the International Federation of Gynecologists and Obstetricians, and is a Fellow of the Royal Society of Canada.

BERNARD M. DICKENS LL B, LL M, Ph.D. (Law-Criminology), LL D (Medical Jurisprudence) (London), a member of the English Bar and the Ontario Bar, is the Dr William M. Scholl Professor of Health Law and Policy in the Faculty of Law, the Faculty of Medicine, and the Joint Centre for Bioethics at the University of Toronto. He is legal articles co-editor of the *Journal of Law, Medicine and Ethics*, co-editor of ethical and legal issues of the *International Journal of Gynecology and Obstetrics*, and a member of editorial boards of several journals including the *American Journal of Law and Medicine* and *Medicine and Law*. His writing includes about 350 publications, including books, chapters in books, articles, and reports, primarily in the field of medical and health law. He was a member of the Board of Governors of the American Society of Law, Medicine and Ethics, and is a former Society President. He is now a member of the Board of Governors of the World Association for Medical Law, and an Association Vice President. He is a Fellow of the Royal Society of Canada.

MAHMOUD F. FATHALLA MD (Cairo), Ph.D. (Edinburgh); Honorary Fellow of the American College of Obstetricians and Gynecologists; Fellow ad eund. Royal College of Obstetricians and Gynecologists; Dr Honoris Causa (Uppsala, Sweden); Dr Honoris Causa (Helsinki, Finland); Dr Honoris Causa (Toronto, Canada); Professor of Obstetrics and Gynaecology and former Dean of the Medical School, Assiut University, Egypt; former Director of the UNDP/UNFPA/WHO/World Bank Special Programme of Research, Development and Research Training in Human Reproduction; former Senior Advisor, Biomedical and Reproductive Health Research, the Rockefeller Foundation; Chairman of the WHO Global Advisory Committee on Health Research; Past President of the International Federation of Gynecology and Obstetrics; former Chairman of the International Medical Advisory Panel of the International Planned Parenthood Federation; author of more than 150 scientific publications; co-editor of the FIGO Teaching Manual in Human Reproduction (English, French, Spanish); editor of the first World Report on Women's Health in 1994; author of *From Obstetrics and Gynecology to Women's Health—The Road Ahead* (New York, London: Parthenon, 1997).

PART I

Medical, Ethical, and Legal Principles

1

Introduction and Overview

Understanding of reproductive health has advanced significantly in the last decade. The field of reproductive health is different from other fields of health care. The inputs from society at large, and the consequences for that society, vary markedly from other areas of medicine and health, not least because human reproduction is the means by which each society perpetuates itself and its traditions. No society, no religion, no culture, and no system of national law has been neutral about issues of human reproduction. Advancing reproductive health, much more than other fields of health, requires inputs from health care providers, health policy makers, legislators, lawyers, human rights activists, women's groups, and the society at large.

Health professionals tend to be relatively uninformed of how the laws by which they are bound have developed, and of the range of legal arguments they may invoke to advance their purposes. Similarly, laws that relate to reproductive health have often been developed ideologically, with little health-related understanding of how they are likely to affect or obstruct necessary clinical care of patients and the reproductive well-being of communities. Legal management of matters affecting reproduction and reproductive choice, whether by legislators, legal administrators or practitioners or judges, is undertaken with little perception of their medical or societal implications for reproductive health. Further, health care providers and administrators, and legislators, tend to work within familiar local frameworks of law and health policy, without specific regard to the significance of human rights principles applicable to reproductive health to which their states have committed themselves.

Health care providers, health policy makers, and lawyers address reproductive health from different perspectives. A primary reason for writing this book is to explain these different perspectives in ways that facilitate dialogue and collaboration among different groups, in order to enhance formulation of reproductive health laws and policies, and to expand and improve the quality of reproductive health services.

This book aims to equip practitioners of broadly defined disciplines that affect health to understand how medical knowledge, ethics, and law, including the part of law that encompasses human rights values, can interact with each other to improve reproductive and sexual health. The purpose is not so much to deepen understanding of origins and responses to reproductive and sexual ill-health, but rather to widen it.

The identification of reproductive and sexual health as a topic worthy of attention and a goal worthy of commitment is of recent origin. The first international adoption of a definition of reproductive health dates only to 1994, at the United Nations' International Conference on Population and Development (ICPD), held in Cairo. This book promotes the view that reproductive and sexual health is a topic that is not only legitimate, but that compels the urgent attention of health care professionals and allies in other fields committed to the achievement of individual and communal health in just and humane societies. It is aimed to inform those familiar with medical and health aspects of human reproduction and sexuality, who work in governmental and non-governmental organizations and private health care practice, about ethical, legal, and human rights dimensions of health care practice. It is also aimed to inform lawyers, human rights activists, ethicists, and others about medical factors relevant to the protection and promotion of reproductive and sexual health.

There is no single discipline, perspective, standard of practice, or ethic that will resolve the many dilemmas, often amounting to crises, in the protection of reproductive and sexual health. For instance, adolescents' unwanted pregnancies cannot be reduced through sex education and access to contraception if girls and young women are at risk of sexual abuse by men, such as those having family, institutional, or other authority over them. Similarly, there is no single level of abstraction that can base comprehensive policies. Failures of reproductive and sexual health have to be addressed at all levels, including at the individual clinical care level, health system and public health levels, and the underlying level of socio-economic conditions and resources. There is also an international level of approach, through policies of intergovernmental and international agencies concerned with health care in particular and worldwide economic, environmental, and other equity in general. Further, the promotion of reproductive and sexual health engages the instruments of national and international public-sector administration, but also concerns private-sector agencies at all levels, from private health care practitioners in clinics to multinational commercial corporations that engage in research, development, and marketing of health care services and products.

A motivating factor in writing this book is the recognition that reproductive and sexual ill-health does not occur in a vacuum, but is conditioned by cultures, laws, and values. It is not the purpose of the book to prescribe solutions to transcending problems of social injustice, but to equip readers to identify key questions and how they can contribute to answering them to advance the reproductive and sexual health of the patients and communities they are committed to serve.

Part I of the book is foundational, addressing basic elements in medical care of reproductive and sexual health, the operation of health systems, ethical analysis, the origin and operation of laws, human rights analysis and the implementation of legal and human rights principles to advance health and well-being. Because the book is intended for multidisciplinary use, many readers will be familiar with the materials in one or more of these chapters. Accordingly, each chapter is intended to be self-contained, since readers may prefer first to address the materials with which they are less familiar. The book is not like a novel, to be read from the beginning in sequence. Readers can begin with any chapter in Part I, and then move to others of their choice before addressing the case studies in Part II that bring together the elements in Part I, reinforced by the data and materials presented in Part III.

Chapter 2 of Part I deals with how the concept of reproductive health has been fashioned in response to the fragmentation of existing services related to health in reproduction and the medical aspects of sexuality. Its focus is that reproductive health implies that people are able to have a satisfying and safe sex life, the capability to reproduce, and the freedom to decide if, when, and how often to do so. The succeeding chapter defines a health care system as the mechanism in any society that transforms or metabolizes inputs of knowledge, human and financial resources into outputs of services relevant to the health concerns in that society. It emphasizes that the promotion of health is not the domain of the health care system alone, since other social systems bear upon the effective, humane, and equitable operation of the health system in each society.

Chapter 4 presents the basic materials of ethical analysis, addressing the origins of the modern concept of pluralistic bioethics and approaches to bioethical orientations, principles, and levels of analysis. Application of ethical assessment is related to applications of law and principles of human rights. Chapter 5, which deals with legal origins and principles, draws heavily on materials most familiar to the authors, but provides a foundation for legal analysis and perception that readers can apply to the legal systems with which they are most familiar to establish comparisons and contrasts. For instance, the contribution that lawyers and legal analysis can make to promotion of reproductive and sexual health may be comparable across different jurisdictions, although the raw materials of the law may differ, sometimes significantly.

Human rights principles are addressed in Chapter 6, identifying first the sources and nature of human rights, particularly those most relevant to reproductive and sexual health. Key human rights are then specified, and amplified on the basis of authoritative interpretations, including consideration of how they may be applicable to reproductive and sexual health. The final, seventh chapter of Part I addresses how legal and human rights principles may be applied, particularly at national but also at international levels. The focus is not simply on development of legal claims to overcome adversaries through conflict, but to achieve success through encouragement and facilitation of compliance with human rights values and collaboration with governmental and other agencies in commitment of their resources to the equitable advancement of reproductive and sexual health.

Part II of the book works through a series of representative case studies that health care providers may face, particularly in resource-poor settings. The studies identify medical, ethical, legal, and human rights aspects of the cases, showing how analysis of these aspects can produce approaches through clinical care, health care systems management and social action to address the underlying conditions from which the cases emerge. The purpose of these exercises is not to present definitive analyses and solutions, but to present readers with methods of analysis illustrating applications of the medical, ethical, legal, and human rights materials outlined in Part I. The hope is to equip readers to undertake their own analyses relevant to their own circumstances, and to develop approaches, at different levels, that they consider feasible and suitable in their localities and circumstances. This includes readers' capacity to adopt different analyses and suggestions from those presented in the case studies.

Behind the case-study approach is the hope that readers will be better able to diagnose the incidence and conditions of the reproductive and sexual ill-health with which they are confronted, by (1) understanding the risk factors that lead to ill-health; (2) understanding the nature and scope of the problems; (3) understanding the conditioning causes of ill-health, including medical causes, health systems causes, legal and policy causes, and underlying causes, including social, cultural, and economic causes. Comprehension of these elements contributes to making an adequate local assessment of why and how particular situations of ill-health have arisen, and means by which they may be resolved and their repetition prevented.

Because the book is designed to present health care providers with general overviews of ethical, legal, and human rights perspectives of reproductive and sexual health care conditions, it has a somewhat abstract character. The case studies in Part II may indicate environments, usually of scarce resources, in which they are situated, but they lack the depth of detail possessed by real-life cases. They propose approaches that are justifiable in principle, but that may be confounded by details of practice that cannot be written into brief case studies. Readers should consider the analyses and proposed approaches against the realities of their local circumstances, and develop their own analyses and approaches that are conditioned by these distinctive circumstances. Proposed solutions to abstract problems may play out differently in practice. Local realities may make certain theoretical approaches impracticable, requiring those who face those realities to be resourceful in different ways. They may also provide opportunities that can be recognized in the immediate circumstances, by those with the vision to see them and the inspiration to take them. The challenge of writing the book will be exceeded by the challenge we hope readers will accept of applying its overviews and explanations in their own real cases, to improve the reproductive and sexual health of those they can influence.

Part III of the book presents selected data and sources of relevant information. They are intended to familiarize readers, from all disciplinary backgrounds and interests, with health information, human rights treaty sources and commitments, and, for instance, key recommendations that human rights monitoring agencies have presented concerning matters of health and equitable access to services.

The central thrust of the book concerns women's health, although it does not underestimate or devalue reproductive and sexual health concerns of men. The medical discipline that is commonly most engaged in issues of reproductive and sexual health is obstetrics and gynaecology, whose patients are women. Accordingly, the book addresses relations between women and men by reference to the natural, biological differences, and the socially structured difference that identifies certain characteristics, capacities, and social roles with women, and different characteristics, capacities, and social roles with men. Social structuring often rests on deeply held cultural, religious, social, and other dispositions that so condition attitudes as to make them appear as self-evident truths or laws of nature that do not require analysis. The different roles discharged by members of the two sexes may be considered not simply a feature of a given society, but the very condition of the society existing. That is, it may be considered basic to a society that men, as leaders, be the physical protectors and bread winners for their families, that women are care-givers to child, elderly, and disabled family members, and that men, as gatekeepers of family economic and other resources, will make the critical decisions for them.

However, social practice commonly departs from these gendered stereotypes. For instance, many families, including those with partners of both sexes, depend on women to discharge the masculine function of providing family sustenance and guidance, and on men to discharge the feminine function of providing care. Accordingly, the book tends to be woman-centred and to reflect the inequality that women frequently experience. Its aim, however, is to show how incorporation of human rights principles can facilitate the pursuit of reproductive and sexual health in circumstances of social justice and equity.

2

Reproductive and Sexual Health

1. *Overview*

The concept of reproductive health has recently emerged in response to the fragmentation of the existing services related to health in reproduction, and to their orientation. With the positive definition of health as a state of complete physical, mental, and social well-being and not merely the absence of disease or infirmity, reproductive health therefore implies that people are able to have a satisfying and safe sex life and that they have the capability to reproduce and the freedom to decide if, when, and how often to do so.

Reproductive health is not just a major health issue; it is also a development issue, and a human rights issue. Because of reasons of impact, urgency, and inequity, reproductive health is a global concern.

A definition of sexual health should include the ability to enjoy mutually fulfilling sexual relationships, freedom from sexual abuse, coercion, or harassment, safety from sexually transmitted diseases, and success in achieving or in preventing pregnancy.

Reproductive health is an important component of health for both women and men, but it is more critical, however, for women. A major burden of disease in females is related to their reproductive function and reproductive potential, and the way in which society treats or mistreats women because of their gender.

Health for women is more than reproductive health. Being a woman has implications for health. Women have specific health needs related to their sexual and reproductive function, collectively expressed in the reproductive health package. Women have an elaborate reproductive system that is vulnerable to dysfunction or disease, even before it functions or after it ceases to function. Women are subject to the same diseases of other body systems that can affect men, but their disease patterns often differ from those of men because of women's genetic constitution, hormonal environment, or gender-evolved lifestyle behaviour. Diseases of other body systems, or their treatments, may interact with conditions of the reproductive system or its function. Because women are women, they are subject to social dysfunctions that impact on their physical, mental, or social health. Examples include female genital cutting (or mutilation), sexual abuse, and domestic violence. Men have reproductive health concerns of their own, but, in addition, their health status and behaviours also affect women's reproductive health.

Determination of health in general, and reproductive health in particular, includes other factors beyond health care services. Lifestyle, behaviour, and socio-economic conditions play an important role in promoting or undermining reproductive health. In addition, our health is, to a certain extent, determined by our genetic constitution.

The World Health Organization (WHO) has proposed a short list of national and global reproductive health indicators, including:

- total fertility rate,
- contraceptive prevalence rate,
- maternal mortality ratio,
- percentage of women attended at least once during pregnancy by skilled health personnel for reasons related to pregnancy,
- percentage of births attended by skilled health personnel,
- number of facilities with functioning basic essential obstetric care per 500,000 population,
- number of facilities with functioning comprehensive essential obstetric care per 500,000 population,
- perinatal mortality rate,
- percentage of live births of low birth weight,
- positive syphilis serology prevalence in young pregnant women attending for prenatal care,
- percentage of women of reproductive age screened for haemoglobin levels who are anaemic,
- percentage of obstetric and gynaecology admissions owing to abortion,
- reported prevalence of women with female genital cutting (mutilation),
- percentage of women of reproductive age at risk of pregnancy who report trying for a pregnancy for two years or more,
- reported incidence of urethritis in men (aged 15–49), and HIV prevalence in pregnant women.

(See Table III.1.1 for data for some of these indicators by country.)

A global overview of reproductive health shows the magnitude of the problem and the health needs. Only 46 per cent of all deliveries worldwide take place in health facilities, 57 per cent of deliveries are attended by skilled personnel, and about 68 per cent of pregnant women receive prenatal care. Every year about 515,000 women die worldwide from causes related to pregnancy and childbirth. Maternity is ranked as the primary health problem in young adult women (ages 15–44) in developing countries, accounting for 18 per cent of the total disease burden. Maternal mortality shows greater disparity among countries than any other public health indicator. For a woman in Africa, the overall lifetime risk of a maternal death is 1 in 16, while for her sister in more developed countries it is 1 in 2,500. Of nearly 8 million infant deaths each year worldwide, around two-thirds occur before the end of the first month. About 3.4 million of these neonatal deaths occur during the first week of life. These deaths are largely a consequence of poorly managed pregnancies and deliveries, or the result of inadequate care of the neonate during the first critical hours of life. In addition, many millions of babies who survive the birth process are so badly damaged that their care will put a major burden on their mothers. Some 25 million low birth weight babies are born each year. It is estimated that in developing countries, 58 per cent of pregnant women and 31 per cent of children under 5 are anaemic.

The number of births a woman is expected to have in her lifetime has decreased and, as a consequence, there has been a decrease in her exposure to the risk of pregnancy and childbirth. Women, as a world average, are now expected to have less than three births in their lifetime. In 1965, only about 9 per cent of all married women of reproductive age in developing countries, or their partners, were using a reliable method of contraception. In 1998, the United Nations estimated contraceptive use to be 55 per cent in less developed regions. There are still large segments of the world's population whose needs of fertility regulation are not met by currently available contraceptive methods and services. It is estimated that at least 100–120 million couples are not using any method of contraception even though they want to space their pregnancies or limit their fertility. Millions of women around the world risk their lives and health to end an unwanted pregnancy. Every day, 55,000 unsafe abortions take place—95 per cent of them in developing countries—and lead to the death of more than 200 women daily (see, for country and regional data on abortion, Table III.1.3).

The World Health Organization estimates that more than 380 million new cases of sexually transmitted infections (not including HIV) occur each year. The human immunodeficiency virus continues to spread around the world, insinuating itself into communities previously little troubled by the epidemic and strengthening its grip on areas where AIDS is already the leading cause of death in adults. It is estimated that, in 2001, 5 million people were newly infected, 40 million were living with the infection, and 3 million died (see, for country data on percentage of pregnant women with HIV/AIDS, Table III.1.1).

Estimates of the worldwide prevalence of female genital cutting (mutilation) range from 85 to 114 million, with an annual rate of increase of about

2 million per year. About 6,000 girls are 'circumcised' every day (see Table III.1.2).

Infertility is an international public health problem. A general estimate is that between 8 to 12 per cent of couples experience some form of involuntary infertility during their reproductive lives. When extrapolated to the global population this means that 50 to 80 million people may be suffering from some infertility problem.

The World Health Organization estimates that 425,000 new cases of cervical cancer are diagnosed each year, mostly in developing countries. Each year about 195,000 die from this largely preventable disease. Cervical cancer, apart from being caused by a sexually transmitted infection with human papilloma virus, is a largely preventable disease, if women have access to appropriate screening programmes.

Although progress has been made, there are still major concerns and short-comings in sexual and reproductive health. Resources have not been forth-coming. An area of major concern is the continued violation of women's human rights, including sexual and reproductive rights. A major challenge that remains ahead, and should continue to bear heavily on our collective conscience, is the neglected tragedy of maternal mortality. Reproductive health is often compromised not because of lack of medical knowledge, but because of infringements of women's human rights. Powerlessness of women is a serious health hazard.

2. *Reproductive Health*

2.1. *The concept*

During the second half of the twentieth century, there was a vast expansion of health technologies and of health services to provide people with certain elements of health care related to reproduction. The services were, however, fragmented and not oriented to respond to the totality of need.

The concept of reproductive health has recently emerged in response to the fragmentation of the existing services related to health in reproduction, and to their orientation. The concept of 'reproductive health' offers a comprehensive, and integrated approach to health needs related to reproduction. It puts women at the centre of the process, and recognizes, respects, and responds to the needs of women and not only to those of mothers.

The concept of reproductive health received great attention in the United Nations International Conference on Population and Development, held in Cairo in 1994. It was endorsed as showing the way forward, as a preferable alternative to narrowly focused family planning programmes.

2.2. *A definition*

One of us (MFF), while working with the World Health Organization (WHO) in 1987, provided a definition for the term 'reproductive health' that was published in 1988. The definition was as follows:[1]

Health is defined in the WHO Constitution as a 'state of complete physical, mental and social well-being, and not merely the absence of disease or infirmity.' Reproductive health, in the context of this positive definition, would have a number of basic elements. It would mean that people have the ability to reproduce, to regulate their fertility; and that women are able to go safely through pregnancy and childbirth; and that reproduction is carried to a successful outcome through infant and child survival and well-being. To this may be added that people are able to enjoy and are safe in having sex.

This definition was adopted, and expanded, in the Programme of Action developed at the International Conference on Population and Development (ICPD) held in Cairo in 1994,[2] and at the International Conference on Women, also sponsored by the United Nations, which was held in Beijing in 1995. The full definition reads:

Reproductive health is a state of complete physical, mental and social well-being and not merely the absence of disease or infirmity, in all matters relating to the reproductive system and to its functions and processes. Reproductive health therefore implies that people are able to have a satisfying and safe sex life and that they have the capability to reproduce and the freedom to decide if, when and how often to do so. Implicit in this last condition are the right of men and women to be informed and to have access to safe, effective, affordable and acceptable methods of family planning of their choice, as well as other methods of their choice for regulation of fertility which are not against the law, and the right of access to appropriate health-care services that will enable women to go safely through pregnancy and childbirth and provide couples with the best chance of having a healthy infant.[3]

In line with the above definition of reproductive health, reproductive health care is defined as the constellation of methods, techniques, and services that contribute to reproductive health and well-being by preventing and solving reproductive health problems. It also includes sexual health, the purpose of which is the enhancement of life and personal relations, and not merely counselling and care related to reproduction and sexually transmitted diseases.

---

[1] M. F. Fathalla, 'Promotion of Research in Human Reproduction: Global Needs and Perspectives', *Human Reproduction*, 3 (1988), 7–10.

[2] UN, *Population and Development, i. Programme of Action Adopted at the International Conference on Population and Development, Cairo, 5–13 September 1994* (New York: United Nations, Department for Economic and Social Information and Policy Analysis, ST/ESA/SER.A/149, 1994) (hereinafter Cairo Programme), para. 7.2.

[3] UN, Department of Public Information, *Platform for Action and Beijing Declaration. Fourth World Conference on Women, Beijing, China, 4–15 September 1995* (New York: UN, 1995), para. 94.

2.3. *A global concern*

Reproductive health is not just a major health issue. It is also a development issue, and a human rights issue.

The *impact* of reproductive health is not limited to the individual, family, and society at large. It extends across national boundaries to the world as a whole. Two areas in reproductive health have, in particular, such a major impact: the ability to regulate and control fertility and safety from sexually transmitted diseases (STDs). Inability of individuals, and particularly of women, in developing countries to regulate and control their fertility is not only affecting the health of the people immediately concerned, but has implications for global stability and for the balance between population and natural resources and between people and environment, and is a violation of women's human rights. Communicable diseases have an impact that transcends national boundaries. Of all communicable diseases, sexually transmitted diseases, including HIV infection, are least amenable to control by erecting national barriers. People with other communicable diseases are less likely to travel than people with STDs, which are sometimes described as air-borne diseases, to indicate the importance of air travel in their transnational spread. Only a global coordinated effort will control them.

There are different ways to define *urgency*. It is used in the present context to indicate a problem which will get much worse through delay and may even become irreversible. Again, this sense of urgency is clear in both areas of fertility regulation and STDs. By their very nature, they constitute a problem that multiplies and not only continues to exist. Any unwanted birth that could not be averted can result in the future in generations of new births. Any person with an STD infection has the potential of infecting several others. Our action or inaction to implement women's rights, including their right to health, in these critical decades will be a decisive factor in the world future.

Inequity in reproductive health is the third compelling reason for international concern about social injustice. There is no area of health in which inequity is as striking as in reproductive health.

3. *Sexual Health*

In the evolution of *Homo sapiens*, the temporal relationship between sex and reproduction has been severed. It must have taken our ancestors a long time to realize any relationship between the sexual act and the event of pregnancy resulting in birth; it was probably not until they began to observe domesticated animals that the relationship was recognized. In our fellow mammals, the female will only be attractive to the male and receptive to his advances if she is ovulating and ready to conceive. In our fellow primates, the female never fails to advertise the fact when she is ovulating. External sexual organs undergo a change in size or colour that is clearly visible and that makes her sexually attractive to the male. At other times, she will have little or no appeal for him. The sexual receptivity of the human female has been completely emancipated from hormonal control. The human female has also succeeded through evolution to hide external evidence of ovulation. The dissociation of the act of sex from reproduction appears to be a purposeful act of nature aimed at increasing the pair bond. Sex was meant by nature for its own sake, not just as a tool for reproduction.[4]

With the worldwide trend for the adoption of the norm of a small family, reproduction is receding further into the background, and the role of sex in our lives is going to evolve further. It will be elevated from an act of reproductive instinct to an expression of love and a confirmation of human bonding. As such, sex will be an increasingly important component in our psycho-social well-being, and decreasingly directed towards reproduction.

With the positive definition of health as a state of complete physical, mental, and social well-being and not merely the absence of disease or infirmity, a definition of sexual health should include the following components:[5]

- the ability to enjoy mutually fulfilling sexual relationships;
- freedom from sexual abuse, coercion, or harassment;
- safety from sexually transmitted diseases; and
- success in achieving or in preventing pregnancy.

4. Reproductive Health: A Woman's Concern

4.1. Gender differentials in health

Reproductive health is an important component of health for both women and men, but it is more critical, however, for women. A major burden of disease in females is related to their reproductive function and reproductive potential, and the way in which society treats or mistreats women because of their gender. While men are more prone to die because of what one may call their 'vices', women often suffer because of their natural physiological role in the survival of the species, and the tasks related to it. In a study on investment in health, reported by the World Bank, ranking of the five main causes of the disease

---

[4] M. F. Fathalla, 'Introduction', in J. Becker and E. Leitman, *Introducing Sexuality within Family Planning: The Experience of Three HIV/STD Prevention Projects from Latin America and the Caribbean* (Quality/Candidad/Qualité. 8: 1–2; New York: Population Council, 1997).

[5] M. F. Fathalla, *From Obstetrics and Gynecology to Women's Health: the Road Ahead* (New York and London: Parthenon, 1997), 33–48.

Table I.2.1. Major disease burdens, 1993

Rank	Females	Males
1	Maternity	HIV infection
2	Sexually transmitted diseases	Tuberculosis
3	Tuberculosis	Motor vehicle injuries
4	HIV infection	Homicide and violence
5	Depressive disorders	War

burden in young adults (15 to 44 years) in developing countries showed the gender differential illustrated in Table I.2.1.[6]

4.2. *The unfair burden on women in reproductive health*

Maternity can be a distinctive joy but also a major health burden for women. In some other aspects of reproductive health where responsibility is shared between men and women, the burden, for both biological and social reasons, falls particularly heavily on women. This applies to the burdens of sexually transmitted diseases, fertility regulation, infertility, and, for instance, child nursing and early rearing.

According to the World Bank study quantifying the burden of disease, sexually transmitted diseases (STDs) rank as the second major cause of the disease burden in young adult women in developing countries, accounting for 8.9 per cent of the total disease burden in that age group.[7] Among males of the same age group, STDs (excluding sexually induced HIV infection) are not among the first ten causes, and account only for 1.5 per cent of the disease burden. For a mix of biological and social reasons, women are more likely to be infected, are less likely to seek care, are more difficult to diagnose, are at more risk of severe disease sequelae, and are more subject to social discrimination and other consequences. The most effective method available for protection against STDs, the condom, is controlled by men. A simple and effective method of protection, that a woman can use without needing her partner's cooperation, does not yet exist.

The modern revolution in contraceptive technology provided women with reliable methods of birth control, which they can use independently of co-operation of male partners. This independence was at a price. Women had to assume the inconveniences and risks involved. The role and responsibility of

---

[6] World Bank, *World Development Report: Investing in Health* (New York: Oxford University Press, 1993), at 223.
[7] Ibid.

Table I.2.2. Contraceptive use, 1999

Contraceptive use	Percentage
Female sterilization	19
Intrauterine device	13
Pill	8
Male sterilization	4
Condom	4
Other supply methods	3
Non-supply methods	8

the male partner have receded as contraception has come to be considered a woman's business. The percentage of contraceptive use, worldwide, among couples of reproductive age, as estimated by the United Nations, is shown in Table I.2.2.[8]

Women therefore assume a disproportionate responsibility for contraception in comparison to men. Not only do women have an undue burden of responsibility in fertility regulation, but the methods that women have available for use are those associated with potential health hazards. The importance of male participation and responsibility has become much greater with the emergence of the Acquired Immune Deficiency Syndrome (AIDS) pandemic and the increasing prevalence of sexually transmitted infections, where the use of the condom is the only effective strategy for protection, other than abstinence.

Responsibility for infertility is commonly shared by the couple, as demonstrated in an analysis of data compiled in a large WHO multinational study.[9] The burden of infertility, however, for biological and social reasons, is unequally shared. The infertility investigation of the female partner is much more elaborate than of the male partner, and is associated with more inconvenience and risk. The burden of treatment also falls mostly on the female partner. Even for male infertility, the promise of successful management is now shifting to assisted reproduction technologies, such as intra-cytoplasmic sperm injection (ICSI), where the female assumes the major burden. The psychological and social burden of infertility in most societies is much heavier on the woman. A woman's status is often identified with her fertility, and her failure to have children can be seen as a social disgrace or a cause for divorce.

---

[8] UN, *World Contraceptive Use 1998* (New York: UN Population Division, Department for Economic and Social Affairs, 1999), ST/ESA/SER.A/175.

[9] P. J. Rowe and T. M. M. Farley, 'The Standardized Investigation of the Infertile Couple', in P. J. Rowe and E. M. Vikhlyaeva (eds.), *Diagnosis and Treatment of Infertility* (Berne: Hans Huber, 1988), 15–40.

The suffering of the infertile woman, and of any woman in an infertile marriage, can be very real.

Perinatal (foetal and early neonatal) morbidity and mortality should be recognized as a disease burden on women. Health statistics classify perinatal mortality as a category on its own, a condition that affects both males and females. Perinatal mortality and morbidity are outcomes of pregnancy and delivery for women. They should be appropriately added to the count of the disease burden on women. Women make major investments of themselves in pregnancy and childbirth. The unfavourable perinatal outcome of a pregnancy can be a frustration or an additional burden on the woman for the care of an unhealthy infant and child.

4.3. *Women's health is more than reproductive health*

A woman is not a womb, but has a womb. Health for women is more than reproductive health. Being a woman has implications for health. Health needs of women can be broadly classified under four categories.[10] First, women have specific health needs related to their sexual and reproductive function, collectively expressed in the reproductive health package. Second, women have an elaborate reproductive system that is vulnerable to dysfunction or disease, even before it functions or after it ceases to function. Third, women are subject to the same diseases of other body systems that can affect men, but their disease patterns often differ from those of men because of women's genetic constitution, hormonal environment, or gender-evolved lifestyle behaviour. Diseases of other body systems, or their treatments, may also interact with conditions of the reproductive system or function. Fourth, because women are women, they are subject to social dysfunctions that impact on their physical, mental, or social health. Examples include female genital cutting, often warranting the judgemental description of mutilation, sexual abuse, and domestic violence.

5. *Men Have Reproductive Health Needs Too*

> The objective is to promote gender equality in all spheres of life, including family and community life, and to encourage and enable men to take responsibility for their sexual and reproductive behaviour and their social and family roles.
>
> (Programme of Action of the United Nations' International Conference on Population and Development, Cairo, 1994, paragraph 4.25)[11]

---

[10] Fathalla, *From Obstetrics.*   [11] Cairo Programme.

Not only do men have reproductive health concerns of their own, but their health status and behaviours also affect women's reproductive health. Men's reproductive health needs include sexuality, protection against sexually transmitted infections, infertility prevention and management, and fertility regulation. Protection against prostatic hypertrophy and prostatic cancer is another concern. Men can play a positive role in promoting women's reproductive health by sharing the responsibility of family planning using a male method, by supporting their partners in using female contraception and deciding on the appropriate family size, and by responsible sexual behaviour, including the use of condoms to protect their partners. Young men need to be educated to respect women and treat them as equals, to support efforts to enhance the status of women, and to prevent gender-based violence.

6. *Determinants of Reproductive Health*

It can be said that four factors (that can be referred to as the four 'Ps'), contribute to the determination of health in general, and reproductive health in particular: providence, people, politicians, and providers of health services.[12]

Providence determines our genetic constitution, including diseases to which we are more susceptible. Whether we are born with two X chromosomes or with one X and one Y chromosome will determine our sex. Gender plays no small part in the determination of our health.[13]

People's lifestyle behaviour can promote or undermine their own health. Their behaviour can even affect other people's health.

The socio-economic conditions of the society in which we are born and in which we live is another determinant of our health. Politicians and legislators play an important role in the shaping of societies. By controlling the resources that can be allocated to health, they are, consciously or unconsciously, making decisions on who shall live and who shall die. Laws and policies can advance women's rights and health, and can obstruct women's autonomy and choice in decisions regarding their reproductive and sexual health.

Providers of health care, until the last century, had really very little to offer to restore health. Advances in medical knowledge now equip health care providers with means to protect, maintain, and restore health, to an extent that was never believed possible before.

Improvement in reproductive health necessitates the understanding of these determinants, which operate to different extents in different reproductive

---

[12] Fathalla, 'Promotion of Research'.

[13] World Health Organization, *Gender and Health: Technical Paper* (Geneva: WHO, 1998), WHO/FRH/WHD/98.16.

health problems, and in different communities. Health care professionals should not limit their concerns to their clinical duty and physician/client relationship. They should look at the health care system obligations and how they are fulfilled. They should also be part of the social action to address underlying conditions.

Barriers to improving women's health are often rooted in social, economic, cultural, legal, and related conditions that transcend health care considerations. Social factors, such as lack of literacy and of educational or employment opportunities, deny young women alternatives to early marriage and early childbearing, and economic and other means of access to contraception. Women's vulnerability to sexual and other abuses, in and out of marriage, increases risks of unwanted pregnancy and unsafe abortion. Social, religious, and economic customs become embedded in the law, and historically have been claimed to provide a justification for discrimination against women. Social science and legal research, particularly research that takes a gender approach, can be helpful to understanding how these underlying socio-legal causes affect and injure women's status and autonomy, and hence their reproductive health.

Legal research can analyse laws that affect reproductive health and the degree to which they are or are not implemented. It can help to identify how laws advance or compromise women's interests in their personal, family, and public lives, with indirect effects on their reproductive health.

The case studies featured in Part II will reflect how these different approaches are needed to advance sexual and reproductive rights and health in specific situations.

7. *Reproductive Health Indicators*

The World Health Organization proposed the following short list of national and global reproductive health indicators:[14]

1. Total fertility rate: total number of children a woman would have by the end of her reproductive period if she experienced the currently prevailing age-specific rates throughout her childbearing life.

2. Contraceptive prevalence: percentage of women of reproductive age (15–49) who are using, or whose partner is using, a contraceptive method at a particular point in time.

3. Maternal mortality ratio: annual number of maternal deaths per 100,000 live births. A maternal death is defined as: 'the death of a woman while

[14] WHO, *Reproductive Health Indicators for Global Monitoring* (Geneva: WHO, 2001), WHO/RHR/01.19, 1–51.

pregnant or within 42 days of termination of pregnancy, irrespective of the duration and site of the pregnancy, from any cause related to or aggravated by the pregnancy or its management but not from accidental or incidental causes'. The maternal mortality rate (annual number of maternal deaths per 100,000 women of reproductive age) is another measure which reflects both the risk of death among pregnant and recently pregnant women, and the proportion of all women who become pregnant in a given year. It therefore can be reduced either by making childbearing safer (as is true for the ratio, above) and/or by reducing the number of unwanted pregnancies.

4. Antenatal care coverage: percentage of women attended, at least once during pregnancy, by skilled health personnel (excluding trained or untrained traditional birth attendants) for reasons related to pregnancy.

5. Births attended by skilled health personnel: percentage of births attended by skilled health personnel (excluding trained or untrained traditional birth attendants).

6. Availability of basic essential obstetric care: number of facilities with functioning basic essential obstetric care per 500,000 population. Basic essential obstetric care should include parenteral antibiotics, oxytocics (drugs that stimulate uterine contraction to prevent and treat haemorrhage after delivery), sedatives for eclampsia (convulsions), and the manual removal of the placenta and retained products.

7. Availability of comprehensive essential obstetric care: number of facilities with functioning comprehensive essential obstetric care per 500,000 population. Comprehensive essential obstetric care should include essential obstetric care plus surgery, anaesthesia, and blood transfusion.

8. Perinatal mortality rate: number of perinatal deaths per 1,000 total births. Perinatal deaths occur during late pregnancy (at twenty-two completed weeks' gestation and over), during childbirth, and up to seven completed days of life.

9. Low birth weight prevalence: percentage of live births of low birth weight (<2,500 g).

10. Positive syphilis serology prevalence in pregnant women: percentage of pregnant women, 15 to 24 years old, attending antenatal clinics, whose blood has been screened for syphilis, with positive serology for syphilis.

11. Prevalence of anaemia in women: percentage of women of reproductive age (15–49 years old) screened for haemoglobin levels who are anaemic (with levels below 110 g/l for pregnant women, and below 120 g/l for non-pregnant women).

12. Percentage of obstetric and gynaecology admissions owing to abortion: percentage of all cases admitted to service delivery points providing in-patient obstetric and gynaecological services, which are due to abortion, spontaneous and induced, but excluding planned terminations of pregnancy.

13. Reported prevalence of women with female genital mutilation (FGM): percentage of women interviewed in a community survey, reporting themselves to have undergone FGM.

14. Prevalence of infertility in women: percentage of women of reproductive age (15–49 years old) at risk of pregnancy (not pregnant, sexually active, non-contracepting and non-lactating) who report trying for a pregnancy for two years or more.

15. Reported incidence of urethritis in men: percentage of men aged 15 to 49 interviewed in a community survey reporting episodes of urethritis in the last twelve months.

16. HIV prevalence in pregnant women: percentage of pregnant women aged 15 to 24, attending antenatal clinics, whose blood has been tested for HIV, who are sero-positive for HIV.

17. Knowledge of HIV-related prevention practices: the percentage of all respondents who correctly identify all three major ways of preventing the sexual transmission of HIV and who reject three major misconceptions about HIV transmission or prevention.

In selecting these indicators, WHO took into consideration that a good indicator must be ethical, useful at the national and international levels, scientifically robust, representative, understandable, and accessible. To be ethical, an indicator must require data that are ethical to collect, process, and present, paying regard to the rights of the individual to confidentiality, freedom of choice in supplying identifiable data, and informed consent regarding the data required. To be useful at the national and international levels, an indicator must be able to act as a 'marker of progress' towards improved reproductive health status. To be scientifically robust, an indicator should be a valid, specific, sensitive, and reliable reflection of that which it purports to measure. To be representative, an indicator must adequately encompass all the issues or population groups it is expected to cover, including minority groups and adolescents. To be understandable, an indicator must be simple to define and its value must be easy to interpret in terms of reproductive health status. An accessible indicator is one for which the data required are already available or relatively easy to acquire.

The list of proposed indicators is not comprehensive, and indicators for other areas still need to be developed, including indicators for quality of care, and indicators to monitor ICPD targets for comprehensive sexual and reproductive health care.

8. A Global Overview of Reproductive Health

8.1. Safe motherhood

8.1.1. *Availability of essential basic and comprehensive health care*

Experience in the past two decades indicates that, as a rough minimal standard, at least 15 per cent of all births in the population will need to take place in either a basic or comprehensive care facility.[15] In addition, the efficiency of the service should be such that the case fatality rate among women with obstetric complications in these facilities should not exceed 1 per cent. According to statistics collected by the World Health Organization, 46 per cent of all deliveries worldwide take place in health facilities.[16] Even in the less developed regions of the world, the figure is 40 per cent, with a range between regions of 26 to 78 per cent.

Health facilities for the most part are there. But we face three problems. First, these health facilities are very unevenly distributed. Many parts in countries are deprived of these facilities. Second, the 40 per cent of women who deliver in these facilities often do not include all or even most of the 15 per cent who really need emergency obstetric care. Facilities are over-utilized by those not in need, and under-utilized by those in need. Third, the quality of the service, whether in terms of equipment or skilled personnel, often leaves much to be desired. Making emergency obstetric care accessible to all women is not an impossible mission. In most cases, it does not mean building new facilities. It means a more rational allocation of available resources with more for those in more need, together with a modest infusion of new resources to upgrade existing facilities, facilitate transport, and improve the skills and performance of health personnel.

8.1.2. *Deliveries by skilled birth attendants*

By skilled birth attendants, we mean health professionals who have the necessary training to detect, and early diagnose, life-threatening complications, and, when needed, refer women to where they can get the necessary help. The World Health Organization estimates that, on average, 57 per cent of deliveries in the world today are attended by skilled personnel.[17] The figure is 99 per cent for more developed regions. But already 53 per cent of deliveries in less developed regions are attended by skilled personnel, with a range between

[15] United Nations Children's Emergency Fund (UNICEF), WHO, and UN Population Fund, *Guidelines for Monitoring the Availability and Use of Obstetric Services* (New York: UNICEF, 1997), 25.

[16] WHO, *Coverage of Maternity Care: A Listing of Available Information* (Geneva: WHO, Family and Reproductive Health, 4th edn., 1997), WHO/RHT/MSM/96.28. at 10.

[17] Ibid.

34 per cent and 86 per cent for different regions. There are more variations between and within countries. There will probably never be enough obstetricians to attend deliveries of all women—not that this is necessary, or necessarily desirable. But in situations where skilled attendants are in shortage, obstetricians should assume the role of team leaders and trainers, delegate responsibilities to other categories of health professionals, and provide the necessary training, support, and supervision.[18] Midwives have an important role to play in making motherhood safe for all women.

Table III.1.1 includes country data on births attended by skilled personnel.

8.1.3. *Access of pregnant women to prenatal care*

On average, about 68 per cent, or more than two-thirds, of pregnant women in the world receive prenatal care, according to WHO data.[19] The figure for less developed regions is 65 per cent, ranging from 52 to 73 per cent between different regions. Much of the traditional practice of prenatal care is not evidence-based. If prenatal care is limited to evidence-based interventions, resources will be freed to expand the availability of the services and also make them more cost-effective.

Table III.1.1 includes country data on antenatal coverage.

8.1.4. *Maternal mortality*

Although maternal deaths are now very rare events in developed countries, they unfortunately remain common events in developing countries. Revised 1995 estimates of maternal mortality indicate that, every year, about 515,000 women die from causes related to pregnancy and childbirth, a rate of over 1,400 maternal deaths each day, and little short of one death every minute.[20] A 1993 World Bank report ranked maternity as the primary health problem in young adult women (ages 15–44) in developing countries, accounting for 18 per cent of the total disease burden.[21] Women who die are in the prime period of their lives. As mothers, their deaths have major health and social impacts on their families. Moreover, maternal mortality should be viewed as only the tip of an iceberg of maternal morbidity and acute or chronic suffering. For every maternal death, there are many women who survive serious illness with continued suffering and incapacity, such as through problems associated with obstetric fistulae.

---

[18] M. F. Fathalla, 'The Hubert de Watteville Memorial Lecture. Imagine a World Where Motherhood is Safe for All Women: You can Help Make it Happen', *Int. J. Gynecol. Obstet.*, 72 (2001), 207–13.

[19] WHO, *Coverage of Maternity Care*.

[20] WHO, *Maternal Mortality in 1995: Estimates Developed by WHO, UNICEF, UNFPA* (Geneva: WHO, 2001), 2, 42–7. WHO/RHR/01.9.

[21] World Bank, *World Development Report* (1993).

Maternal mortality in developing countries is also a tragedy in terms of equity and social justice. Of the 515,000 total number of maternal deaths, only about 2,800 take place in more developed countries, while 512,000 take place in less developed countries. Over half of these maternal deaths, 273,000, occur in Africa, compared with a total of only 2,200 maternal deaths in Europe.

The WHO revised estimates indicate that the global figure for the maternal mortality ratio (number of maternal deaths per 100,000 live births) is 400.[22] For individual countries, ratios vary from below 10 maternal deaths per 100,000 live births (such as in Australia, Canada, Spain, and Sweden) to over 1,500 (such as in Burundi, Ethiopia, Rwanda, Sierra Leone, and Somalia). Maternal mortality ratios show greater disparity among countries than any other public health indicator.

The inequity is even more dramatic by reference to the lifetime chance of maternal death. Maternal mortality is a recurrent risk. Lifetime risk reflects the probability of maternal death faced by an average woman over her entire reproductive life-span. Like the maternal mortality rate, it reflects both a woman's risk of dying from a pregnancy-related cause, as well as her risk of becoming pregnant. However, it also takes into account the accumulation of risk with each pregnancy. For a woman in Africa, the overall risk is 1 in 16, for a woman in Asia it is 1 in 110, for a woman in Latin America and the Caribbean it is 1 in 160, and for a woman in more developed countries taken as a whole it is 1 in 2,500.[23] A woman from the South goes through the journey of pregnancy and childbirth burdened with a heavy luggage of social injustice, which she accumulated as a girl not considered to be her brother's equal, as a woman denied control of her fertility, and as a pregnant mother whose interests as a woman are considered by her family, community, and even health care providers to be secondary to the interests of her foetus.[24]

Table III.1.1 includes country data on maternal mortality ratio.

8.1.5. *Perinatal mortality*

While infant mortality declined markedly during the early 1980s and late 1990s, most of this improvement was among older infants. Of nearly 8 million infant deaths each year, around two-thirds occur during the neonatal period, before the age of one month; 3.4 million of the neonatal deaths occur within the first week of life.[25] Moreover, for every neonate who dies, at least one other infant is a stillbirth. These deaths are largely a consequence of inadequate or inappropriate care during pregnancy, delivery, or the first critical hours after birth. In addition, many millions of babies who survive the birth process are so

[22] WHO, *Maternal Mortality*.   [23] Ibid.
[24] M. F. Fathalla, 'The Long Road to Maternal Death', *People*, 14 (1987), 8–9.
[25] WHO, *Reduction of Maternal Mortality: A Joint WHO/UNFPA/UNICEF/World Bank Statement* (Geneva: WHO, 1999), 18.

badly damaged that their care will put a major burden on their mothers. Some 25 million babies each year are born weighing less than 2,500 g.[26] Low birth weight babies are at high risk of infection, hypothermia and asphyxia, and impaired growth and development, putting a heavy burden in child care on women.

Table III.1.1 includes country data on perinatal mortality rate, and on low birthweight.

8.1.6. *Anaemia*

Iron deficiency and anaemia contribute to increased maternal and newborn mortality, impaired health and development, limited learning capacity, impaired immune function, and reduced productive capacity. It is estimated that in developing countries 58 per cent of pregnant women and 31 per cent of children under 5 years of age are anaemic.[27] While anaemia may not cause maternal death directly, it may contribute toward death from other causes. For instance, anaemic women may not tolerate blood loss to the same extent as healthy women. In pregnant women with sickle cell anaemia, deaths may result from the effects of embolism, or bacterial infections during the last four weeks of pregnancy, labour, and the first week after delivery.

Table III.1.1 includes country data on anaemia in pregnant women.

8.2. *Fertility by choice*

8.2.1. *Total fertility rate*

Every pregnancy should be a wanted pregnancy. Fertility by choice, thanks to the contraceptive technology revolution, has already led to a significant decrease in total fertility rates and the number of births a woman is expected to have in her lifetime, and as a consequence, a decrease in her exposure to the risk of pregnancy and childbirth. Women, as a world average, are now expected to have less than three (2.9) births in their lifetime.[28] In less developed regions, the average is 3.2 (3.7 excluding China). In more developed regions, the average is 1.5.[29]

Table III.1.1 includes country data on total fertility rate.

[26] WHO, *Low Birth Weight: A Tabulation of Available Information* (Geneva: WHO, 1992), WHO/MCH/92.2, 12.

[27] WHO, *Evaluation of the Implementation of the Global Strategy for Health for All by 2000, 1979–1996. A Selective Review of Progress and Constraints* (Geneva: WHO, 1998), WHO/HST/98.2, at 166, 174.

[28] Population Reference Bureau, *World Population Data Sheet: Demographic Data and Estimates for the Countries and Regions of the World* (Washington, DC: Population Reference Bureau, 2000).

[29] Ibid.

8.2.2. *Contraceptive prevalence*

In 1965, only about 9 per cent of all married women of reproductive age in developing countries, or their partners, were using a reliable method of contraception. In 1998, the United Nations estimated world contraceptive use to be 58 per cent, 55 per cent in less developed regions, and 70 per cent in more developed regions.[30] There are, however, marked regional variations, from 20 per cent in Africa, to 66 per cent in Latin America and the Caribbean, to 83 per cent in China. There are still large segments of the world's population whose needs for fertility regulation are not met by the currently available methods and services. It is estimated that at least 100–120 million couples are not using any method of contraception even though they want to space their pregnancies or limit their fertility.[31]

Table III.1.1 includes country data on contraceptive prevalence.

8.3. *Abortion*

Millions of women around the world risk their lives and health to end an unwanted pregnancy. According to WHO, every day, 55,000 unsafe abortions take place—95 per cent of them in developing countries—and lead to the death of more than 200 women daily.[32]

The moral and religious controversies about abortion tend to obscure its dimensions as a clinical and public health problem. At least 70,000 women die from complications related to unsafe abortion every year, according to World Health Organization estimates.[33] Worldwide, unsafe abortions account for 13 per cent of all maternal deaths, but in some countries up to 60 per cent of all maternal deaths are due to unsafe abortion. WHO estimates that more than half of the deaths caused by induced abortion occur in South and South-East Asia, followed by sub-Saharan Africa. Table I.2.3 shows the WHO estimates for global and regional mortality due to unsafe abortion for the period 1995–2000. WHO data show that the global case fatality rate associated with unsafe abortion is probably 700 times higher than the rate associated with legal induced abortion in the USA; in some regions, it is well over 1,000 times higher. Even in developed regions, this rate is eighty times higher for an unsafe abortion than for a legal abortion procedure. Table III.1.3 includes regional and certain country data on unsafe abortion.

Making contraceptive methods widely available and accessible is the best approach to decrease the number of unwanted pregnancies, and hence the

---

[30] UN, *World Contraceptive Use.*   [31] WHO, *Evaluation.*
[32] WHO, *Unsafe Abortion: Global and Regional Estimates of Incidence of and Mortality due to Unsafe Abortion with a Listing of Available Country Data* (Geneva: WHO, 3rd edn., 1997), WHO/RHT/MSM/97.16, 3–14.
[33] Ibid.

Table I.2.3. Global and regional mortality due to unsafe abortion,
1995–2000

Area	Estimated no. of unsafe abortions (000)	Estimated no. of deaths due to unsafe abortion	Case fatality rate (deaths per 100 unsafe abortions)
World total	20,000	78,000	0.4
More developed regions	900	500	<0.1
Less developed regions	19,000	77,500	0.4

number of induced abortions. It should be kept in mind, however, that contraceptive methods vary in their effectiveness. With the exception of complete
abstinence, all methods of contraception are associated with failure rates.
Contraceptive failures account for a significant proportion of cases of induced
abortion. Based on estimates of the range of failure rates of the different contraceptive methods and the estimated number of users worldwide, the yearly
number of accidental pregnancies due to contraceptive failure was estimated
to range from 8,860,000 to 30,310,000.[34]

Women exposed to the risk of sexually transmitted infections face a
dilemma in the selection of a method of contraception. Effective methods of
contraception do not offer protection against infection. Protective methods
against infection are less reliable as contraceptives. Using a dual method is an
option, but it may not always be affordable and practical. The availability of
safe pregnancy termination services can allow more women to use barrier
methods for protection against sexually transmitted infections.

Emergency contraception has been greatly under-utilized. It will probably
prevent at least 75 per cent of unplanned pregnancies.[35] Within seventy-two
hours of unprotected sex, a woman can use a regimen of oral pills in two doses.
Within five days, she can have a copper intra-uterine device inserted.

From a medical point of view, the distinction between contraception and
abortion is clear. Pregnancy is only considered established with the completion
of implantation of the ovum in the lining of the uterus. A woman with a fertilized ovum floating in her Fallopian tube or uterus is not pregnant. A method
that acts before complete implantation is a method of contraception. A
method that acts after complete implantation is a method of abortion. This is
the medical point of view. From an ideological point of view, people can argue
about when life begins. Life is a continuity, and life can only begin from life,

[34] S. J. Segal and K. D. LaGuardia, 'Termination of Pregnancy: A Global View', *Baillieres Clin. Obstet. Gynaecol.* 4 (1990), 235–47.
[35] WHO, *Emergency Contraception: A Guide for Service Delivery* (Geneva: WHO, 1998), WHO/FRH/FPP/98.19, 1–59.

. Sexually transmitted diseases, yearly incidence

ransmitted diseases	Millions
	12
⊃ccal infection (gonorrhoea)	62
,ydial infections including	89
⸱phogranuloma (venereum)	
᷄. ᷄croid	2
Trichomoniasis	170
Anogenital herpes	20
Anogenital warts	30

meaning living gametes and other cells. It depends on where an individual wants to draw the line, and on the purpose for which a line is proposed. Similar arguments concern the beginning of personhood, human identity, genetic uniqueness, and individuality. The theoretical potential to clone human cells to produce human tissues, organs, and living beings adds further dimensions to arguments about the nature of human life.

8.4. *Sexually transmitted infections*

8.4.1. *Not including HIV*

The WHO 1996 estimates for the yearly incidence (in millions) of sexually transmitted diseases, not including HIV infection, are shown in Table I.2.4.[36] The prevalence patterns of STDs in developing countries are up to 100 times those in developed countries for syphilis, ten to fifteen times higher for gonorrhoea, and three times higher for chlamydial infection. Incidence is also higher in developing countries. Among developing countries, the rates in Africa are generally higher than those of Asia and Latin America.

8.4.2. *HIV infection*

At the United Nations General Assembly Twenty-Sixth Special Session (UNGASS) in June 2001, world governments expressed their deep concern that the global HIV/AIDS epidemic, through its devastating scale and impact, constitutes a global emergency and one of the most formidable challenges to human life and dignity, as well as to the effective enjoyment of human rights, which undermines social and economic development throughout the world and affects all levels of society—national, community, family, and individual. They noted with profound concern that, by the end of the year 2000, 36.1 million

[36] WHO, *The World Health Report 1998: Life in the 21st Century. A Vision for All* (Geneva: WHO, 1998), at 45–6, 78–9.

Table I.2.5. HIV/AIDS epidemic, 2001 (million)

People affected	People newly infected with HIV in 2001	People living with HIV in 2001	AIDS deaths in 2001	Total no. of AIDS deaths
Total	5.0	40.0	3.0	18.8
Adults	4.3	37.2	2.4	15.0
Women	1.8	17.6	1.1	7.7
Children <15 years	0.8	2.7	0.5	3.8

people worldwide were living with HIV/AIDS, 90 per cent in developing countries and 75 per cent in sub-Saharan Africa. They noted with grave concern that all people, rich and poor, without distinction of age, gender, or race, are affected by the HIV/AIDS epidemic, further noting that people in developing countries are the most affected and that women, young adults, and children, in particular girls, are the most vulnerable.[37]

Table I.2.5 shows global estimates (in millions) of the HIV/AIDS epidemic as of December 2001.[38] AIDS has orphaned at least 10.4 million children currently under 15 (that is, they have lost their mother or both parents to the epidemic). The total number of children orphaned by the AIDS epidemic is forecast to more than double by 2010.

The diversity of HIV's spread worldwide is striking. But in many regions of the world, the HIV/AIDS epidemic is still in its early stages. While sixteen sub-Saharan African countries reported overall adult HIV prevalence of more than 10 per cent by the end of 1999, there remained 119 countries of the world where adult HIV prevalence was less than 1 per cent. Low national prevalence rates can, however, be very misleading. They often disguise serious epidemics that are initially concentrated in certain localities or among specific population groups and that threaten to spill over into the wider population.

Table III.1.1 includes available country data on HIV infection.

8.5. *Female genital cutting (circumcision/mutilation)*

Estimates of the worldwide prevalence of female genital cutting or mutilation (FGM) range from 85 million to 114 million, with an annual rate of increase of about 2 million per year. About 6,000 girls are 'circumcised' every day.[39]

[37] UN, *Final Declaration of Commitment on HIV/AIDS: United Nations General Assembly Twenty-Sixth Special Session, Adopted 27th June 2001* (New York: UN, 2001), Doc. A/s-26/L2.
[38] UNAIDS, *AIDS Epidemic Update: December 2001* (Geneva: UNAIDS, 2001), UNAIDS/01.74E-WHO/CDS/CSR/NCS/2001.2, 1–29.
[39] N. Toubia, 'Female Genital Mutilation and the Responsibility of Reproductive Health Professionals', *Int. J. Gynecol. Obstet.* 46 (1994), 127–35.

The practice of female genital cutting, in one form or another, continues to exist in around forty countries, mostly in East and West Africa, and parts of the Arabian Peninsula. The variation in prevalence between countries ranges from 5 to almost 98 per cent. With immigration, it is now also practised in Europe and North America. More detail on this harmful practice is provided in the case study in Part II, Chapter 2.

Table III.1.2 includes available country data on female genital cutting.

8.6. *Infertility*

Definitions of infertility widely vary; some measures are based on failure to conceive after twelve months of contraceptively unprotected intercourse, while others are based on twenty-four months of failure to conceive. A general estimate is that between 8 to 12 per cent of couples experience some form of involuntary infertility during their reproductive lives.[40] When extrapolated to the global population, this means that 50 to 80 million people may be suffering from some infertility problem.

There would probably always be a certain percentage of couples who would be infertile, because of reasons we cannot prevent, we cannot treat, or we do not know. This is what is referred to as core infertility, the percentage of which is probably not more than 5 per cent, and could be much less. A prevalence of infertility higher than that is considered as acquired infertility, which generally indicates that there are causes in the community for adding a new layer of infertile couples. In certain parts of sub-Saharan Africa, the prevalence of infertility may be as high as 30 per cent or more. The most important cause of acquired infertility is pelvic infection as a result of sexually transmitted diseases (such as chlamydia or gonorrhea), unsafe abortion, or puerperal (after delivery) infection.

8.7. *Cervical cancer*

There are a number of reasons for including cervical cancer (and not all genital cancers) in this overview on reproductive health. The vast majority of cervical cancer cases are caused by a sexually transmitted infection, with the human papilloma virus (HPV). The infection is generally asymptomatic and is easily transmitted. Women are generally infected at a young age, from their teens to their thirties. The risk of getting HPV and cervical cancer in those who first had intercourse around age 15 has been shown to be double the risk in those who first do so after age 20.[41]

---

[40] J. J. Sciarra, 'Infertility: An International Health Problem', *Int. J. Gynecol. Obstet.* 46 (1994), 155.
[41] WHO, *World Health Report 1998*.

It takes the disease twenty years or more to develop. During this long period, precancerous lesions can be detected and easily and effectively treated, leading to the prevention of the development of cervical cancer. The World Health Organization estimates that 425,000 new cases of cervical cancer are diagnosed each year, mostly in developing countries. Each year about 195,000 women die from this largely preventable disease.[42]

Screening and treatment of precancerous lesions are cost-effective interventions. It has been suggested that cervical cancer screening (defined as screening women every five years, with standard follow-up for identified cases) costs about US$100 per disability-adjusted life year (DALY) gained, compared with about US$2,600 per DALY for treatment of invasive cancer and palliative care.[43]

The classical methods of screening for cervical precancerous lesions are taking a smear from the cervix and examining it cytologically, together with colposcopy (visualization of the cervix under high magnification). New approaches are being explored for application in low-resource settings. These include visual inspection of the cervix after painting it with acetic acid, and HPV testing. New approaches are also being explored for the treatment of precancerous lesions, such as cryotherapy and the loop electosurgical excision procedure. These approaches allow the possibly immediate treatment of any suspected lesion, rather than waiting for the pathologic report for the cytologic smear and tissue biopsy. The possibility of a vaccine against HPV is also being pursued.

9. *Progress and Challenges*

Since the international commitment to reproductive health was made in Cairo in 1994, we can say that progress has been made, but we still fall short.[44] Family planning programmes have moved away from demographic-driven quotas and targets towards a needs-driven, woman-centred, broadly defined reproductive health approach. Silence has finally been broken on sensitive but vital issues in reproductive health. We have discovered that sex is a three, not a four-letter word. Sex and sexuality are ceasing to be taboos. Sex is being recognized for what it is, an important psycho-social component of the well-being of

[42] Ibid.
[43] J. Sherris and C. Herdman, 'Preventing Cervical Cancer in Low-Resource Settings', *Outlook*, 18 (Sept. 2000), 1–8.
[44] UN, General Assembly, *Report of the Ad Hoc Committee of the Whole of the Twenty-First Special Session of the General Assembly: Overall Review and Appraisal of the Implementation of the Programme of Action of the International Conference on Population and Development*, A/S-21/5/Add.1 (New York: UN, 1999), 1–23.

women and men. Adolescents are making their voices heard and their needs expressed. Female genital cutting is no longer kept behind sound-proof walls of culture and tradition. Unsafe abortion, a major public health problem, is widely discussed, and action is being taken. With due respect to the widely divergent views on the issue of abortion, an issue cannot be kept under the carpet when every year 20 million women are risking their health and even life in the process.[45] Another example of breaking the silence is that the pervasive violence against women, in all its forms, is rightly making its way up international and national agendas of attention and preventive efforts.

Although progress has been made, there are still major concerns and short-comings. Resources have not been forthcoming. The record of countries has been uneven. It is deplorable that armed conflicts or the threat of armed conflicts are deflecting badly needed resources in poor countries from enhancing human lives to destruction of human lives. There is a genuine concern about the impact of economic restructuring, particularly that programmes of structural adjustment in the health sector are leaving the poor and disadvantaged, predominantly women and children, without a safety net.

Another area of major concern is the continued violation of women's human rights, including sexual and reproductive rights.[46] Women are subjected to discrimination even before they are born; and as young innocent girls they begin to face the harsh reality that they are not boys' equals.

A major challenge that remains ahead, and should continue to bear heavily on our collective conscience, is the neglected tragedy of maternal mortality. Maternal mortality should not be lumped with nor ranked against other disease problems. Maternity is not a disease. It is the means by which the human species is propagated. Society has more of an obligation to prevent maternal deaths than to prevent deaths from diseases. The neglected tragedy of maternal mortality poses the basic question of how much societies consider the life of a woman to be worth.[47] When societies invest less in girls than in boys and underestimate the economic contribution of women, and when only a few women are in positions of decision-making, it should be no surprise, in resource-poor settings, that a low priority is given to allocating the necessary resources to save the lives of mothers. Women, worldwide, should mobilize for the right to safe motherhood, basically the woman's right to life.[48] It is true that women in the North have mostly forgotten what maternal mortality is. But for

---

[45] WHO, *Unsafe Abortion*.

[46] R. J. Cook and M. F. Fathalla, 'Advancing Reproductive Rights beyond Cairo and Beijing', *International Family Planning Perspectives*, 22 (1996), 115–21.

[47] M. F. Fathalla, 'How Much are Mothers Worth?', *International Federation of Gynecology and Obstetrics (FIGO), Proceedings of the XIII World Congress of Gynecology and Obstetrics, Singapore, 15–20 September 1991* (London: Parthenon, 1992), 203–9.

[48] Fathalla, 'Imagine a World'.

their sisters in the South, the journey of pregnancy and childbirth is still dangerous, and many do not return.

The health professions cannot remedy deficiencies in reproductive and sexual health alone. Improving reproductive and sexual health needs action beyond the health sector. The noble task of reproducing our species has not brought societal rewards to women. On the contrary, it has often led to their subordination, and worse to gender discrimination practices which, among other consequences, adversely impact on their health. A majority of women and girls in the world today still live under conditions that limit educational attainment, restrict economic participation, and fail to guarantee them equal rights and freedoms, as compared to men.

The International Federation of Gynecology and Obstetrics' 1994 World Report on Women's Health concluded that improvements in women's health need more than improved science and health care.[49] They require state action, long overdue, to correct injustices to women. Reproductive health is often compromised not because of lack of medical knowledge, but because of infringements on women's human rights. Powerlessness of women is a serious health hazard.

[49] M. F. Fathalla, 'Women's Health: An Overview', *Int. J. Gynecol. Obstet.* 46 (1994), 105–18.

3

Health Care Systems

1. Overview

The health care system can be defined as the mechanism in any society that transforms or metabolizes inputs of knowledge, and human and financial resources, into outputs of services relevant to the health concerns in that society. Health is not the domain of the health care system alone. Other systems (or sectors) in every society have a bearing on the health of the population, which may be, and in fact in many cases are, more important than that of the health care system. Society grants the health care system the 'legitimacy' to function and the resources to operate. In this 'social contract', society expects a return. The highest expectation is the human right to health, 'the right of everyone to the enjoyment of the highest attainable standard of physical and mental health'.

Reproductive health care is a part of general health care. There are, however, special considerations and special challenges which set it apart from general health care. Reproductive health care providers deal with mostly healthy people, they deal mostly with women, they often have to take into consideration the interests of more than one 'client' at the same time, and they have to deal and interact with society.

In spite of major expansions and improvements in health care and development, health care systems have been unable to meet the health needs of large segments of the world population. Shortcomings of health care systems vary from country to country and even within the same country. Among shortcomings that need to be addressed are an imbalance in available services, inefficient utilization, and lack of responsiveness to women's expectations and perspectives. Basically, one can differentiate three patterns of inefficiency: deficiency, under-utilization, and over-medicalization. These patterns of inadequacy apply to the whole field of health care, but they are particularly prominent in the area of reproductive health.

Lack of awareness or gender blindness frequently leads to gender bias in the health care system and to the prioritization of male interests in decision-making. The mainstreaming of gender concerns is vital in policy formulation, health planning, health service delivery, monitoring, and evaluation.

For implementation of reproductive health care, the health care system needs to unpack the reproductive health package. This has to be handled with care, because some components are fragile and more sensitive than other. Different components of the package pose different challenges in implementation. The system is challenged to meet new and emerging needs, to serve new customers and to develop cost-effective interventions for currently expensive and less affordable services.

Laws and policies may facilitate or inhibit women's access to reproductive health care. Systems of health law and policies that restrict women's reproductive choices are usually based on historical connections between sexuality and morality. Many restrictive policies reflect the idea that women's sexuality and access to birth control endanger morality and family security. Providers and their professional associations may invoke laws, particularly human rights laws, to advocate for better reproductive health services on behalf of their patients.

Health care systems now represent one of the largest sectors in the world economy. However, the resources devoted to health care systems are very unequally distributed, and not at all in proportion to the distribution of health problems. Lack of resources is not always a valid excuse for governments not to invest in health. There is no country that is so poor that it cannot do something to improve the reproductive health of its people. Dollar for dollar spent on health, many countries are falling short of their performance potential. The result is a large number of preventable deaths and lives stunted by disability. The impact of the failure is borne disproportionately by the poor. Setting priorities among health problems for allocation of resources is not an easy task. Priority-setting has to take into consideration not only the magnitude of the burden of disease, but also the availability of cost-effective interventions. In setting priorities, it should be recognized that reproductive health is special and cannot be simply ranked with disease problems. Although we may not know exactly how much money it will cost to provide reproductive health services for all, we have a better idea about what it will cost in women's lives and health if we do not make reproductive health care universally available.

The United Nations in 1999 reaffirmed that governments should strive to ensure that, by 2015, all primary health care and family planning facilities are able to provide, directly or through referral, the widest available range of safe and effective family planning and contraceptive methods; essential obstetric care; prevention and management of reproductive tract infections, including sexually transmitted diseases, and barrier methods (such as male and female condoms and microbicides if available) to prevent infection.[1] By 2005, 60 per cent of such facilities should be able to offer this range of services, and by 2010, 80 per cent of them should be able to offer such services.[2]

---

[1] UN, General Assembly, *Report of the Ad Hoc Committee of the Whole of the Twenty-first Special Session of the General Assembly: Overall Review and Appraisal of the Implementation of the Programme of Action of the International Conference on Population and Development*, A/S-21/5/Add.1 (New York: UN, 1999), para. 53.

[2] Ibid.

e System and the Right to Health

trace their origin to the mystical beginnings of medicine.
:d history, societies have sought relief from physical and
·ough the institutionalization of roles, the functions of
ninister to the suffering. Health personnel and health fac-
1 the context of a 'health care system'. The health care
system can thus be defined as the mechanism in any society that transforms or
metabolizes inputs of knowledge, and human and financial resources, into
outputs of services relevant to the health concerns in that society.

The health care system is one of several differentiated systems that serve
needs of societies. It has to compete with these other systems for often scarce
resources. The competition is not only at the level of governments (and donors)
when they are allocating resources to different sectors, but also at the level of
the family and individuals when they make decisions on how much to spend
on health.

Health is not the domain of the health care system alone. Other systems
(or sectors) in every society have a bearing on the health of the population and
may be, and in fact in many cases are, more important than that of the health
care system. Agriculture (nutrition), education, housing, transportation and the
general economic level, among other factors, all have their bearing on health.

In recognition of the role of other systems in health, the World Health
Organization uses the term 'health system' to include all the activities whose
primary purpose is to promote, restore, or maintain health.[3] Health care
services fall within these boundaries. So does home care of the sick, which is
how somewhere between 70 and 90 per cent of all sickness is managed. Other
interventions like road and environmental safety improvement are also part of
the system. Beyond the boundaries of this definition are those activities whose
primary purpose is other than health—education, for example—even if these
activities have a secondary, health-enhancing benefit.

Society grants the health care system the 'legitimacy' to function and the
resources to operate. People are investing in the system, whether directly by
out-of-pocket payments, indirectly by paying insurance premiums and social
security contributions, or almost unknowingly when their paid taxes are used
to finance the system. In this 'social contract', society expects a return. Social
expectations from the health care system vary and are affected by the value
system of a society. The highest expectation is the human right to health.

The human right to health is recognized in numerous international instruments (Pt. III, Ch. 4). Article 25.1 of the Universal Declaration of Human

---

[3] WHO, *The World Health Report 2000. Health Systems: Improving Performance* (Geneva:
WHO, 2000), at 5.

Rights affirms that: 'everyone has the right to a standard of living adequate for the health of himself and of his family, including food, clothing, housing and medical care and necessary social services'. According to the International Covenant on Economic, Social and Cultural Rights, in Article 12.1, State Parties recognize 'the right of everyone to the enjoyment of the highest attainable standard of physical and mental health'.

The right to health is an inclusive right, extending not only to timely and appropriate health care but also to the underlying determinants of health, such as access to safe and potable water and adequate sanitation, an adequate supply of safe food, nutrition, and housing, healthy occupational and environmental conditions, and access to health-related education and information, including on sexual and reproductive health. A further important aspect is the participation of the population in all health-related decision-making at the community, national, and international levels.

The right to health is not to be understood as a right to be *healthy*. The right to health contains both freedoms and entitlements. The *freedoms* include the right to control one's health and body, including sexual and reproductive freedom, and the right to be free from interference, such as the right to be free from torture, non-consensual medical treatment, and experimentation. By contrast, the *entitlements* include the right to a system of health protection that provides equality of opportunity for people to enjoy the highest level of health (see Pt. III, Ch. 6, Sect. 3).

The health care system has obligations to people's right to health. It has the obligations to respect, to protect, and to fulfil the right to health. It has to respect and protect the 'freedoms' and to fulfil the 'entitlements' embodied in the human right to health. The health care system can be held in violation of the right to health through *acts of commission* and through *acts of omission*. The obligation to respect requires the system to refrain from interfering directly or indirectly with the enjoyment of the right to health. The obligation to protect requires the system to prevent third parties from interfering with the freedom of people to enjoy their right to health. The obligation to fulfil requires the system to ensure that people have access to a system of health care that provides equal opportunity for everyone.

Further discussion on the implications of the human right to the highest attainable standard of health is presented in Chapter 6.

3. *Special Considerations in Reproductive Health Care*

Reproductive health care is a part of general health care. There are, however, special considerations which set it apart from general health care. Reproductive health care providers deal with mostly healthy people, they often have to take into consideration the interests of more than one 'client' at the same time, they deal mostly with women and they have to deal and interact with society. These special considerations have ethical, legal, and human rights implications.

3.1. *Dealing with healthy people*

Reproductive health care providers respond to needs of healthy subjects, related to their physiological, sexual, and reproductive functions (including the prevention of unwanted pregnancy and the prevention of sexually transmitted infections). This has several implications.

Different from other disciplines in medicine, reproductive health care is more health-oriented than disease-oriented. Promotive and preventive health care are major components of reproductive health care.

Dealing with healthy people implies a change in the provider–patient relationship, from a giver–recipient relationship to a more participatory type of health care. Counselling is the description for a good part of reproductive health care. There is no other field of medicine in which participation of the 'patient' in health care decisions is as much desired and practised. The ethical principle of respect, a minimal standard for ethical conduct, includes autonomy of capable persons. While in other fields of medicine, *patients* are required to give their *informed consent* to the treatment proposed by the health care provider, freely and without undue pressure or inducement, in the case of reproductive health care, *clients* have to make *informed choices and decisions*.

The risk/benefit ratio is different when a drug or device is used for a healthy subject, to prevent a condition which may or may not happen, from what it is when a drug or device is used by a person suffering from a disease which in itself carries a risk. The risk/benefit ratio is also different from another aspect. Often, very large numbers of people are involved in receiving a treatment, so that rare adverse effects assume more importance. Safety and efficacy of drugs and devices are regulated by government agencies, and are subject to laws of product liability. Reproductive health products, in terms of regulation and law, are seen as different from products developed and marketed to treat patients with diseases. In dealing with healthy people, the temptation to over-medicate for normal life events would be resented, but in reproductive health care of women it has often been accepted, sometimes without valid scientific evidence, by the health profession.

3.2. *Dealing with more than one 'client'*

Different from other health professionals, reproductive health care providers often deal with, or have to take into consideration, more than one 'client' at the same time. This other party to a treatment decision could be a woman's male partner, or her foetus. The interests of the different parties may coincide and may diverge, or even conflict. Beneficience, the ethical duty to do good and maximize good, underpins the provision of much medical treatment and health care. As will be discussed in Chapter 4, beneficience poses an ethical challenge when what one person seeks as beneficial for herself may have adverse implications for others.

3.3. *Dealing mostly with women*

Providers of reproductive health care deal mostly with women, who have often been subordinated to their societies' needs and have been under-valued. Providers, who are mostly men, should set a male model in respecting women and treating them as equals. They must not only respect women, but also be sensitive to their concerns and perceptions. The profession must encourage and promote the participation of women in their health care, and be sensitive to their perspectives. Respect for women should be shown in providing them with confidentiality, privacy, and access to all information they need to make well-informed decisions about their health. It is true that a majority of women in many parts of the world are illiterate, but they are fully capable of making sound decisions. An illiterate person in a rich society is a person who, in spite of the opportunity, cannot read and write. In poor societies, illiterate persons are those who were not given the opportunity to read and write. Poor people have a very narrow safety margin for error in making decisions about their lives and, consciously or subconsciously, they know that. Women, literate or illiterate, rich or poor, given the information and the right to choose and decide, will make the right decisions for themselves and their families, and for the community at large.

   As explained by the General Recommendation on Women and Health of the Committee on the Elimination of Discrimination against Women, lack of respect for confidentiality of women seeking reproductive health care can deter women from seeking advice and treatment and thereby adversely affect their health and well-being (see Pt. III, Ch. 6, Sect. 2, para. 12(d)). Women will be less willing, for the reason of unreliable confidentiality, to seek medical care for diseases of the genital tract, for contraception, or for incomplete abortion and in cases where they have suffered sexual or physical violence.

   Women have been excluded from historical sources of moral authority, and under-represented in learned professions of medicine and law, and in legislative assemblies. The voices of women, and their perspectives, have often not been taken into consideration in laws, policies, and regulations governing sexual and reproductive health care for women.

3.4. *Dealing with society*

Reproductive health care providers have to deal and interact with their society
at large. No society has ever been neutral about sexual and reproductive issues.
No other health profession has to deal with such emotionally charged health
issues as sexuality and abortion. As new health technologies develop, new
issues arise for which society may or may not be well prepared. Enforcing
perceived interests of the society may violate women's human rights. Fertility
control is a case in point.

4. *Shortcomings in the Performance of the Reproductive Health Care System*

Health reforms, commonly referred to as health sector reform, have been
taking place in many countries over the last decade. This has been in response
to a general dissatisfaction with the performance of the system. In countries
which have undergone structural adjustment, the main drivers have been constraints on government expenditure and donor conditionalities. In economies
in transition, health systems are being reconstructed as a response to economic liberalization and the need to move away from command and control
management models. In general, there have been a rethinking of the role of
governments, moves towards decentralization, emphasis on cost recovery, and
an expanded role of the private sector. The impact of health sector reform on
reproductive health services is a matter for concern,[4] and its human rights
implications are discussed in Part I, Chapter 6.

A well-functioning system should respond adequately to the health care
needs of the population. In spite of major expansions and improvements in
health care and development, health care systems have been unable to meet
the health needs of large segments of the world population. Shortcomings of
health care systems vary from country to country and even within the same
country. Among those that need to be addressed are an imbalance in available
services, inefficient utilization, and lack of responsiveness to women's expectations and perspectives.

4.1. *Imbalance in the health care system*

4.1.1. *Health facilities*

There is a growing consensus that a better balance of services is needed among
health facilities at various levels. Within provinces or districts, health facilities

---

    [4] H. Standing, 'Gender and Equity in Health Sector Reform Programmes: A Review', *Health
Policy and Planning*, 12 (1997), 1–18.

typically consist of the sub-centre (a clinic or dispensary) at the periphery, then the health centre, and up to the district (rural) or provincial hospital. In many countries, the upper end of the system, consisting of large, urban hospitals serving a small and relatively affluent portion of the total population, is unduly preponderant with a virtual monopoly over resources.[5] This makes the balanced development of more basic health care facilities impossible. Those concerned for health service coverage for an entire population urge that a strong brake be placed on further development of large hospitals, in order to free resources for a rapid expansion of a network of smaller primary health care institutions.

The area of reproductive health suffers most from this unbalanced structure. Reproductive health care differs from other types of medical care in that it is not an occasional need for an unfortunate few. It is a universal requirement of all healthy people who need, among other services, fertility regulation, protection against sexually transmitted infections, and safe motherhood. To provide universal access to this care, a better balanced structure is required in health care systems.

4.1.2. *Human resources*

Regarding human resources for health, there are four kinds of imbalances that may be encountered in health care systems:[6]

1. under-supply (or over-supply) of a specific category of personnel for a country's health needs;
2. mismatch between training and job requirements, especially inadequate preparation of providers for their potential role in promoting health;
3. poor 'mix' of categories (usually too few nurses per doctor);
4. poor geographical distribution of existing providers, seen as a marked disparity in access to basic services not only between under-served and other areas/populations within almost every country, but also among countries, and among medical specialties.

The WHO estimates the number of physicians per 10,000 population, during the period 1994–6, to have been as follows:[7]

- 13.2 for the world;
- 24.6 for developed market economies;
- 34.6 for economies in transition;
- 7.4 for all developing countries;
- 1.0 for least developing countries; and
- 8.9 for other developing countries.

---

[5] WHO, *Evaluation of the Implementation of the Global Strategy for Health for All by 2000, 1979–1996: A Selective Review of Progress and Constraints* (Geneva: WHO, 1998), WHO/HST/ 98.2. at 64–76, 168–77.

[6] Ibid.   [7] Ibid.

Comparable figures for nurses were as follows:

- 36 for the world;
- 81.8 for developed market economies;
- 87.7 for economies in transition;
- 7.2 for all developing countries;
- 2.7 for least developed countries and
- 8.5 for other developing countries

4.1.3. *Hospital beds*

There are large disparities in hospital bed availability both within countries, availability being much greater in the larger cities than in most rural areas, and between countries at different economic levels of development. According to WHO estimates in 1994, the number of hospital beds per 10,000 population was:[8]

- 37 in the world;
- 96 in developed countries;
- 15 in developing countries; and
- 7 in least developed countries.

4.2. *Inefficiency in the health care system*

Basically, one can differentiate three patterns of inefficiency: *deficiency*, *under-utilization*, and *over-medicalization*.[9] These patterns of inadequacy apply to the whole field of health care, but they are particularly prominent in the area of reproductive health.

Deficiency is only partly due to lack of resources. It is also due to inefficient allocation of resources. According to a WHO evaluation of the implementation of the global strategy of health for all, the coverage of health care services in developing countries is deficient, with a distinct urban bias. Levels of coverage of maternal health care remain inadequate in most developing countries. In developed market economies and economies in transition, well over 90 per cent of pregnant women receive antenatal care and are assisted by a person trained in midwifery during childbirth.[10] In the least developed countries, only 50 per cent receive antenatal care, and only 30 per cent deliver with the help of

---

[8] WHO, *Evaluation of the Implementation of the Global Strategy for Health for All by 2000, 1979–1996: A Selective Review of Progress and Constraints* (Geneva: WHO, 1998), WHO/HST/98.2. at 64–76, 168–77.

[9] M. F. Fathalla, 'Health Needs and Problems of Women of the World and the Present Inadequate Health Care System', in H. Ludwig and K. Thomsen (eds.), *Gynecology and Obstetrics: Proceedings of the XIth World Congress of Gynecology and Obstetrics* (Berlin and Heidelberg: Springer-Verlag, 1986), 33–6.

[10] WHO, *Evaluation*.

a skilled birth attendant. In other developing countries the figures are about 70 and 60 per cent respectively. Levels of post-partum coverage are particularly low: below 30 per cent for many developing countries.

In 1965, only about 9 per cent of all married women of reproductive age in developing countries, or their partners, were using a reliable method of contraception. Today, this figure is approaching 60 per cent.[11] In spite of this increase in the use of fertility regulation over the past thirty years worldwide, there remain marked differences between the developed and developing parts of the world, and among regions within the developing part. There are still large segments of the world's population whose needs of fertility regulation are not met by the currently available methods and services. In 1990, it was estimated that 200 million couples were using methods of family planning that they considered unsatisfactory or unreliable, contributing to the estimated 30 million unintended pregnancies that occur each year among people practicing contraception.[12] In addition, at least another 100–120 million couples were not using any method of contraception even though they wanted to space their pregnancies or limit their fertility. Finally, contraceptive choices available to couples in developing countries are often very limited, with heavy reliance on permanent methods (male and female sterilization), which account for nearly 50 per cent of use.

The *under-utilization* of the health care system is a distressing phenomenon in some developing countries. Culturally inappropriate, alien, socially non-relevant health care services are bound to be rejected. Where different societies have their own traditions of disease prevention and sickness care, the introduction of the concepts and technologies of modern scientific medicine will be most effective only through adaptation and accommodation to these existing systems. Health care professionals find it easy to blame patients when they do not utilize the service, and advocate their better education. It is less palatable to health professionals, but more true, to fault the health care system. The question should not be why patients do not accept the services they offer, but rather why health professionals do not offer patients the services they will accept.

Over-medicalization of the health care system is becoming typical of affluent societies. Technology utilization is lurching from appropriate use into indiscriminate use. The thirst for technology and medical over-consumption are raising the costs of health care to staggering heights. Women are also voicing their concerns about the over-medicalization of physiological events in their lives. There is a need to keep normal labour normal.[13]

---

[11] Ibid.   [12] Ibid.

[13] M. F. Fathalla, 'Health Care Systems: The Seven Sins', in P. Belfort, J. A. Pinotti, and T. K. A. B. Eskes (eds.), *Advances in Gynecology and Obstetrics: The Proceedings of the XIIth World Congress of Gynecology and Obstetrics, Rio de Janeiro, October 1988, iv. Maternal Physiology and Pathology* (New York and London: Parthenon, 1988), 3–13.

4.3.   *Inadequate responsiveness to women's expectations and perspectives*

4.3.1. *A health system that cares*

It is not enough for the health care system to be properly in place and for it to provide modern services. People's perceptions of the services and their rightful expectations also matter.

Among other important criteria in assessing the performance of the health care system, and the respect paid to the right to health, are respect for the dignity of the person, not humiliating or demeaning persons, confidentiality or the right to determine who has access to one's personal health information, access to social support networks—family and friends—for people receiving care and autonomy to participate in decisions about one's health. It is not overall perception that matters, but each instance of care. It can be that some people are treated with courtesy, while other groups in the population are humiliated.

Most of these elements do not have cost implications. There is thus scope for improving this aspect of the performance of the health care system without the need to infuse any significant amount of new resources.

The Platform for Action of the Fourth World Conference on Women, 1995, commented that

> The quality of women's health care is often deficient in various ways, depending on local circumstances. Women are frequently not treated with respect, nor are they guaranteed privacy and confidentiality, nor do they always receive full information about the options and services available. Furthermore, in some countries, over-medicating of women's life events is common, leading to unnecessary surgical interventions and inappropriate medication.[14]

Throughout human history, medicine has been recognized as a profession for both care and cure. This was the way it was when the medical man or woman was also the religious or spiritual guide and/or the magician. This was also how it continued to be when the medical profession diverged from religion and from magic. A reader of the history of medicine would realize that our physician ancestors, for the major part of human history, had really little in their hands that could influence the process of disease or prevent deaths. Their treatments had an equal chance, in many cases more than an equal chance, of being more harmful than useful. In spite of the clumsy performance of our ancestor physicians in the function of cure, they continued to command respect and prestige in the societies they served, and societies continued to

---

[14] UN, Department of Public Information, *Platform for Action and Beijing Declaration: Fourth World Conference on Women, Beijing, China, 4–15 September 1995* (New York: UN, 1995), para. 103.

invest in their activities. This was because they did so well in the function of care. Their pastoral/supportive function may be described as the provision of psychological help and 'tender loving care' to anxious patients. This psycho-emotional support and reassurance more than compensated for the shortcomings in treatment.

Unfortunately, the personally supportive, pastoral aspects of medical care tend to be squeezed out by our thirst for technology. 'Pride' in the application of scientific knowledge and biomedical technology is now creating an 'emotional gap' in the care of patients. Machines now stand between doctors and their patients.[15]

The loss of the physicians' caring function is no more evident than in the field of reproductive health. In exercising normal functions, women are often in need of more care than cure. They are receiving instead depersonalized, mechanized, mystery-clouded medical services. Women are protesting at being objectified in one of their fundamental physiological roles, and they are right to do so.

4.3.2. *Women as ends and not means*

A major shortcoming in reproductive health care within the health care system was in the philosophy with which services were provided. Women were considered as means in the process of reproduction, and as targets in the process of fertility control. Services were not provided to women as ends in themselves. Women benefited from the process, but were not at its centre. They were objects, and not subjects.

The needs of women in reproduction have been traditionally addressed within the concept of maternal and child health (MCH). The needs of women were submerged in their needs as mothers. MCH programmes and services have played, and continue to play, an important role in promotive, preventive, and curative health care of mothers and children. MCH services tend to focus on a healthy child as the desired outcome. While mothers care very much for this desired outcome because of the investment they make in the process of reproduction, this focus resulted in less emphasis being put on caring about the health risks to which mothers are liable during pregnancy and childbirth, and on putting in place the essential obstetric services and facilities to deal with them. As a result, the tragedy of maternal mortality in developing countries has now risen to dimensions that can no longer be ignored.

Despite all their benefits to the quality of life of women, family planning programmes have left women with some genuine concerns as well as unmet needs. Women have more at stake in fertility control than men have. Contraceptives

---

[15] M. F. Fathalla, 'When Medicine Rediscovered its Social Roots', *Bulletin of the World Health Organization*, 78 (2000), 677–8.

are meant to be used by women to empower themselves by maximizing their choices, and controlling their fertility, their sexuality, their health, and thus their lives. Family planning, however, can be used, and has been used by governments and others, to control rather than to empower women. The family planning movement has been largely demographically driven. As far as policy makers were concerned, women were often considered as targets. Some governments were so short-sighted as not to see that when women are given a real choice, and the information and means to implement their choice, they will make the most rational decisions for themselves, for their communities, and ultimately for the world at large.[16]

With women as only means and not ends, health care related to reproduction has been fragmented, and important health needs have been left unmet. The concept of MCH focuses special attention on women when and if they are reproducing, to ensure that society gets a healthy child, but often neglects women's other reproduction-related health needs. Infertility may not be a serious hazard as far as physical health is concerned, but can be a major cause of mental and social ill-health, so that infertility denies 'health' as understood by the World Health Organization. It is not fair that a society should provide care to women who are capable of reproduction, but should neglect the suffering of those who are unable to conceive. Sexual intercourse exposes women to the risk of unwanted pregnancy. It also exposes many women to another serious or more serious risk, that of sexually transmitted infections, including HIV infection. If a family planning programme has an exclusive demographic focus, it may not see the point of meeting this important need for women's protection. Women's reproduction-related health needs are not limited to the reproductive years of their lives. The girl child, the adolescent girl, and the mature adult and older woman have health needs related to their future or past reproductive function. Men have their reproductive health needs too, and male participation and responsibility are important for women's health.

The societal attitude of looking at women as means to produce children and not ends is even more pervasive. Services offered to women often have something of a 'veterinary' quality. Proponents of the education of girls cite the advantages that such education will have for the survival and health of their children, and the impact education will have on reducing birth rates. Nutrition of women is justified because of the needs of the foetus and the nursing child. Even with the tragedy of maternal mortality, a justification put forward for investment in keeping mothers alive is that their survival is critical for the survival of their children.

[16] M. F. Fathalla, 'The Impact of Reproductive Subordination on Women's Health–Family Planning Services', *American University Law Review*, 44 (1995), 1179–90.

4.3.3. *A fragmentary response to a totality of needs*

The concept of reproductive health illustrates that health in reproduction is a package. People cannot be healthy if they have one element of health but miss another. Moreover, the various elements of reproductive health are strongly inter-related. Improvements in one element can result in potential improvements in other elements. Similarly, lack of improvement in one element can hinder progress in other elements.

Pelvic infection, for example, accounts for about one-third of all cases of infertility worldwide, and for a much higher percentage in sub-Saharan Africa.[17] The resultant infertility is also the most difficult to treat. The magnitude of the problem of infertility will not be ameliorated except by a reduction of sexually transmitted diseases (STDs), by safer births that avoid post-partum infection, and by decreasing the need for or the resort to unsafe abortion practices.

Infant and child survival, growth, and development cannot be improved without good maternity care. Proper planning of births, including adequate child spacing, is a basic ingredient of any child survival package. Unless adequately controlled, STDs, and in particular HIV infection, can impede further progress in child survival.

Fertility regulation is a major element in any safe motherhood strategy. It reduces the number of unwanted pregnancies, with a resultant decrease in total exposure to the risks of pregnancy, and decreases the number of unsafe abortions. Proper planning of births can also decrease the number of high-risk pregnancies.

The different needs in reproductive health are not isolated from each other. They are simultaneous or consecutive, related needs. Adolescent health care serves as a good illustrative example. Adolescents need sex education, and at the same time they need to protect themselves against STDs and against unwanted pregnancies, while preserving their fertility potential. If they become pregnant, they need to be safeguarded from the special hazards of pregnancy and childbirth, and to be helped to care for their infants and children.

According to a recent WHO evaluation, related reproductive health interventions often come to be delivered over time as separate and discrete activities, rather than as a comprehensive response to people's needs at different stages of their lives.[18] Thus, for example, family planning clinics often function independently of those catering to other aspects of maternal and child health. A woman attending a clinic session for child immunization cannot, at the same

---

[17] World Health Organization, 'Infections, Pregnancies and Infertility: Perspectives on Prevention', *Fertil. Steril.* 47 (1987), 964–8.
[18] WHO, *Evaluation*.

time, obtain care for her own health needs; she will be asked to come back on a different day, or even to go to a different health facility.

5. *Mainstreaming the Gender Perspective in the Health Care System*

Sex is determined by individuals' biological characteristics. Gender is the term used to distinguish those features of females and males that are socially constructed from those that are biologically determined. Women and men are differentiated by social characteristics, on the one hand, and by biological characteristics on the other. Gender issues are not just of concern to women. Men's health too is affected by gender divisions in both positive and negative ways. Despite their commonalities, women and men have their own particular needs, and these different needs have to be met in a gender-sensitive approach.

The Committee on the Elimination of Discrimination against Women (CEDAW), established under the UN Women's Convention, has issued a General Recommendation on Women and Health that explains how different kinds of risk factors may affect women and men. These factors include:

- biological factors that vary between women and men according to their reproductive functions, such as pregnancy and childbirth;
- socio-economic factors that can vary according to sex, race, and age, such as widely prevalent marriages of adolescent girls;
- psycho-social factors that can vary according to sex, such as post-partum depression; and
- health system factors such as maintaining legal and practical obstacles to access to services and denying confidentiality when women seek services (see General Recommendation, Pt. III, Ch. 6, Sect. 2, para. 12).

Lack of awareness, or gender blindness, frequently leads to gender bias and to the prioritization of male interests in decision-making. The mainstreaming of gender concerns is vital in policy formulation, health planning, health service delivery, monitoring, and evaluation.[19]

Chapter 6 in Part I includes further discussion on the human right to non-discrimination as it relates to sex and gender.

6. *Challenges in the Implementation of Reproductive Health Care*

For implementation of reproductive health care, the health care system needs to unpack the reproductive health package. This has to be handled with care,

[19] UN, *Women and Health—Mainstreaming the Gender Perspective into the Health Sector: Report of the Expert Group Meeting 28 September–2 October 1998, Tunis* (New York: UN, 1999), UN Publication Sales No. 99.IV.4, 1–64.

because some components are fragile and more sensitive than others. Different components of the package pose different challenges in implementation.[20]

One part of the package includes traditional services with which health care systems already have experience. These include maternal and child health services and family planning. The challenge will be how to expand the coverage and improve the quality of the services.

In other parts of the package, the system is challenged to meet new and emerging needs. Among the new needs, we have to face the new pandemic of HIV/AIDS, the dilemma of unsafe abortion, gender-based violence, and sexual abuse in all its offensive forms. The challenge is how to approach sensitive and socially divisive issues, how to overcome tradition and social barriers to improved care, and how to influence human behaviour.

In another part of the package, the system is challenged to serve new customers. Among the new customers the system is challenged to reach and serve are men, adolescents, and, unfortunately, the growing number of displaced persons and refugees. Services, including information and education, need to be tailored to serve the needs of these new customers. At 1.05 billion worldwide, today's is the biggest-ever generation of young people aged between 15 and 24, and this age group is rapidly expanding in many countries.

Another part of the reproductive health care package stands out because the services needed are more expensive, and to some countries may seem to be unaffordable. These include treatment of HIV-positive pregnant women to prevent transmission of the infection to the foetus and newborn; infertility management; and detection and management of reproductive cancers. The challenge is to develop and test new cost-effective interventions that can be implemented in resource-poor settings.

7. *Health Care Systems and the Law*

7.1. *Legal principles governing health care delivery*

Laws and policies may facilitate or inhibit women's access to reproductive health care. Most systems have core principles of medical law that protect the right to informed and free decision-making by patients, their privacy and confidentiality, the competent delivery of services and the safety and efficacy of products. Systems vary, however, in the extent to which these principles are applied to reproductive health services, including obstetric care. Moreover, the enforcement of laws that entitle women to obstetric services, and that oblige governmental or other agencies to deliver them, and to create accountability

[20] M. F. Fathalla, 'Reproductive Health for All: A Commitment towards the New Millennium', *European Journal of Contraception and Reproductive Health Care: Millennium Edition*, 4 (1999), 212–16.

for their absence, also vary significantly across national boundaries. Laws may oblige husbands to provide their wives with necessary health care, but are difficult to enforce when families are impoverished.

The core principles of medical law governing health care delivery assume more importance in the case of reproductive health care. Women sometimes refuse to seek health services that are available, because they believe that their medical confidentiality will not be sufficiently respected. This may be particularly so in smaller communities where personal relationships among patients and clinic personnel exist in social life outside the clinic setting. Women's perceptions that their confidentiality may be breached might be usefully addressed by ensuring that clinic policies on legal duties of confidentiality are carefully explained to all those seeking health care. Careful training of health professionals on how to protect confidentiality, both by themselves and by their assistant personnel, particularly in sensitive matters of reproduction and sexuality, will equip them to avoid breaches that occur in good faith or through negligence. Emphasis on professional duties of confidentiality, through professional disciplinary committees and/or courts, would reduce the risk of individual breaches, and also instruct members of professions in their ethical and legal responsibilities of confidentiality. Safe motherhood would be promoted through assuring women that they can trust that reproductive health services will be delivered in professional confidence.

There may be other deterrents to women, or some sub-groups of women, seeking obstetric services. For example, indigenous women experiencing obstetric complications may refuse to go to governmental hospitals for fear of being sterilized post-partum without their consent. Moreover, suspicion and fear of improper practices may persist long after they have been eradicated.

7.2. *Obstructive laws*

Laws and policies may facilitate or inhibit women's access to reproductive health care. Health professionals have to abide by the laws in their countries. They, however, have two obligations. First, they have to understand the limits of the law, which may not be as restrictive as sometimes perceived. Second, where the laws appear to be dysfunctional in practice, and contributing adversely to women's health, health professionals have an obligation to work with the legal profession, women's groups, and other progressive forces in the society to demonstrate the need for legal reform.

Laws governing reproductive health care are not generally contained within a separate body of law. General laws have to be applied. There are exceptions where countries develop laws with a particular goal in reproductive health care. For instance, countries may reform laws that criminalize abortion. Countries may adopt laws to prohibit female genital cutting. Countries

have also adopted laws and policies to regulate access to medically as
reproduction.

Laws that obstruct women's access to information and care can function
as causes of maternal mortality. Preventing access to services are laws that
criminalize medical procedures that only women request and that may be indicated to save their lives and health, such as those that govern contraception
and abortion. While often tied to social or religious concerns, these criminal
laws put women at risk when they prohibit or deter performance of treatment
necessary to save the lives of pregnant women. When tested in courts, many
of these restrictively worded laws are interpreted to have exceptions where
procedures are undertaken in good faith to preserve women's lives or health,
but unless so interpreted, their prohibitive language and severe punishments
deter physicians from undertaking therapeutic interventions in pregnancy.
Laws that prohibit medical procedures but that do not have clearly stated or
indeed any exceptions where women's lives or physical and mental health are
at risk can be shown to violate human rights requirements.

Another dysfunction found in laws and health regulations or policies is
that they require unnecessarily high qualifications of health service providers
for reproductive health care. Different from health care for other disease
systems, which is required by relatively small numbers of people, the need for
reproductive health care is a universal need by all people. Such laws are often
enacted in the belief that they are necessary for women's protection. However,
they frequently unduly obstruct care, or make it unavailable because of limits
of facilities, personnel, or women's financial means to meet unnecessarily
high costs. Such regulations may apply to maternity services. Requirements in
terms of special facilities or qualifications of personnel may restrict access to
pregnancy termination services, where these services are not against the law.

Some countries have codified laws that entrench women in roles subservient
to their brothers and husbands. They require, for instance, that women
requesting health services obtain their husbands' authorization, or that adolescent girls seeking health services obtain parental authorization, thereby
obstructing medically indicated care and placing women and girls at risk.
Often, permission is impossible to receive, or women are afraid or embarrassed
to seek it.

Systems of health law and policies that restrict women's reproductive
choices are usually based on historical connections between sexuality and
morality. Many restrictive policies reflect the idea that women's sexuality and
access to birth control endanger morality and family security. Legislation
against the provision of contraceptive services and means has historically been
expressed in terms of preservation of morality. Some national laws still characterize the provision of birth-control information and contraceptives as an
offence against morality.

...etter place to begin to impart an awareness of human ...ity than in the small world of the doctor–patient rela-
...e human rights principles have been articulated and ...has been the tradition since Hippocrates that those who ...profession of health care should commit themselves to maintaining the highest standards of personal integrity and competence and to having compassion for those placed in their care. Medical students have traditionally been asked to recite a version of the Hippocratic Oath on graduation.

When Eleanor Roosevelt spoke to the United Nations on the tenth anniversary of the Universal Declaration of Human Rights, she said: 'where, after all, do universal human rights begin? In small places, close to home—so close, so small that they cannot be seen on any map of the world . . . unless these rights have meaning here, they have little meaning anywhere.'

Human rights laws have been gender blind. They tended to focus on the public sphere of men and to miss the private sphere in which most women live and have specific concerns. As will be discussed in Chapter 6, human rights are applicable to situations in sexual and reproductive health.

7.3.2. *Compliance with human rights law*

Members of the health profession have been involved in the past in violations of human rights. Although eugenics programmes are usually associated with Nazi Germany, they could, and did, happen everywhere.[22] The eugenics movement, including demands for sterilization of people considered unfit, blossomed in the United States, Canada, Britain, Scandinavia, and other countries.

Members of the health profession have been involved in atrocities and torture.[23] The Truth and Reconciliation Commission looked specifically at the role of the health professions in human rights abuses in apartheid South Africa.[24] Human rights abuses have also been committed in the name of medical research.[25]

---

[21] J. Leaning, 'Editorials, Human Rights and Medical Education', *British Medical Journal*, 315 (1997), 1390–1.

[22] D. J. Kevles, 'Eugenics and Human Rights', *British Medical Journal*, 319 (1999), 435–8.

[23] B. Loff and S. Cordner, 'Learning a Culture of Respect for Human Rights in Apartheid South Africa', *Lancet*, 352 (1998), 1800, 1852–3.

[24] P. Sidley, 'South African Doctors Demand Action on "Unethical" Colleagues', *British Medical Journal*, 319 (1999), 594.

[25] A. M. Hornblum, 'They are Cheap and Available: Prisoners as Research Subjects in Twentieth Century America', *British Medical Journal*, 315 (1997), 1437–41.

7.3.3. *Advocacy for human rights*

Providers and their professional associations may invoke laws, particularly human rights laws, to advocate for better reproductive health services on behalf of their patients. When resources that patients require are denied, providers should learn to use human rights principles to make reasoned representations to institutional, governmental, private insurance, and other agencies that allocate resources, explaining why such agencies should serve their patients' needs. Human rights laws may thereby operate to strengthen systems of health care.

The General Assembly of the International Federation of Gynecology and Obstetrics (FIGO), in its meeting in Washington, DC, on 5 September 2000, adopted a resolution on 'women's rights relating to reproductive and sexual health'.

The resolution affirmed 'that improvements in women's health need more than better science and health care; they require state action to correct injustices to women'. The resolution called upon FIGO member societies to make their expertise available to health, educational, and legal professional associations and to collaborate with women's and human rights groups to promote a working partnership, in order to foster compliance with human rights relating to reproductive and sexual health, by:

Proposing and promoting guidelines for obstetrician/gynecologists for the respect of these rights;

Playing an active role in educating the public, and making expertise available to policy makers and legislators, about the health dimension of women's rights and their impact on society at large; and

Proposing national standards for the respect of these rights.[26]

The resolution called upon all members of the profession to respect and protect women's rights in their daily practice, including women's sexual and reproductive rights.

8. *The Question of Resources*

8.1. *Overall resources*

Health care systems now represent one of the largest sectors in the world economy. Global spending on health care was estimated to be about $2,985 billion in 1997, or almost 8 per cent of world gross domestic product.[27] The

---

[26] International Federation of Gynecology and Obstetrics (FIGO), *FIGO Resolution on Women's Rights Related to Reproductive and Sexual Health* (London: FIGO, 2000) at http://www.figo.org/default.asp?id=/00006118.htm, last accessed 14 May 2002.

[27] WHO, *World Health Report 2000*.

International Labour Organization estimates that there were about thirty-five million health workers worldwide a decade ago. Employment in health services now is likely to be substantially higher.

The level of financial resources a country devotes to the health sector depends on a variety of factors. Important determinants include income levels, the relative priority given to health in comparison with other sectors, the price of inputs such as labour, and the size of the private-for-profit sector.

Per capita spending on health services reflects the level of resources made available for health. According to WHO estimated figures for 1995, the total health expenditure per capita in US$ was as follows.[28]

- 2,701 in developed market economies;
- 122 in economies in transition;
- 177 in middle income developing countries;
- 23 in low income developing countries; and
- 8 in least developed countries.

Government health expenditure as a percentage of total government expenditure was estimated for 1995 to be as follows:

- 15.6 for developed market economies;
- 3.6 for economies in transition;
- 5.0 for middle income developing countries;
- 1.1 for low income developing countries; and
- 5.5 for least developed countries.

The resources devoted to health care systems are very unequally distributed, and not at all in proportion to the distribution of health problems. The World Health Organization estimated that in 1990 the developed market economies accounted for over 86 per cent of all health spending. The USA alone, constituting only 5 per cent of the world's population, accounted for 41 per cent of total expenditures, while sub-Saharan Africa, with 10 per cent of the world's population, accounted for only 1 per cent.[29]

Within governments, many health ministries focus on the public sector, often disregarding the—frequently much larger—private finance and provision of care. A growing challenge is for governments to harness the energies of the private and voluntary sectors in achieving better levels of health systems performance, while offsetting the failures of private markets.

The relative mix of public and private financing for health services reveals both the extent to which governments have the resources to intervene in the health sector, and (particularly in the richer world) governments' views on the appropriate level of public involvement. For example, in the USA in 1995,

---

[28] WHO, *Evaluation*.   [29] Ibid.

58 per cent of total health spending came from private sources, while in Norway the figure was only 6 per cent.[30] While the USA gives greater weight to consumer choice and market mechanisms, leaving tens of millions of its population without access to affordable services, Norway believes that intervention to ensure access for all takes priority. Contrary to what some people may think, the poorest countries rely the most on private financing, with an average of 59 per cent (compared to 30 per cent for developed market economies, 22 per cent for economies in transition, 49 per cent for middle income economies, and 46 per cent for developing countries). With the inability or failure of governments to finance comprehensive health services for the entire population, the private sector often grows by default. Since the debt crisis in the early 1980s, many governments have been forced to introduce user charges for drugs and visits to public health facilities. The World Health Organization estimated that in half of the world's countries, health spending from private sources increased from 37 per cent in 1990 to 42 per cent in 1992.[31]

Lack of resources is not always a valid excuse for governments not to invest in health. There is no country that is so poor that it cannot do something to improve the reproductive health of its people. A look at military expenditure · shows how resources are abused even in poor developing countries. As a United Nations Development Programme (UNDP) report reveals, their military expenditures rose three times as fast as those of industrialized countries between 1960 and 1987—from $24 billion to $145 billion—including a staggering $95 billion a year in some of the world's poorest countries.[32] In developing countries, the chances of dying from social neglect (from malnutrition and preventable diseases) are thirty-three times greater than the chance of dying in a war from external aggression.

External support for the health sector amounted to approximately 3 per cent of total health expenditures in developing countries in 1990, with 38.5 per cent of the total (equal to $2.45 per capita) going to Africa.[33] Almost half of donor aid is spent on the development of infrastructure through grants for hospitals and health services. The other 50 per cent is directed towards specific health programmes, particularly leprosy, onchocerciasis, HIV and STD infections, and blindness conditions. External aid is particularly important in countries in a state of conflict, or in the immediate aftermath of conflict such as Mozambique and Angola. In Cambodia, aid accounted for 60 per cent of total government expenditure in 1990.

Contrary to a popular belief, the proportion of official development assistance (ODA) allocated for population programmes, including reproductive

---

[30] Ibid.   [31] Ibid.

[32] UN Development Programme, *Human Development Report 1994* (New York: Oxford University Press, 1994), 47–60.

[33] WHO, *Evaluation*.

health, is only a small fraction of the total, estimated in 1993 to be an average of just 1.4 per cent.[34]

8.2. *Fair allocation of resources*

The critical measure of the performance of the health system in a country is its achievement relative to resources. Each health system should be judged according to the resources actually at its disposal, not according to other resources that could have been put at its disposal. Dollar for dollar spent on health, many countries are falling short of their performance potential. The result is a large number of preventable deaths, and lives stunted by disability. The impact of the failure is borne disproportionately by the poor.

Fair financing in health systems means that the risks each household faces due to the costs of healthcare are distributed according to ability to pay rather than to the risk of illness. According to the *World Health Report 2000*, 'the way health care is financed is perfectly fair if the ratio of total health contribution to total non-food spending is identical for all households, independently of their income, their health status or their use of the health system'.[35] It is not enough that the health care system should be good. It should also be fair.

8.3. *Priorities in the allocation of resources*

Setting priorities among health problems, for allocation of resources, is not an easy task. It has to take into consideration not only the prevalence of the health problem but also its seriousness. Seriousness does not mean only the risk of mortality. It has also to take into consideration the risk of morbidity or disability, short- and long-term. The age at which the health problem strikes should also be factored in the equation. A health problem that affects only old people is different from one that affects people in the prime of their lives. The World Bank in a 1993 report tried to quantify all the above considerations, to arrive at an estimate of the burden of disease expressed as 'disability-adjusted life years' (DALYs) lost for each health problem.[36]

Estimation of the burden of disease is not enough to make decisions on the priority for allocation of resources. Much will depend on the availability of cost-effective interventions to deal with the particular health problem. The World Bank considers that an intervention is cost-effective if it can substantially control the problem at a cost of less than $100 per DALY saved.

---

[34] UN Population Fund, *Population Issues Briefing Kit 1997* (New York: UN Population Fund, 1997), at 22.

[35] WHO, *World Health Report 2000*, at 36.

[36] World Bank, *World Development Report—Investing in Health* (New York: Oxford University Press, 1993), 59–71, 223.

For young women (aged 15–44) in demographically developing countries, maternity ranked as the number one cause of the disease burden (accounting for 18 per cent of the disease burden). Sexually transmitted diseases ranked as number two, accounting for 8.9 per cent of the disease burden. Both conditions can be controlled by cost-effective interventions.

8.4. *Reproductive health is special*

Using the DALYs for estimation of the burden of disease has to take into consideration that reproductive health is special in a number of ways. Mortality and physical disability are not the only costs a woman may pay for a health problem. A woman with an unwanted pregnancy may not die and her pregnancy may leave her with no physical disability. But from a woman's perspective, the condition is serious enough that every year almost 20 million women risk their health or life by undergoing an unsafe abortion for an unwanted pregnancy. A woman with infertility may have no disease condition but her suffering, in many communities, is real, judging by what she is willing to go through, in terms of discomfort, risk, and cost, to have a wanted child. A woman may be raped but she may have no serious injuries or physical health sequelae.

The impact of a reproductive health problem often goes beyond the persons concerned. Sexually transmitted infections are not just a disease burden on the person affected. They can be transmitted to others. They can also pass from mother to foetus. Survival and health of a mother impacts on the health and survival of her children. Unwanted pregnancy impacts on the whole family, community, country, and even the world at large.

In the counting of DALYs, conditions of perinatal mortality and morbidity are counted as paediatric health problems. In fact, however, they are part of the burden of disease on women, who have made a major investment of themselves in the pregnancy and who will suffer for the care of a disabled child.

Finally, maternity is not a disease, to be ranked for priority with other disease problems. Maternity is the means of propagation of our species. It is a risky business which women undertake. Women have a right to be protected when they go through risks for survival of our species.

8.5. *The cost of not providing reproductive health services*

Although we may not know exactly how much money it will cost to provide reproductive health services for all, we have a better idea about what it will cost in women's lives and health if we do not make reproductive health care universally available. The following are some of the costs.[37]

---

[37] UN Population Fund, *The Right to Choose: Reproductive Rights and Reproductive Health* (New York: UN Population Fund, 1999), 2–3.

- 515,000 women—almost one every minute—each year will die worldwide from causes related to pregnancy.
- 70,000 women each year will die as a result of unsafe abortion; an unknown number will suffer from infection and other adverse health consequences.
- In developed countries (where average desired family size is small), of the 28 million pregnancies occurring every year, an estimated 49 per cent will be unplanned, and 36 per cent will end in abortion. In developing countries (where average desired family size is still relatively large), of the 182 million pregnancies occurring every year, an estimated 36 per cent will be unplanned, and 20 per cent will end in abortion.[38]
- Six out of ten women in many countries will have a sexually transmitted disease (STD). All will face a higher risk of infertility, cervical cancer, or other serious health problems.
- Based on 2001 estimates, there will be nearly 5 million new cases of HIV infection.[39] Every minute of every day, ten people will become newly infected with HIV. One in seven of those who became infected during 2001 was a child under the age of 15 years. The vast majority was in sub-Saharan Africa, and most children have acquired the virus from their mothers.
- 2 million young girls will be at risk of female genital cutting. The international community and individual governments have condemned the practice, yet it remains widespread in many countries, and is spreading to immigrant communities.
- Rape and other forms of sexual violence will continue to increase. Unfortunately, the stigma of rape keeps all but a very small percentage of cases from being reported.
- An increasing number of refugees will be denied access to a basic package of reproductive health care.
- The 'Day of 6 Billion' was observed in 1999. Human numbers will certainly reach 7 billion, but whether world population then goes on to 8, 10, or 12 billion will depend on policy decisions and individual actions, within the reproductive health approach, in the next decade. Whatever its size, over 90 per cent of the net addition will be in today's developing countries.[40]

---

[38] Alan Guttmacher Institute, *Sharing Responsibility—Women, Society and Abortion World-wide* (New York and Washington: Alan Guttmacher Institute, 1999), 1–56.

[39] UNAIDS, *AIDS Epidemic Update: December 2001* (Geneva: UNAIDS, 2001), UNAIDS/01.74E-WHO/CDS/CSR/NCS/2001.2, at 1.

[40] UN Population Fund, *The State of the World Population 1998: The New Generations* (New York: UN Population Fund, 1998), 1.

9. *The Commitment*

'All countries should strive to make accessible through the primary health-care system, reproductive health to all individuals of appropriate ages as soon as possible and no later than the year 2015.'[41] The solemn commitment to make reproductive health care universally available no later than the year 2015 was a consensus approved by the governments of 179 countries, in their meeting under the umbrella of the United Nations in Cairo, 5–13 September 1994. It should be noted that the commitment about reproductive health was not made in a conference about health. It was made in a conference about population and development. Reproductive health is not only a serious health issue; it is a development issue.

Concern about reproductive health at the international level is a reflection of our increasing global consciousness. The great technological revolution in transport and communication has made the world smaller and brought it closer together. Moreover, we have realized, more than ever before, how interdependent we are, and that the attainment of health and development by people in any one country directly concerns and benefits every other country.

Five years after the Cairo International Conference on Population and Development, where the commitment to reproductive health was made, the United Nations General Assembly discussed in its Twenty-First special session on 30 June–2 July 1999, an overall review and appraisal of the implementation of the Programme of Action of the 1994 Conference. The United Nations General Assembly reaffirmed the commitment to the goal of reproductive health for all, and stated that

At least 40 per cent of all births should be assisted by skilled attendants where the maternal mortality is very high, and 80 per cent globally by 2005; these figures should be 50 and 85 per cent, respectively by 2010 and 60 and 90 per cent by 2015.

The gap between the proportion of individuals using contraceptives and the proportion expressing a desire to space or limit their families should be reduced by half by 2005, by 75 per cent by 2010, and by 100 per cent by 2015. Recruitment targets or quotas should not be used in attempting to reach this goal.

To reduce the vulnerability to HIV/AIDS infection, at least 90 per cent of young men and women, aged 15–24, should have access by 2005 to preventive methods such as female and male condoms, voluntary testing, counseling and follow-up, and at least 95 per cent by 2010. HIV infection rates in persons 15–24 years of age should be reduced

---

[41] UN, *Population and Development*, i. *Programme of Action adopted at the International Conference on Population and Development, Cairo, 5–13 September 1994* (New York: UN, Department for Economic and Social Information and Policy Analysis, ST/ESA/SER.A/149, 1994).

by 25 per cent in the most affected countries by 2005, and by 25 per cent globally by 2010.[42]

The reaffirmed international consensus about making reproductive health care universally available is, however, not enough to make it happen. The will has to be backed by the wallet. The necessary resources must be mobilized.

---

[42] UN, General Assembly, *Report of the Ad Hoc Committee of the Whole of the Twenty-First Special Session of the General Assembly: Overall Review and Appraisal of the Implementation of the Programme of Action of the International Conference on Population and Development*, A/S-21/5/Add.1 (New York: UN, 1999), paras. 53, 58, 64, 70.

4

Ethics

1. *Overview*

In the course of the last half-century, medical ethics or bioethics has become a major field of enquiry at scholarly and professional levels. It is not the preserve of any individual discipline, but is a multidiscipline or interdiscipline with contributions from philosophy, biology, medicine, health care science, law, nursing, and, for instance, religious studies. The field has generated an immense literature and several weighty subdivisions, such as medical research ethics and genetics ethics. It is enriched by contributions from several leading textbook writers and in proliferating general and more specialized journals, and by well-indexed paper and electronic bibliographies.

The intensive literature in the field encompasses a number of core areas and an expanding range of novel concepts, constantly fuelled by new achievements and newly perceived prospects and possibilities related to human biology. Accordingly, there is widening recognition of positive and negative implications of these achievements, prospects, and possibilities for individual health, social welfare, and interactions within families, communities, national economies, and dealings among different countries and cultures.

The purpose of this chapter is to present a very generalized overview of the structure of bioethical analysis, related to the pursuit of reproductive and sexual health. As an overview or distillation, it will not anchor particular perspectives or perceptions in the writing of particular authorities, and is not scholarly in the academic sense of consciously drawing its individual contents from identified works. Rather, it integrates perceptions, sensitivities, and experiences from the general body of literature, particularly texts that are at the basis of modern teaching in the field (see Select Bibliography).

The duty to act ethically lies at the very origins of the medical profession in many cultures. The Hippocratic Oath includes more on the ethics of the physician's conduct than on the science or efficiency that a physician should apply. Because reproductive health care involves factors of human reproductive biology, the ethics that applies to it is often described as 'bioethics'. Bioethics in a narrow sense is a subdivision of the body of ethics that applies to relations between health care providers and recipients of their care. It is generally regarded more widely, however, as a multidisciplinary field of enquiry, both academic and professional, that addresses ethical issues in clinical practice and health care, biomedical research involving humans and animals, health policy, and the environment.

Reproductive health care often presents medical, ethical, and bioethical issues in particularly challenging forms. For instance, dilemmas may arise between ethical principles of the relationship between a health care provider and a patient, and ethical principles that apply to health care providers as members of their communities. A patient may seek contraceptive protection in an abusive sexual relationship, for example, and also require confidentiality regarding her suffering abuse, perhaps fearing that criminal proceedings against an abusive partner will jeopardize the patient's domestic, economic, or other security. The health care provider may feel, however, that failure to act to prevent the abuse amounts to complicity or partnership in it, and leaves the patient and perhaps dependent children at risk of injury, even though appropriate action would violate the patient's request for confidentiality.

Further, compliance with individuals' requests for reproductive health services that practitioners are capable of providing may conflict with a particular practitioner's religious faith or the practitioner's sense of the best interests of the patients themselves or of social order. In deciding whether or not to comply in delivery of requested services, practitioners may have to confront and define their personal ethics and their personal and professional contributions both to their patients' health, and also to the character and conscience of their communities. In addressing concerns of everyday professional practise, ranging from meeting the needs of vulnerable individuals to responding to the confidential requests of influential individuals concerning sensitive matters, reproductive health care practitioners face ethical and bioethical questions.

Frequently, such practitioners face these questions in more acute forms than arise simply from the inherently unequal relationship between one who possesses the power of medical knowledge and a patient requesting assistance based on that knowledge. Practitioners also face ethical issues from the most ancient, such as how abortion is to be approached, to the most modern, such as appropriate employment of advanced reproductive technologies including the creation of human embryos outside a woman's body to relieve the effects of infertility. They must resolve conflicts that arise when the ancient and the modern collide. An example arises when hormonally stimulated superovulation results in multiple pregnancies that are best managed by selective reduction, which aborts the lives of some foetuses but is intended to preserve pregnancies and the lives and health of patients and of the children they will deliver.

2. *The Origins of Bioethics*

The word 'bioethics' appeared in the 1960s, and is popularly attributed to Van Rensselaer Potter, an American biochemist and scientific researcher at the University of Wisconsin, who combined 'bio', representing biological knowledge or the science of living systems, with 'ethics', representing knowledge of human value systems. The first institutional use of the word was in 1971, when what is now usually called the Kennedy Institute of Ethics was founded at Georgetown University in Washington, DC, as the Joseph and Rose Kennedy Institute for the Study of Human Reproduction and Bioethics.

Notwithstanding the relatively modern and primarily North American origins of bioethics, the value systems that assess developments in human medicine and biology have ancient roots. They are traceable to value systems described by philosophers of Classical Greece such as Aristotle and Plato, and to teachings of religious advocates of medical ethics of later centuries. Conscientious care for the sick has long been the inspiration of Christian physicians and nurses, and many hospitals bear the names of Christian saints. Similarly, the twelfth-century Jewish teacher, physician, and philosopher Maimonides (Moses ben Maimon) advanced scholarship in medical ethics based on Jewish law. The modern medical school and hospital at Al-Azhar University in Cairo draw on the inspiration of the orthodox Islamic university founded in the year 972, associated with the mosque of Al-Azhar. Women herbalists and caregivers to the sick provided conscientious comfort in pre-Christian Europe, but knowledge of their motivations and *modus operandi* had been lost by the beginning of the eighteenth century following centuries of their persecution as witches by the Christian Church in Europe and North America.

The modern field of bioethics is new enough that several of its founding figures remain active contributors to its literature, especially in the USA, and have reflected on its origins. Perhaps the broadest account has been offered by Daniel Callahan. In 1969, he was a co-founder and became the director of the Hastings Center, established at Hastings-on-Hudson in New York state, initially named the Institute of Society, Ethics and the Life Sciences. He has written that:

Bioethics can surely be spoken of as a child of the 1960s . . . Four developments were important: the opening up of once-closed professions to public scrutiny, which happened strikingly with medicine; the fresh burst of liberal individualism, putting autonomy at the top of the moral mountain; the brilliant array of technological developments in biomedicine, ranging from the [contraceptive] pill and safe abortions to control the beginning of life to dialysis and organ transplantation to hold off the end of life; and the renewed interest within philosophy and theology in normative ethics, pushing to one

64   *Medical, Ethical, and Legal Principles*

side the positivism and cultural relativism that seemed for a time in the 1940s and 1950s to have spelled the end of ethics as a useful venture.[1]

The historian David Rothman has added the influence of concerns about biomedical research and experimentation with humans in the mid-1960s to causes of the emergence of modern bioethics,[2] and the philosopher Albert Jonsen has claimed that the birth occurred in the US in Seattle at about the same time, when a dialysis committee was empowered to make decisions about access to the then scarce and costly means of mechanical dialysis, thereby deciding who might survive and who would not.[3]

A more narrow but relevant account, by Warren Reich, claims that bio-ethics evolved in Western countries in reaction to the tendency of religions to approach medical developments through their own narrow doctrines and theologies. A particular obstacle to the natural development of perceptions based on scientific understanding was the conservatism of the Roman Catholic Church and its political power in several regions of the world. Its inflexibility was compounded in 1870 when the Church adopted the doctrine of papal infallibility. This froze evolving debate, since any different thinking became a defiance of papal authority amounting to heresy and a scandal. Reproduct-ive and sexual health issues were of particular significance in development of the modern interdiscipline of bioethics, since it concerned matters on which the Roman Catholic Church was rigid and prohibitive. Reich has observed that:

Fertility control was the major issue that spawned bioethics, more than any other single issue—certainly more than any high-technology-related issue in medicine. It was an issue that directly affected hundreds of millions of people; it dealt with quintessen-tially human suffering and fulfillment; it had been medicalized by Margaret Sanger specifically to bring medical authority to bear on the issue; and it was the topic of exten-sive debates over a period of at least three decades prior to the rise of bioethics—not only by specialists but by the general public as well. The debates were interdisciplinary, involving ethical, religious, legal, and social controversy on the levels of social policy as well as personal ethics and ecclesiastical authority. The theologians, who were the first ethicists working in bioethics, cut their teeth on contraception/sterilization and abor-tion debates; and in a very real sense, much of the great energy that was turned toward bioethics around 1970/71 was energy that was diverted from the then-increasingly futile church debates on fertility control.[4]

[1] D. Callahan, 'The Social Sciences and the Task of Bioethics', *Daedalus*, 128 (1999), 275–94 at 278.
[2] D. Rothman, *Strangers at the Bedside: A History of How Law and Bioethics Transformed Medical Decision Making* (New York: Basic Books, 1991).
[3] A. Jonsen, *The Birth of Bioethics* (New York: Oxford University Press, 1998).
[4] W. T. Reich, 'The "Wider View": André Helleger's Passionate, Integrating Intellect and the Creation of Bioethics', *Kennedy Institute of Ethics Journal*, 9 (1999), 25–51 at 37.

3. *The Role of Bioethics*

Religiously inspired care-givers to the sick provide services
their religious beliefs and sacred teachings, and those inspi
philosophies may invoke their philosophical convictions to
passionate conduct towards sick and suffering individuals.
describe themselves or to be described by others as bioethi
bioethics is essentially secular, pluralistic, and multidisciplin... ... some leaders
in bioethics come from religious or philosophical traditions, but many others
are primarily physicians, nurses, biologists, lawyers, and, for instance, his-
torians or anthropologists. Bioethicists are interested in working with others
outside their disciplines to determine the values that should underlie the
provision of medical care in particular and health care in general. They make
assessments not simply on the basis of religious authority or philosophical
claims, but through scientific knowledge and disciplinary interactions.

Bioethics has been recognized to address two fundamental questions,
namely what should individuals and human communities do, permit, tolerate, or prohibit in biology, particularly affecting existing and future human
beings, and how should decisions be made to determine what conduct is mandatory, permissible, tolerable, or prohibited. Bioethics addresses basic issues
in the human, institutional, and social management of human birth, sickness,
and death, but has come to popular attention through technological developments. These have concerned techniques for assisted conception or assisted
reproduction to overcome infertility, effective means to limit or remedy unplanned and undesired conception, mechanical means to assist or replace organ
functions, tissue and organ transplantation to prolong or enhance life, and, for
instance, medical means that may terminate life.

Bioethicists determine information from a range of scientific and non-
scientific fields of knowledge, following the maxim that good ethics depends
on good facts, and propose appropriate conduct in medical care and provision
of health services. They often work in and through committees in hospitals
and other health care facilities or medical research institutes, as members of or
consultants to committees. Governmental and other public-sector agencies,
and also private-sector bodies, are increasingly creating ethics committees that
make or recommend decisions on issues of bioethical concern.

Bioethics presents language and concepts in which to express ideas about
right conduct in medical care and health policy, and in which to dissent from
others' views and preferences. In offering language of criticism, bioethics also
offers language of explanation and justification. The different orientations,
prioritized principles, and levels of bioethical analysis outlined below, when
taken together, do not necessarily lead to self-evident conclusions. Bioethical
analysis does equip commentators and decision-makers in medical care and

...th policy to explain and defend their conclusions, and to respectfully dis-agree with those of others without facing the accusation that they are defying the teaching authority of an institutional or hierarchical leader. Concepts of bioethics empower individuals and institutions to react to others' conduct and observations in a common language, and to invite and engage in compre-hensible, civil discussion about ends and means in medicine and health care. Adversaries may recognize each other as following different ethical reasoning rather than as being unethical because their views diverge.

4. *Bioethical Orientations*

Several different ethical orientations guide bioethical conclusions. Historical orientations continue in effect today, and reflect the philosophical origins of bioethics.

4.1. *Duty-based bioethics*

Duty-based (or deontological) bioethics is attributed to natural reason or nat-ural law, and distinguishes vice from virtue as a matter of the inherent quality of an act or proposal. Natural law, propounded for instance by Aristotle, was incorporated into doctrine of the Roman Catholic Church in the thirteenth century by St Thomas Aquinas to harmonize reason and faith as divine gifts. An exponent of secular duty-based ethics was the late eighteenth-century German philosopher Immanuel Kant, who taught, for instance, that humans are to be treated as ends in themselves, never only as means towards ends. Duty-based bioethics tends to be absolutist, unaccommodating of ethical relativity and pluralism. The Roman Catholic Church once prohibited the reading of Kant's writings.

Duty-based bioethicists believe that good cannot come from evil, and that an end that is good in itself does not justify the use of inherently wrongful means. For instance, Roman Catholic bioethicists believe that artificial con-traception such as by use of condoms is wrong. They have therefore opposed condom distribution programmes that are intended to contain sexually trans-mitted HIV infection. They consider it desirable that infection be reduced, but only by inherently virtuous means, such as abstinence and self-control. Similarly, Kantians may be troubled by a couple's decision to continue con-ception and births of daughters until they conceive a son who will marry, inherit family land and bring a wife to his home who will give care to the couple in their old age. The fear is that the son, and later his wife, would be regarded only as a means to serve the existing couple's ends of securing shelter and care. In the former case, preventable HIV infection might occur, and in the latter, if the son were not conceived, the couple, particularly the widowed wife, might face poverty and homelessness in old age, due to their daughters' lack of inheritance and economic rights. However, duty-based bioethicists feel no liability for the consequence of their teachings and policies contributing to human suffering. They consider that a beneficial end does not justify unethical means, and that unethical means cannot become ethical simply because they may produce a result desirable or good in itself.

4.2. *Consequentialist or utilitarian bioethics*

Consequentialist or utilitarian bioethics recognizes moral responsibility for the consequences of individuals' bioethical choices, and judge good or right conduct as that which is useful to promote and maximize human well-being or happiness. Ethical conduct serves and maximizes desirable outcomes, and conduct is wrongful if it causes or contributes to harmful or undesirable consequences, judged by communal, democratic, or political assessments of welfare. Consequentialist or utilitarian ethics, unlike duty-based ethics, does not aspire to be universal or enduring, but presents a pragmatic response to varying circumstances.

For instance, by this bioethical orientation, birth control programmes are considered proper to reduce unplanned pregnancies that would result in induced abortion, and induced abortion should be lawful and conducted by doctors or other trained personnel in order to reduce the incidence of unskilled abortion that results in women's death or injury. Similarly, health care providers' conscientious objection to participation in such procedures is considered tolerable only when it does not prevent or obstruct women's access to early, safe, and convenient abortion services. Further, providers who invoke conscientious objections to their own participation, perhaps because of their religious or other duty-based convictions, should be bound to refer applicants for such services to providers who have no objections to performing them.

4.3. *Feminist bioethics*

Feminist bioethics is sometimes described as the ethics of care or of connectedness. This orientation reacts against the exclusion of women from historical sources of moral authority, such as clerical ranks of religions, centres of scholarship including universities and other learned societies, learned professions such as medicine and law, and legislative assemblies. Exclusion of the relevance of women's voices and experiences, half of the accumulated wisdom of humankind, was often deliberate, but is now considered to discredit the moral authority of exclusionary institutions. For example, national population or family health programmes that do not incorporate knowledge of and respect for women's preferences regarding the size of their families are considered ethically inadequate.

Feminist analysis addresses concerns not only of sex, which is biological or genetic, but also of gender, which is socially constructed. For instance, some occupations are male gendered, and others female gendered. Attention is drawn to an incongruity between sex and gender, such as by reference to 'a woman doctor' and 'a male nurse'. Not all women are 'feminists', of course, and not all 'feminists' are women, since the focus of this bioethical orientation is on the ethical incorporation of women's social experiences and realities into the value systems of medical treatment and health care.

Much traditional bioethical discussion of contraception and abortion, for instance, fails to consider the impact that unplanned and undesired pregnancy has on women's enjoyment of their lives. Women's inability to influence medical research agendas, and the medical belief that male physiology is 'normal' and women are different only in their reproductive functions, have contributed to inadequate understanding of women's health needs, including for geriatric care arising from women's longer life expectancy. The role of women as caregivers, to their children, parents, and husbands' parents, as well as to others who are sick or elderly, is often devalued or completely disregarded, for instance in discharging patients from medical facilities. It is inadequately recognized that 'home care' and 'community care' mean women's care, and that women are often expected to forgo alternative goals and satisfactions to provide it, and condemned if they decline.

4.4. *Other bioethical orientations*

Other bioethical orientations exist, such as communitarianism, which seeks to advance human community as a good in itself, but proponents usually acknowledge the seniority of orientations addressed above, and aim to show that their approach is preferable. Casuistry is favoured, for instance, by those who believe that cases should be resolved on their particular merits and not by appeals to universal rules. Similarly, advocates of virtue ethics identify the virtues that human and institutional agents in biomedical settings should observe and foster, such as compassion, trustworthiness, sound judgement or discernment, and conscientiousness or integrity, which supplement virtues Hippocrates commended such as modesty, sobriety, patience, promptness, and loyalty.

5. *Principles of Bioethics*

In order to escape the contradictions and restrictive orthodoxies of competing ethical orientations, some bioethical analysts have identified a small number of key principles of bioethical analysis that are common to different orientations. These appeared most visibly as three principles in the Belmont Report (1979) of the US National Commission for the Protection of Human Subjects of Biomedical and Behavioral Research, since the principle of Non-Maleficence (Do No Harm) was considered implicit in the principle of Beneficence (Do Good). However, the authoritative US bioethicists Tom Beauchamp and James Childress[5] and the British authority Raanan Gillon[6] consider this principle explicitly separate, and address four principles.

The description 'principlism', meaning an application of principles of bioethics, is often applied by critics to condemn the mechanical application or prioritization of a narrow range of perceived principles of bioethics that are believed to be shared by many adherents to different distinctive bioethical orientations. However, a limited number of key principles brings coherence and rationality to ethical discussion, and allows comparisons and contrasts in a common currency,[7] in preference to the medical ethics of the 1960s, which K. Danner Clouser described as 'a mixture of religion, whimsy, exhortation, legal precedents, various traditions, philosophies of life, miscellaneous moral rules, and epithets'.[8] The four principles are presented here in a conventional sequence, but none has priority over others, and much bioethical controversy concerns which should be given priority over others to resolve particular problems.

5.1. *Respect for persons*

Respect for persons seems a minimal standard for ethical conduct, but its absence often leaves civil bioethical discussion unachievable. The abortion conflict is insoluble, for instance, when abortion opponents characterize advocates of women's choice as child-killers, and the latter characterize the former as Nazis, bigots, or religious zealots. This principle includes the following.

5.1.1. *Autonomy of capable persons*

This principle sometimes seems to transcend all others, particularly in the US, where strong individualism and a limited role for social agencies organized through government are emphasized. Patient autonomy is served for instance by ethical requirements that patients' consent to treatment be adequately

    [5] T. L. Beauchamp and J. F. Childress, *Principles of Biomedical Ethics* (New York: Oxford University Press, 5th edn., 2001).

    [6] R. Gillon (ed.), *Principles of Health Care Ethics* (Chichester: John Wiley & Sons, 1994).

    [7] J. H. Evans, 'A Sociological Account of the Growth of Principlism', *Hastings Center Report*, 30/5 (2000), 31–8.

    [8] K. D. Clouser, 'Bioethics and Philosophy', *Hastings Center Report*, 23/6 (1993), s. 10–s. 11 at s. 10.

informed and freely given, without undue pressure or inducement. The principle often prevails over the duty to do no harm in that it upholds patients' informed but poor choices, and condemns any compromise of patients' autonomy as paternalism or as infantilization of patients. The principle is increasingly invoked in support of patients' rights to determine the size of their families and to medically assisted conception and reproduction when needed.

5.1.2. *Protection of persons incapable of autonomy*

Protection against harm or distress of children is uncontentious, although imposing elective treatments over children's resistance is questionable, since use of forceful constraints may be harmful. Nevertheless, reasonable pressure to allow administration of some therapies and preventive care, such as vaccination against childhood diseases, is often supported because of the highly favourable risk-to-benefit ratio. Female circumcision or genital cutting is often opposed under this principle in countries where it has not customarily been practised and in some where it has been, and non-religious male circumcision has similarly been questioned. Criteria by which to assess the need for protection can be contentious where adolescents and some adults are concerned, particularly where their low intellect, low income, low social status, or, for instance, low self-esteem expose them to personal and social vulnerability, including sexual exploitation, and to dependency. Normally capable adults may be vulnerable to exploitation, for instance, when physicians on whom they depend for therapeutic care ask patients to participate in their risk-bearing reproductive and other medical research.

An overlap among ethical principles is evident in that an explanation of the protective aspect of respect for persons could serve as well to explain the principle of beneficence, and illustrate non-maleficence. Conduct can be ethically justified according to more than one principle.

5.2. *Beneficence*

Beneficence, the ethical duty to do good and maximize good, underpins the provision of much medical treatment and health care. The quest for improved medical therapies and effective preventive health care accords with this principle. It may be limited, however, by patients' autonomy to choose poorly and the choice of individuals who could benefit from care deciding not to seek it. Where poverty limits potential patients' access to care, charitable aid may assist them. Religiously inspired health care providers and service funders have enjoyed an honourable history of assistance to the poor, under the motivation of beneficence. Beneficence poses an ethical challenge when what one person seeks as beneficial for herself may have adverse implication for others.

Obstetricians may encounter difficulties when care a pregnant woman requests for herself may inadvertently harm her foetus. Medical care appropriate and beneficial for a woman who is not pregnant, for instance, may have unknown effects or known teratogenic effects for a later conceived child *in utero*. An ethical dilemma concerning treatment of pregnant women may arise that is sometimes described as a maternal–foetal conflict, although women usually want care that is appropriate for both themselves and the children they will deliver. Medical research to develop therapies beneficial for women, for instance, has been limited by investigators' fear that unproven agents such as drugs might prove harmful. Researchers have been told that research should not be undertaken on women who might be or become pregnant, lest foetal harm may be caused. However, the women's health advocates require research that will develop beneficial treatments for women, except when experimental drugs or other treatments have scientifically been proven harmful to foetuses *in utero*. That is, beneficial research should not be deterred by unproven speculation about harm or by lack of evidence of safety for foetuses of a test treatment. Women can make decisions for themselves, with relevant information, regarding the risks and benefits of treatment and research.

5.3. *Non-Maleficence*

Non-Maleficence incorporates the foundational medical ethic Do No Harm. The principle requires an extended understanding of the senses in which medical treatment and health care can cause harm. The practical application of Non-Maleficence requires the distinction to be drawn between 'harms' and 'wrongs', because it may be incorrectly reasoned that a practice is not wrong if it causes no harm. It is often wrong to cause and even to risk causing harm, in the sense of injury, pain, disability, or distress. Harm may also consist, for instance, in damaged self-esteem or causing people to feel that they have been used, exploited, or treated disrespectfully.

There may be wrong, however, even where there is no injury, pain, disability, or distress. This is sometimes described as causing 'harmless wrong', which is nevertheless unethical, and may constitute a human rights violation. For example, when women receive gynaecological examinations in a medical school's hospital or clinic, they may agree to several medical students observing their examinations. If a student were to disguise a non-student friend in a white coat, with a stethoscope or similar device indicating that he was a medical student, and bring him in unobserved among genuine medical students to attend an examination, the woman who agreed to the medical students' presence and was unaware that a disguised intruder was present would not have been harmed. She would, however, have been wronged. She would have been deceived, her good will would have been betrayed, and she would have been used, by the medical student and the friend, as an object of sport, curiosity, and perhaps salacious satisfaction. Conduct that is not directly harmful may nevertheless be ethically wrong.

In a historical instance of wrongdoing in the USA, for instance,[9] the effectiveness of contraceptive drugs that appeared promising but were not fully tested was shown when Mexican-American women living in Texas unable to afford such drugs requested them from a family planning clinic that offered free supplies to some women. Women who were told they would receive contraceptive pills were secretly randomized, so that some received them but others, a matched control group, were given placebo pills. The birth rate among women who received the inactive pills proved significantly higher than among women who had received the drug that was being tested, showing effectiveness of the tested drug. Women in the placebo group had no right to receive contraceptive pills, and so were not denied treatment to which they were entitled, and nothing that they might otherwise have used. However, they might have behaved differently if not believing they had contraceptive protection, and they were deceived. These women were used without their consent and without compensation in research of which they were not informed. Today this study is considered to have been unethical for breach of the principle of Non-Maleficence.

A consequence of research being considered liable to injure a subject's child *in utero*, demonstrated by recognition of foetal harm from use of the drug Thalidomide, was that it became usual to exclude women of reproductive age from studies that might affect fertility or an unborn child. A more recent approach, however, is that refusal to employ a fair proportion of available resources on studies to advance the health care of women, including those of reproductive age, is considered unethical. Women continue to use pharmaceutical products whose effectiveness and safety were not tested on women research subjects, because the products were tested and approved for marketing at a time when including women of reproductive age in drug studies was considered ethically improper or at least questionable.

Today, failure to include women of reproductive age in testing of products intended or liable to be used, in therapeutic or preventive health care, by women of reproductive age is considered an unethical breach of the principle of Non-Maleficence, in that it risks causing harm through inadequate testing. The earlier policy of exclusion also treated women disrespectfully as being unable, as competent and informed adults, to make their own decisions on whether to enter medical studies. Non-Maleficence means not only not doing harm, but also not doing wrong, which includes treating people as objects or

---

[9] J. P. Kahn, A. C. Mastroianni, and J. Sugarman (eds.), *Beyond Consent: Seeking Justice in Research* (New York: Oxford University Press, 1998), at 2263.

means to ends and impersonally, even when they are not exp(physical injury or harm.

5.4. *Justice*

Justice is the ethical principle that the law and legal instit
courts aim to serve. Bioethics is less concerned with punitive or compensatory
justice than with distributive justice. Punitive justice provides means by which
wrongdoers may become liable to suffer punishment. Compensatory justice
requires those who have injured others' interests, even unintentionally and
with no wrongful purpose, to compensate them appropriately. Whether laws
are just or unjust is a matter of communal or democratic judgement. Lawyers
have no better sense of this than non-lawyers. Lawyers' contribution to justice
is their understanding of just processes of trial and legal decision-making,
often called due process of law.

Distributive justice is concerned with fairness, and ensuring that all people
receive the rights to which they are entitled. This requires that like cases
be treated alike, for instance in the allocation of scarce resources, and that
different cases be treated to show the differences. Bioethical concerns focus
on criteria of likeness and difference, since cases that seem different by some
criteria appear alike by others. For instance, it was once believed that only
men could exercise social authority, as leaders of political, military, religious,
professional, and educational institutions, and only women could care for
children and disabled and elderly persons. Therefore, social activities became
separated on grounds of gender, male-gendered activities being undertaken
by people of male sex, female-gendered activities being assigned to people of
female sex. In health care, for instance, medical care and surgery were masculine activities, so that a 'woman doctor' was identified by her sex. Simliarly,
nursing was feminine, so that 'male nurses' were described as such. Today,
however, it is recognized that males can discharge both male- and female-
gendered activities, and that women undertake both types of activities too.
Women serve competently and effectively as political, military, religious,
professional, and educational leaders, and men are competent care-givers to
others. Accordingly, policies or practices of excluding persons from occupational or vocational roles on the grounds of their personal sex are now widely
considered unjust and so unethical.

As against this, however, distributive justice requires recognition of biological differences between the sexes where they are ethically significant. Women's
lives, for instance, unlike men's, are endangered by closely spaced and frequent
pregnancies. Women's access to means of birth-spacing is ethically necessary,
as are accessible, safe, and timely means to terminate pregnancies that are dangerous to women's lives and continuing health. Legal and other rules, which in

past were developed principally by institutions that did not include and often deliberately excluded women, that obstruct women's access to necessary reproductive health care and management of pregnancy violate the ethical principle of justice. This recognition is seen in the progressive relaxation of prohibitive abortion laws.

6. *Levels of Bioethical Analysis*

Ethical orientations and principles can be applied at different levels or pitches of analysis. Positions that are ethically defensible at one level of analysis may be indefensible at another. Health care practitioners who believe their conduct to be ethical may therefore be surprised and distressed to face condemnation from critics who assess their conduct from a different analytical level than they have applied. For instance, a physician who has acted in what he or she con-scientiously determines to be a patient's best health interests, such as by steril-izing a woman in the course of delivering another of her unwanted children without seeking her prior consent, may be condemned for acting paternalist-ically. Disrespecting patients as persons worthy of information and capable of choice among various options infantilizes and demeans them. Similarly, a religiously devout physician who intrudes into an unmarried adolescent's life by informing her parents that she is choosing an immoral way of living, because she has requested contraceptive assistance, is liable to be condemned for violation of the patient's confidentiality. Accordingly, actors should select the ethical level on which to justify their conduct, and be able to explain the grounds on which other levels of ethical analysis were considered inappropri-ate. Equally, commentators on others' conduct should explain the grounds on which they claim that their level of analysis is preferable to others, and be able to recognize that conduct they condemn at one level may be ethically explicable at another. Four levels of ethical analysis may be recognized.

6.1. *The microethical level*

This level of analysis applies ethical criteria to how one person treats another. At this analytical level, each person pays each other his or her ethical due. For instance, a health care provider respects a patient's right of informed choice whether or not to accept proposed care. Reciprocally, the patient respects the provider's right not to undertake a form of treatment the provider considers to be counter-therapeutic or futile, because of the 'Do No Harm' commitment, or to which he or she has a conscientious objection. The provider respects the patient's conscientious choice by transfer of the patient's care to another provider if the patient still requests that treatment. A provider acts unethically by withholding information of the legal availability of a treatment option to which the provider has a personal conscientious objection.

It is similarly unethical to not disclose information of an accessible but scarce or expensive form of care that would advance a patient's health interests under the conviction that the care would provide a greater benefit to another patient. For a health care provider whose help a patient has requested unilaterally to subordinate that patient's interests to those of another violates a microethical responsibility. Health care systems or institutions that require physicians to act as gatekeepers or allocators of public, institutional, or other resources in their clinical treatment of patients present the physicians with conflicts of duty, and the probability that they will be compelled to violate one or other of those duties, and perhaps both.

6.2. *The macroethical level*

This level of analysis applies ethical criteria to how one group of persons such as members of a community collectively treats other communities, and individuals such as members of the group itself and non-members. Bioethics have been slow to develop at this level, in part perhaps because of their origin in the US, which has not created a uniform right of all citizens to receive necessary health care. In many countries elsewhere, however, most have variants of a national health system that attempts to achieve equity in access to medical services between resource-rich and resource-poor communities, members of majority and minority populations and residents of urban, suburban, and rural areas. Many public health medical services, such as control and treatment of communicable diseases, including sexually transmitted diseases, HIV infection, and, for instance, tuberculosis, reflect a communal, macroethical commitment to achieve and maintain healthy populations. Public health engineering services such as regarding sanitation, drainage, and sewerage, purification of domestic water supplies, and control of air-borne pollutants are similarly responses to macroethical concerns about the quality of the environment a community enjoys. Provision of family planning services serves the goals of those who receive them, but also the public purpose of allowing communities to have no more than the number of children they want.

The ethical principle of justice applies at a social or macroethical level. Even if parties to settlement of a dispute each believe that the terms of settlement are fair, they can know the terms are just only by comparison with settlements of similar disputes. This is why justice requires access to previous judgements or terms of settlement in other cases, the giving of reasons for decisions that explain the grounds on which other cases are found to be alike or different, and, in many legal systems, a preoccupation with precedents to ensure that like facts result in applications of the same laws.

6.3. *The mesoethical level*

Ethical analysis at this level falls somewhere between the microethical and macroethical levels. Mesoethics are a concern of governmental, institutional, and private-sector resource managers and administrators, since they address administrative or bureaucratic resource allocation among competing demands. Mesoethics implicate principles of beneficence and distributive justice, such as when a finite health care budget is subject to legitimate claims on behalf of paediatric, geriatric, maternity, emergency, and other services. Authorities allocating resources among primary, secondary, and tertiary health care facilities are similarly responsible for mesoethical choices. Allocations have to address a spectrum of health care services. These range from basic preventive and therapeutic services, such as mass immunization against childhood diseases and oral rehydration therapy, an inexpensive and effective treatment for children at risk of preventable death from loss of body liquids due to diarrhoea, to multiple organ transplantation, variants of *in vitro* fertilization and very costly similar interventions dependent on high levels of scientific and/or surgical skill. The spectrum therefore goes from inexpensive treatments for mass populations to very costly interventions that serve relatively few patients, but prolong or enhance their lives.

Bioethicists have become increasingly engaged with mesoethical, particularly resource-allocation concerns. For instance, contrasting the relatively few health care resources given to disorders of children and adolescents in some economically developed countries with the high proportion of resources applied to elderly patients who suffer from multiple age-related disorders, some have developed an ethic of intergenerational justice.[10] This advocates devotion of a major proportion of resources to remedy or alleviate disorders among younger people, in order to promote every person's prospects to achieve advanced age in tolerable health. That is, relatively inexpensive care for the bulk of younger patients is favoured over very costly treatment of a small number of gravely ill elderly persons, reflecting a utilitarian ethical orientation of pursuing the greatest benefit of the greatest number of patients.

6.4. *The megaethical level*

Issues addressed at the megaethical level transcend national health issues that may be considered by macroethics. They include such considerations as the effects on human health of environmental degradation and pollution, but a medically more direct bioethical concern for the health of human populations is the international HIV/AIDS pandemic. Concerns also include ecological

---

[10] D. Callahan, *Setting Limits: What Kind of Life* (New York: Simon & Schuster, 1990).

impacts of failures to contain population growth. Overpopulation
pollution-generating, impoverished, and unhealthy megacities (that is,
with populations in excess of 10 million persons), the large majority of which
are in resource-poor countries. At this point, however, bioethics is superseded
by ethical concerns that include but go far beyond considerations of human
biology.

Policies can often be ethically defended at more than one level of analysis,
as in the provision of family planning services, which is justifiable at both
microethical and macroethical levels. Further, apparent inconsistencies or
contradictions in policies may be resolved by reference to different levels of
analysis. For instance, some feminist scholars who oppose state intervention
by restrictive abortion laws, also advocate laws to punish disclosure of foetal
sex, in order to prevent women from having sex-based abortions. Their fear
is that women will select, or be compelled, to terminate pregnancies of female
foetuses, reinforcing discrimination against girl children and perpetuating the
devaluation of women in their communities.

Commentators have pointed to the apparent inconsistency or paradox
of seeking to preserve women's right to terminate pregnancies for minor or
trivial reasons, but to bar or obstruct the right that women want to exercise for
reasons that are important in their lives and families or to their health. A
woman who has delivered three or four daughters, for instance, may be willing
to complete another pregnancy, perhaps later in her reproductive life, to have
a son but not another daughter. Advocates of these policies may explain, however, that the abortion decision is, in principle, a microethical decision to be
made between a woman and her physician. In contrast, the decision to prohibit
sex-based abortion is, in principle, a macroethical decision to be reached at a
societal level, since it affects women's social status, dignity, and respect. It may
also be of megaethical significance in reinforcing the status of women in all
cultures and communities of the world, and reflecting condemnation of sex-
based abortion in international human rights documents.

7. *Reproductive and Sexual Health Ethics*

The restrictive approach to fertility control maintained by the Roman
Catholic Church, reflecting its deontological orientation, that persuaded several influential activists in the 1970s to contribute to the newly established field
of bioethics as a secular enterprise, maintains its full vigour. This has been
evidenced in Church opposition to liberalizing initiatives taken at international conferences on population, development, and women's rights. Ethical
divisions continue regarding proper medical, scientific, and biotechnological
means to preserve individuals' reproductive health and capacity, and to

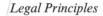

...er their fertility and the safety to themselves, their
...their sexual behaviour. Human sexuality is a conten-
... of ethical decision-making for the Roman Catholic
...se its reasoning has been developed by celibate priests
...ience of human sexuality is through concepts of sin.
...by its principle of infallible leadership, considers sexual
...il and proper only when directed towards reproduction
...exual intercourse is considered permissible only within
he... ...age. Infertile people, such as postmenopausal women, may
marry provid... ...at sexual intercourse remains open in principle to the transmission of human life, perhaps through miraculous divine intervention. The
use of artificial means of contraception, whether of transitory or permanent
effect, is prohibited. Claiming to be the centre of the only true and Universal
Church, the Vatican does not limit its prohibitions to believers in the Church.
It actively opposes employment of reproductive practices that violate its teachings wherever their application is proposed or accepted.

Studies in sociology have shown that, in human as opposed to animal populations, sexuality serves purposes in addition to reproduction of the species,
particularly human bonding and the establishment and stability of private and
family life. There is growing acceptance that sexuality is a natural part of
human life, and that the claim to sexual intimacy is legitimate and should be
actively accommodated where voluntary. Studies have also shown the wide
variety of sexual practices in which human beings participate, extending far
beyond the heterosexual reproductive intercourse that some duty-based ethicists consider alone to be 'natural'.

In addition to sociological evidence demonstrating the need to accommodate reproductive and sexual health, the World Health Organization and
associated agencies have provided pragmatic reinforcement through estimates
that, worldwide each year, approximately 515,000 women die of complications of pregnancy,[11] amounting to over 1,400 maternal deaths each day, that
over 7 million women who survive childbirth suffer serious health injuries, and
that a further 50 million suffer adverse health effects.[12] Over 99 per cent of these
consequences occur in economically developing countries, and most could
be prevented by women's access to reproductive health services, such as to
limit unwanted and untimely pregnancy, and to provide access to emergency
obstetric care. Bioethicists concerned with utilitarian values, who assess theoretical principles by their consequences in practice, have treated these considerations as a basis for remedial action.

[11] WHO, UNICEF, and UN Population Fund, *Maternal Mortality in 1995: Estimates Developed by WHO, UNICEF and UNFPA* (Geneva: WHO, 2001).
[12] UN Population Fund, *The State of the World Population 1999, 6 Billion: A Time for Choices*
(New York: UN Population Fund, 1999).

Accordingly, during the final decade of the twentieth century, a concept of reproductive and sexual health arose, based on the widely endorsed description of 'health' contained in the Constitution of the World Health Organization. This is that health is a 'state of complete physical, mental and social well-being and not merely the absence of disease or infirmity'. The new concept extends this to reproductive and sexual health. The UN International Conference on Population and Development, held in Cairo, in 1994, and the UN Fourth World Conference on Women, held in Beijing in 1995, adopted a comprehensive concept of reproductive and sexual health. The definition is given in Chapter 2 above but, because of its bioethical significance, it warrants repetition. It provides that:

Reproductive health is a state of complete physical, mental and social well-being and not merely the absence of disease or infirmity, in all matters relating to the reproductive system and to its functions and processes. Reproductive health therefore implies that people are able to have a satisfying and safe sex life and that they have the capability to reproduce and the freedom to decide if, when and how often to do so. Implicit in this last condition are the right of men and women to be informed and to have access to safe, effective, affordable and acceptable methods of family planning of their choice, as well as other methods of their choice for regulation of fertility which are not against the law, and the right of access to appropriate health-care services that will enable women to go safely through pregnancy and childbirth and provide couples with the best chance of having a healthy infant.

Accordingly, reproductive health care is to be understood as the cluster of methods, techniques, and services that contribute to reproductive health and well-being. This involves both preventing and remedying reproductive health disabilities. The purpose of sexual health included in this definition is the enhancement of life and personal relations, which includes but goes beyond counselling and care related to reproduction and sexually transmitted diseases.

This definition encompasses contraception, sterilization, and abortion. The qualifying phrase 'which are not against the law' allows legal limitation of delivery of such services in countries that find restriction of reproductive autonomy ethically defensible. The definition also covers access to medically assisted reproductive means, including by technologies designed to remedy infertility and to allow infertile couples to overcome childlessness, such as by different techniques collectively described as *in vitro* fertilization (IVF). Treatment of sexually transmitted diseases, which may be a source of infertility, has become of growing importance due to the international HIV/AIDS pandemic. In most situations, infection is spread by sexual intercourse and the population group showing the most rapidly rising rate of infection consists of young women.

Delivery of reproductive and sexual health services raises profound ethical issues at every level of analysis. At the microethical level are relations between patients and health service providers, particularly those who have conscientious objections to delivery of lawful services their patients request. Ethical codes frequently provide that practitioners who would decline to provide a lawful health service on conscientious grounds, such as abortion or sterilization, will inform in advance any people who are seeking health care services. Further, if their existing patients request such services, they will make reasonable efforts to refer them to alternative practitioners who are willing and able to provide them. At the macroethical level are issues of whether and by what means a society may prohibit private voluntary sexual and reproductive practices, or compel women to continue pregnancies against their will. It is widely accepted that police and other public officers have no place in citizens' bedrooms, monitoring contraceptive or other private sexual practices to bar or compel reproductive choices.

Those who claim otherwise bear a heavy ethical burden of persuasion. They may discharge the burden for instance to prevent incest or sexual exploitation of vulnerable people. States may ethically claim an interest in unborn human life, and demonstrate that interest through provision, for instance, of prenatal care services and dietary supplements for pregnant women. States that claim to protect human life from conception may be hard-pressed, however, to justify promoting the interests of foetuses over those of pregnant women on ethical grounds. Women do not forfeit their own rights on becoming even voluntarily pregnant. States cannot credibly claim that their interests in unborn human life ethically supersede the choices women must make among competing interests in their individual lives, such as caring for their born children, parents, and others who depend on them.

A principle-based or deontological orientation may claim that every human being, foetus, and embryo has inherent value, and that none may be knowingly sacrificed for the benefit of even hundreds of thousands of others. Democratic governments are accountable for the maximization of health among the populations they serve, and may be required to adopt utilitarian principles, because they are responsible for the consequences of the policies they apply. They may accordingly have to apply macroethical principles and, for instance, promote women's health and welfare through access to fertility regulation. At a minimum, they will permit private purchase of contraceptive means. They may go further, and sponsor contraceptive education to instruct their populations on the advantages and means of contraceptive practice. To go further still, they may actively provide contraceptive means to those unable to purchase them, or to all who are covered by publicly funded health services irrespective of their personal means.

Mesoethical decisions concern such matters as the distinction between reproductive and sexual health care services that governments will make available without charge to recipients, and other services that will be 'luxury' services available only to those with private means to pay for them. Public health interests may be served in a variety of utilitarian ways. These include provision of antibiotic and other routine treatment of curable sexually transmitted diseases, to reduce public financial and other costs of widespread infection, and also provision of contraceptive means. Those too poor to purchase these means may be unable to provide the children they would bear with the material resources that children require to thrive, presenting public authorities with a choice of funding social services for them or suffering the effects of numbers of deprived and unhealthy children. Treatment of infertility due to illness, by simple medical or surgical means, may be publicly funded in the same way as treatment for other illnesses. However, medically assisted reproduction to overcome infertility may be considered more cosmetic, and denied public or institutional funds or subsidies, except perhaps in countries that urgently want to promote their population growth. Alternatively, funders may approve providing treatment of primary infertility, affecting people who have no children, but not of secondary infertility, affecting people who have living children but now want additional children they find themselves unable to conceive.

Megaethical issues concerning reproductive and sexual health include world population growth and distribution, and economic and other consequences of sexually transmitted diseases, particularly HIV/AIDS. International funding of family planning programmes for resource-poor countries is opposed by conservative religious bodies whose deontological orientation family planning services offend, and by anti-abortion opposition in wealthy countries whose political decision-makers identify family planning with abortion. Opponents within resource-poor countries may also raise the principle of justice, to point out that the proportion of the world's resources absorbed by a child in an economically developed country is vastly higher than the proportion absorbed by a child in an economically undeveloped or underdeveloped country. If population growth is considered to endanger international resource availability, for instance, of food or non-renewable energy, they argue that family limitation programmes should focus on the world's developed countries.

In some developing countries with high populations, such as India, many and perhaps most of the population have not yet reached their reproductive years, and threaten a population explosion when they do. The pressure of rapidly rising population growth is sometimes perceived to endanger national and international stability, and risk international conflicts over territorial possessions, especially of fertile land. Population movements, particularly by illegal immigration, into more economically advanced countries, are similarly perceived to risk urban strife in those countries. National populations are often enriched, however, by the arrival of diverse immigrants. Further, in countries with ageing indigenous populations, where fewer younger workers support a rising population of retired people, an influx of a young immigrant workforce may be welcomed, even at a cost of introducing cultural changes to which elderly residents find it difficult to adapt.

Pragmatic questions concern whether an effect of the HIV/AIDS pandemic will be to halt and even to reverse population growth in some countries, due to rising death rates of younger people and children, and whether ethical duties exist to fund preventive research and provision of care. This reflects a background issue, at every level of ethical analysis, namely whether ethical rights to reproductive and sexual health services are positive rights or no more than negative rights. Negative rights are 'rights to be left alone', by state and other agencies and officers, freely to undertake conduct and obtain services of one's choice. Where rights to reproductive and sexual health services are negative rights, individuals may obtain contraception, sterilization, and abortion services, and IVF and other medically assisted means of reproduction, without state or other obstruction. In that obtaining health care services may require the skills to find them, capacity to reach them, and money to purchase them, negative rights may be rights of the educated rather than of the uneducated, of the able-bodied rather than of the disabled or of urban rather than rural residents, and of the rich rather than of the poor. Further, where legal conditions are set for access to services, such as to therapeutic but not non-therapeutic abortion services, negative rights will not exist to services that are made illegal.

Positive rights are rights to be provided, by state or other agencies, institutions, or persons, with provisions or services one cannot obtain without assistance. A person's right, for instance, of access to contraceptive protection is worthless if the person cannot find, reach, or purchase the only services that exist. At the microethical level, where health service providers have a discretion to select whose request for lawful assistance they will accept and reject, rights to their services are only negative rights. Macroethically, societies may decide to make some but not other services available, to all or only to some who request them or who need them. Rights are positive rights for those made eligible to receive them, but at best only negative rights to others. Mesoethical decisions within institutions often mainly concern the services to which they will provide positive rights, other rights being more passively accommodated as negative rights. For instance, a hospital may provide prenatal care for residents of the area it serves at no cost to recipients, and be available to render such care at cost-recovery rates to paying patients who are not residents. At the international, megaethical level, countries and, for instance, commercial companies with the means, acting directly or through international agencies, may create positive rights for resource-poor countries and for groups within their populations, such as to receive therapeutic products at reduced or no cost. Countries and companies may, however, deny general ethical obligations towards any particular country or group of persons.

Ethical duties to persons and populations may arise in reproductive health and other research, however, such as when commercial pharmaceutical companies have conducted studies in particular populations. They may be bound by ethical duties of justice to repay benefits they have derived, by making products available, without charge or at a reduced charge for an appropriate period of time, to the subjects of their studies or the communities from which the subjects who participated in the studies came. This relates to the wider context of research ethics.

8. *Research Ethics*

Medical research enjoys a long and distinguished history, but it has been under ethical scrutiny and sometimes suspicion since the second half of the twentieth century. In recent decades, a major branch of health care ethics in general and of bioethics in particular has arisen that addresses the ethics of research involving human subjects. The requirement that research proposals be submitted in advance to independent panels or boards of multidisciplinary and lay membership, for their review and approval on ethical grounds, has introduced lay people to the world of bioethics, and created a sizeable body of literature, scholarship, and experience in the area of research ethics.

The duty-based or deontological orientation to research recognizes limits to what it is proper to research. Before the mid-nineteenth century, for instance, religious influence in Europe and elsewhere prevented dissection of dead bodies for medical research and education, for fear that opening or dismembering a corpse would cause escape and loss of the deceased person's soul. Today, forms of research into human reproductive biology and certain reproductive technologies and, for instance, stem cell research based on manipulation of human embryos, is condemned by some religious institutions. At the secular level, there is very widespread if not universal opposition to creating independent, genetic duplicate human beings by cloning cells of existing people or, if scientifically possible, of recently deceased people. Similarly, the Kantian imperative that people not be treated only instrumentally, as means to others' ends, underlies much ethical scrutiny of research proposals. Investigators' need to use human subjects as means to achieve their research ends, such as promotion of scientific knowledge or promotion of commercial enrichment, creates the fear that the subjects may be considered only as means, and that their intrinsic value and dignity as human beings may be discounted.

Proponents of an orientation that claims that an end perhaps desirable in itself cannot justify improper means, and that some means of research are unethical, face the challenge of deciding whether therapeutic and preventive health care advances that resulted from improper means of research can be incorporated into their clinical practice. The alternative may be that their patients must be required to bear preventable suffering, in order that wrongful research conduct not seem to be condoned. A utilitarian or consequentialist orientation approves application of techniques such as research on human embryos to advance reproductive knowledge and practice, and approves stem cell research, for instance by the cloning of human embryos, because of its potential to achieve considerable health care benefits. More controversial, however, is the use of medical information acquired by techniques that violated human rights. A leading instance concerns techniques by which members of captive populations and prisoners in concentration camps during the Second World War were literally tested to death by deliberate exposure to extreme temperatures, radiation, and, for instance, lethal infections. A utilitarian orientation to research must resolve the challenge of disapproving wrongful research methods while preserving results that are of scientific value to relieve suffering of innocent patients.

Adherents to feminist orientations face a similar challenge when they insist that research into women's health be conducted with the participation of informed women volunteers who are, or who may become, pregnant. Such research should not involve drugs or other products that have been shown harmful to embryos or foetuses. Adherents have gained influential government support, however, in North America and beyond, in claiming that it is not an ethical reason to exclude women research subjects of reproductive age that it is unknown whether an unproven practice or product is harmful to embryos or foetuses they may carry. The ethical principle to do no harm applies in the therapeutic setting, but in research some controlled risk of harm may ethically be justified and perhaps be necessary to prevent greater injury.

For instance, if an unproven drug is in fact harmful to human embryonic or foetal life, that should be shown as a result of research, rather than being shown, as in the 1960s in the case of the drug Thalidomide, many years after the drug has been prescribed for pregnant women in the belief that it does not cause such harm, with countless hundreds or thousands of children suffering gross defects as a result. Feminist and utilitarian bioethicists would apply macroethical reasoning to claim that minimized injury in research to a small number of embryos or foetuses is justified by the prevention of injury to innumerably more in development of a generally therapeutic product for sick patients.[13] However, those duty-based bioethicists whose primary commitment is to survival of each unborn human life, rather than to development of medical knowledge about the effects of medical interventions before birth, may be more cautious about research that may cause pregnant subjects to lose

---

[13] See T. Stephens and R. Brynner, *Dark Remedy* (Cambridge, Mass.: Perseus Publishing, 2001), on the rehabilitation and therapeutic benefits of Thalidomide.

or to terminate their pregnancies because of harm suffered by their embryos or foetuses.

Following the Second World War, trials of alleged war criminals, particularly at Nuremberg and also at Tokyo, demonstrated abuses of vulnerable people through their involuntary recruitment as subjects of medical research. Following the trial of 'the Nazi Doctors', the Nuremberg Code of 1947, developed in the course of trial proceedings, became a founding document that prescribed conditions for the ethical conduct of medical research. The Code is limited, however, by its origins in reaction to inhumane testing, at times to intended death, of individuals under the control of those who considered them subhuman and disposable. For instance, the Nuremberg Code does not consider conditions under which necessary therapeutic research on mentally compromised or paediatric populations might ethically be undertaken, nor the requirement of maintaining research subjects' confidentiality. A more fully considered, generally compatible code was developed in Helsinki in 1964 by the World Medical Association (WMA). Its Declaration of Helsinki, at first subtitled Recommendations Guiding Physicians in Biomedical Research Involving Human Subjects and most recently resubtitled Ethical Principles for Medical Research Involving Human Subjects, is periodically reviewed and amended when necessary, the fifth amendment occurring at the Fifty-Second General Assembly of the WMA in October 2000 (see Pt. III, Ch. 2).

The Declaration states basic principles of ethical research, addressing principles applicable to all medical research and additional principles for medical research combined with medical care. The Declaration requires that a protocol of a proposed experiment be submitted in advance to a committee that is independent of the investigator and the sponsor of the study 'for consideration, comment, guidance, and where appropriate, approval'. Modern committees include members familiar with the scientific basis of proposals and with applicable ethical and legal considerations and non-specialist members such as community members. The committee should be established and run 'in conformity with the laws and regulations of the country in which the research experiment is performed'.

The Declaration of Helsinki requires medical research to conform to generally accepted scientific principles, be based on thorough knowledge of the scientific literature, and be conducted by appropriately qualified persons acting under competent medical supervision. A scientifically sound proposal may be ethically flawed for a variety of reasons, but a scientifically flawed study is necessarily unethical in that it exposes subjects to risk, loss of privacy, inconvenience, or other disadvantage for no scientific benefit. There must be a proportionate balance of the beneficial objective of the study over inherent risks to subjects. Both predictable benefits and risks should be carefully assessed in advance, and the assessments presented to the independent review committees.

Studies should be discontinued if, in execution, the hazards are found to out-weigh the potential benefits. It is established that 'considerations related to the well-being of the human subject should take precedence over the interests of science and society',[14] in accordance with a microethical level of assessment.

Central to ethical research is adequately informed consent. Competent per-sons make decisions for themselves on whether or not to consent to become subjects of research, and if they are patients they must be free to decline or dis-continue involvement without any loss of entitlement to clinically indicated care. Physicians should be guarded about proposing that their own patients or others in a dependent relationship to them, such as students they instruct and evaluate, should be subjects of their investigations, because of the pressure such persons may be under to please them and maintain the relationships on which they depend. Any invitation to participate in research should come from someone on whom the potential subject feels no dependency. When potential subjects are not competent to make their own informed decisions, informed consent may be given by legal guardians, according to local law, provided that any conflict of interest such guardians may have is properly resolved. Even when such consent is given, research cannot be continued when the potential subjects deny consent to or resist procedures to which they are intended to be subjected. Family members of mentally incompetent institutionalized persons, such as mentally impaired but sexually mature adolescents, should be involved in decisions about their participation in research rather than institutional administrators. Administrators' consent will usually also be required, how-ever, for studies to be conducted in the centres for which they are responsible.

In interventions not intended for individuals' therapeutic care, each subject should be a volunteer, freely giving his or her own informed consent. When patients under treatment volunteer, special care must be taken to ensure that they understand whether they may be denied standard treatments they would ordinarily receive were they not to enter, for instance by being allocated to a group that would receive a different, perhaps unproven, treatment or no active product at all. Where medical research is combined with professional care for the individuals for whom procedures are proposed, an investigator who intends not to seek subjects' informed consent should state the specific reasons in the proposal submitted to the independent review committee. Such investi-gations may be proposed, approved, and undertaken only to the extent that the research is justified by its potential preventive, diagnostic, or therapeutic value for the patient.

In addition to the Declaration of Helsinki, codes of research ethics or guide-lines have been developed by the Council for International Organizations of

---

[14] World Medical Association, Declaration of Helsinki, as amended Oct. 2000, Article 5 (see Pt. III, Ch. 2).

Medical Sciences, an agency co-sponsored by WHO and UNESCO. These guidelines address both biomedical research[15] and epidemiological studies,[16] and focus on ethical duties that arise when studies sponsored by public or private (such as commercial) agencies or by international organizations are undertaken in economically developing host countries. They include elaboration on how the principle of justice applies when study sponsors from wealthy countries undertake research with members of resource-poor populations, particularly in developing countries, from which the sponsors intend to reap commercial, scientific, or other benefits. The principle requires that they grant their research subjects or an appropriate host population, or the host country, a reciprocal benefit. This may be in the form of otherwise unobtainable medical care, free or reduced-cost drugs, such as marketable products that resulted from the study, or other products, services, or opportunities, such as scholarships or training programmes, that the recipients value.

Beyond the several general elaborations of the Declaration of Helsinki are codes specific to particular types of research. For instance, regarding studies to develop a vaccine to prevent HIV/AIDS, the Joint United Nations Programme on HIV/AIDS, called UNAIDS, has produced a guidance document that applies general principles of ethical research to the particular features this type of research possesses.[17]

The Declaration of Helsinki goes beyond considerations for the welfare of only human subjects of research. Its basic principles observe that appropriate caution must be exercised in the conduct of research that may affect the environment, and that the welfare of animals used for research must be respected. Many countries have laws for the protection of animals in general and the proper care of animals to be used in scientific research in particular. Even when investigators are in compliance with the Declaration of Helsinki and comparable ethical codes, they are not relieved from criminal, civil, and other responsibilities under the laws of their own countries. This raises considerations of the relationships between ethics and law.

9. *Ethics and the Law*

Ethics and law are different systems of rule-making and rule-application, but they constantly interact with each other. Law tends to address what must be

---

[15] Council for International Organizations of Medical Sciences (CIOMS), *International Ethical Guidelines for Biomedical Research Involving Human Subjects* (Geneva: CIOMS, 2002).

[16] CIOMS, *International Ethical Guidelines for Ethical Review of Epidemiological Studies* (Geneva: CIOMS, 1991).

[17] UNAIDS, *Ethical Considerations in HIV Preventive Vaccine Research* (Geneva: UNAIDS, 2000).

done, what does not have to be done but may be, and what must not be done. Ethics similarly addresses what should be done, what should not be done, and what it is permissible although not mandatory to do. When law creates legitimate discretions, what may be done is optional, so that both performing an act and not performing it are legal choices, and the law itself provides no direction. Then, the grounds on which that legal choice should be made are governed by ethical considerations.

For instance, when an intellectually mature sexually active adolescent seeks contraception without her parents' knowledge, a physician may lawfully accept her as a patient and preserve her confidentiality, under the legal doctrine of the 'mature minor', or may lawfully decline to accept her as a patient, or make accepting her conditional on her permitting her parents to be informed. If her request for assistance is declined, her confidentiality is still legally required to be preserved. How the legal choice between accepting her and declining is exercised is an ethical matter influenced, for instance, by the principle of beneficence and the adolescent's risk of pregnancy and its outcome in childbirth or abortion. If the practitioner is willing to accept her as a patient, the choice whether the practitioner makes acceptance conditional on her parents being informed is equally an ethical matter. Ethical judgement will be influenced, for instance, by whether she will be beaten or confined by her family, and whether she is voluntarily sexually active with a partner of her choice or is being sexually exploited and victimized by men against whom she cannot protect herself but her family or others could give protection. If the adolescent is not being victimized and the practitioner undertakes confidentiality, however, it would be both illegal and unethical for the practitioner to abuse her disclosure of her voluntary sexual activity to inform her parents or others, such as schoolteachers. This emphasizes the concurrent legal and ethical duty of confidentiality owed by physicians who are engaged by school or education authorities to work in schools.

Sometimes ethics and law coincide or overlap, and at other times they conflict with and contradict each other. Exercise of a legal choice is not necessarily ethical; that is, whether a legal power or right should be exercised is an ethical matter. For instance, a clinic funded to provide services without charge to area residents may be legally empowered to refuse such services to a recent immigrant or refugee, but may be ethically expected to treat such a person as a resident. Equally, an ethical choice of conduct may not be legally permitted, because the law bars an option it would be ethical to exercise. For instance, some physicians have risked legal liability for providing contraceptives when laws have been unethically restrictive. A general ethical expectation is that the law should be observed, although severely oppressive or unconscionable laws may be ethically challenged. Reciprocally, however, the law usually attempts to respect ethical choices, and tries not to compel conduct the medical profession or an individual practitioner considers unethical. For instance, laws usually recognize legal rights of conscientious objection to performing procedures practitioners are otherwise legally required to undertake, such as under contracts with hospitals or clinics.

At times, however, there is conflict. Those who oppose abortion on moral grounds, for instance, often oppose others having any legal permission to facilitate or undertake abortion even though a permissive law does not require opponents of abortion to perform such procedures. Laws that accommodate conscientious objection usually require that practitioners who object will refer applicants for their services to other, reasonably accessible practitioners who do not have such objections. Some objecting practitioners believe this also to be wrongful conduct, however, on the ground that it is as wrong to facilitate abortion as to perform it. Nevertheless, the law usually complies with the principle that individuals should be treated in accordance with their own conscientious preferences among lawful options, and not be limited by those of the medical practitioners whose care they request. Practitioners should not be lawfully compelled to perform procedures to which they ethically object, but a practitioner cannot lawfully limit a patient's ethical choices, or other practitioners' procedures, to those that the practitioner ethically approves.

The law is sometimes employed to enforce an ethical conclusion, by prohibiting conduct that is found ethically erroneous, such as an attempt at cloning a human being, or compelling conduct that is ethically required, such as preserving patients' confidentiality. At first appearances, law may seem to be a more powerful influence than ethics, because its provisions are more authoritatively and accessibly stated by political legislatures and judges, more publicly and systematically exposed by newsmedia reports of laws enacted and court decisions, more practically enforceable through lawyers, courts, and police officers, and more institutionally challengeable and appealable by political and judicial processes.

As against this, however, law that is considered to lack an ethical dimension, to deny ethical options, to cause unethical consequences, or to be ethically bankrupt, is impoverished in its capacity to educate and inspire those it governs to distinguish between right and wrong conduct. Judges often take account of ethical values in interpreting and applying the law, disfavouring choices that would lead to unethical results or permit unethical conduct. Law frames the setting within which ethical choices may be practically exercised, but ethics frames the limits within which law is voluntarily obeyed and respected as an expression of the values and aspirations of the society in which it applies.

Whether ethical conduct should be made legally mandatory is an issue of philosophical debate. If the result of poor ethical choice would be intolerably harmful, such as a physician choosing to leave a woman suffering serious infection or other grave injury from illegal abortion to die, the ethical error can be prohibited by law. For instance, the law can mandate that physicians must complete spontaneous or induced incomplete abortion. A patient in peril might be given a positive legal right to care, since a medical practitioner could be obliged to give treatment, for instance by a practitioner's refusal resulting in liability to a criminal charge for manslaughter or criminal negligence causing death or bodily harm. Within limits, the law can compel obedience, but it cannot necessarily make those it governs exercise sound ethical judgement. If ethical judgement is to be allowed and encouraged, the law may have to accommodate ethical choices, and tolerate all but the most grave ethical errors. Not everything that is ethical need be compelled by law, and not everything that is unethical need be prohibited by law.

Less directive than provisions of the law and more educational for medical and related health care practitioners may be their liability to face professional ethical disciplinary proceedings, brought by their professional associations or their legal licensing authorities. The basis of disciplinary power is law that permits an association or authority to withdraw membership or suspend a licence to practise, or to make retention of a licence conditional, for instance on the practitioner at fault passing or attending a course of instruction on professional ethics. The grounds on which such lawful power would be exercised, however, would be the standards of ethical conduct expected by members of the profession, and the judges of whether a practitioner's conduct had been ethical or unethical would not be lawyers but other practitioners. By these means, the law permits and encourages professionals to be self-regulating, and to set and enforce ethical standards, subject to wider regulation by the law if the standards set are inadequate, or unenforced. For instance, it is not unlawful for physicians to publicize results of research they have undertaken on a product, but if they have a commercial interest in sales of the product or in a commercial competitor against the product, it may be considered a violation of professional ethics for them not to disclose that interest in the publication and other publicity of their research.

10. *Ethics and Human Rights*

It has been seen that law aims to serve the ethical principle of justice. Accordingly, it is not an ethical justification of a policy simply that it is legal. It is not even an ethical justification that a democratic government of a country had a popular mandate to introduce or support the particular law, and that it has been upheld by a country's most significant court according to the country's constitution. These features alone, while legally and politically significant, do not show that the law is ethical. The Universal Declaration of Human Rights,

1948, which was drawn up under the auspices of the United Nations Organization and is the basis of modern human rights concepts, was a reaction against unethical laws enacted more than a decade earlier under an initially democratic government in Germany. These increasingly oppressive laws, which for instance barred Jews from practising as lawyers, were upheld and applied by judges through national courts. Under these laws, innocent individuals lost their occupations, their property, their rights for instance to reproductive choice, and their lives. Law alone does not make practices or policies ethical.

For policies given effect through laws to be ethical, and for health care, legal, and other practitioners to be satisfied that the laws under which they conduct policies and practices are ethical, the policies must conform to ethical standards and meet ethical requirements. The ethical bankruptcy of policies legally enforced in Nazi-dominated countries, such as compulsory sterilization of 'unfit' people and severe prohibition of abortion by women able to bear racially 'pure' children, led to the Universal Declaration of Human Rights in 1948. The governments that sponsored these unethical laws justified them on grounds of the sovereignty of their states, and condemned foreign criticism as objectionable intervention in their domestic affairs. The Declaration recognizes, however, that states themselves, their lawful governments, and others acting under authority of state governments, are not free legally to implement any policies they consider to be moral or in their interests. Policies and laws must conform to at least minimum respect for individuals' ethical rights as human beings, now commonly called their human rights.

The human rights expressed in the Universal Declaration were not created simply from abstract philosophies or novel concepts. Rather, they were declared on the basis of existing principles that countries' leaders had found through experience to be fundamental to civil society and to civilized and humane government, and expressed in many constitutional and other major legal instruments. The 1948 document was described as a 'Declaration' because it declared the best of prevailing values, inspired by ethical traditions and given practical effect through law, which states acknowledge themselves ethically bound to respect.

It has been observed that what ethics are to clinical medicine, addressing individuals' health, human rights are to public health, addressing populations' health, including reproductive health. This is because:

ethics and human rights derive from a set of quite similar, if not identical, core values. As with medicare and public health, rather than seeing human rights and ethics as conflicting domains, it seems more appropriate to consider a continuum, in which human rights is a language most useful for guiding societal level analysis and work, while ethics is a language most useful for guiding individual behaviour. From this perspective, and precisely because public health must be centrally concerned with the structure and function of society, the language of human rights is extremely useful for expressing, considering and incorporating values into public health analysis and response.

Thus, public health work requires both ethics applicable to the individual public health practitioner and a human rights framework to guide public health in its societal analysis and response.[18]

11. *Ethics Review*

The duty of ethical reflection is individual, collaborative, and institutional. Individuals are expected, as intelligent, conscientious persons whose actions are intended to affect the lives of others, to consider the ethical nature of their motivations, conduct, and influence. Colleagues in the provision of care are also expected to address together the ethical implications of their actions. Even sole professional practitioners rarely work in isolation, but usually collaborate with colleagues at different levels. Providers are expected to work with colleagues in ways that are ethical in themselves, and to address the ethical aspects of the practices in which they collaborate. Because individual ethical reflection can be influenced by personal bias, unconscious self-interest, and perhaps undue favour or antipathy conditioned by past experience, providers should be willing to exchange and explain their views with colleagues, at all levels, concerning their guiding ethical perceptions, although each one is a moral agent ethically accountable for what he or she does. That is, collaborative reflection and decision-making do not exonerate individuals of responsibility for their own acts.

The duty of ethical reflection and explanation is institutionalized regarding research involving human subjects. The Declaration of Helsinki, CIOMS International Ethical Guidelines, and additional international, national, institutional, and other formulations of research ethics invariably require independent ethical scrutiny of research proposals. Because of the historical US initiatives and dominance in bioethics, research ethics committees were often described elsewhere as they are in the US and US-derived literature as Institutional Review Boards or IRBs. However, they have become increasingly described differently outside the US, because national variants in other countries do not have the same composition, legal status, powers, or responsibilities as US IRBs.

The usual pattern is that research ethics review committees will have scientifically qualified and non-scientific members, including at least one with

---

[18] J. M. Mann, 'Medicine and Public Health, Ethics and Human Rights', *Hastings Center Report*, 27/3 (1997), 6–13 at 10.

training or credible experience in (bio)ethics, and lay members whose most relevant identification is with potential subjects of research, the whole to include members of both sexes. It is often expected in addition that a committee will include a member with legal knowledge, or at least that a committee will have the advice of or access to a lawyer. However, committee members should not include lawyers employed by the institutions that committees serve as independent agents, or professional counsel to such institutions, because the professional obligations such lawyers have to their employers or clients would present a conflict of interest. The ethical allegiance of members of independent ethical review committees for research proposals is to the potential subjects of the research, but this cannot be the primary commitment of lawyers employed or retained as independent counsel to serve the interests of institutions that sponsor or accommodate research. Institutional lawyers defend their employees' or clients' interests by minimizing risks of harm to research subjects, but have to anticipate the chance of subjects bringing legal complaints, in which case the lawyers will serve the interests of the institutions in opposition to those of such subjects.

Although research ethics committees include members familiar with scientific matters, they do not necessarily bear responsibility for scientific review of the proposals under ethical consideration. Some committees undertake the double responsibility to review the ethical and the scientific integrity and appropriateness of proposals, but many investigators have to satisfy independent scientific and ethical reviewers in separate stages. Nevertheless, members of ethics review committees are free to raise issues of a scientific nature, because a scientifically unsound study cannot satisfy the ethical principle of beneficence, since no adequate benefit can be derived from exposing human subjects to risks, including such relatively mild risks as inconvenience, in a scientifically flawed project.

Research ethics committee guidelines usually provide or imply that committees will be supported by appropriate secretariats and funding. Committee members are usually unpaid, although in economically developed countries some commercial research ethics boards exist, unaffiliated with academic medical centres, whose members may be paid. Further, so-called contract research organizations (CROs) are emerging that are hired by pharmaceutical companies to recruit research subjects, monitor ongoing research, and manage data, which set up ethics review committees whose members are paid a *per diem* fee. Whether unpaid or paid, however, committee members should have their travel and related costs reimbursed, and other communication costs, such as for documentation creation, mail, and electronic mail (e-mail) or telefax (fax) and telephone costs should be covered. Accordingly, research ethics committees should have a budget supplied or underwritten by the institutions they serve as independent bodies and agents, and appropriate administrative support.

In many countries, hospitals, clinics, and comparable health care facilities have general (that is, not research-related) committees to oversee ethical concerns that arise there, and that the practices and policies of the facilities create. These committees are often larger than research ethics committees, since they include representatives of several different stakeholder groups affected by how facilities function, and they have a more diverse mandate. They address such ethical matters as relations between patients and providers, patients and facility administrative personnel, administrators and staff-member and non-staff-member providers, and among different types of providers. They often also consider issues that arise among patients' family-members, providers, and facility administrators. In some countries, particularly those with fewer personnel who have the capacity to provide governmental and private institutions with experienced, independent advice on ethics issues, committees may be charged with both review of general clinical care and the functions of research ethics review. These functions involve different and at times incompatible priorities, however, and may not easily be undertaken by the same committee without difficult conflicts of interest.

Where general institutional ethics review committees do not exist, the advantages of creating them might be considered. They widen the net of facility personnel actively involved in ethical deliberations, often expand and ease relations between facilities and members of the communities in which they are located and serve, provide transparency in ethical deliberation and decision-making, and demonstrate the institutional and professional commitment to ethical practice. They can also serve to bring sources of grievance and friction to the surface, and facilitate complainants' sense of satisfaction that they have been heard. They also add cumulatively to the education and experience of facility administrative personnel, providers, patients, patients' family-members, and, for instance, local community members, in the identification, analysis, and resolution of ethical concerns arising in, and raised by, health care facilities.

5

Legal Origins and Principles

1. *Overview*

Policy is a plan or purpose that a government, an institution, or an individual may select from among options in order to achieve a particular goal. Law is a powerful instrument because of its influence on how people think and act. Law may be used by public officials and by individuals to advance the purpose of reproductive health, but the law as such has no inherent purpose of its own. The law is an instrument that government officers, health care professionals, and individuals may use to advance policies they favour.[1] Reproductive health policies may therefore be advanced by law, but so may other policies that deliberately or accidentally obstruct reproductive health. Laws may be used in different ways to advance policy, and policy may be influenced by various means that a legal system makes available for the application of policy, so that policy and law interact with each other. Before legal means can be employed, however, the challenge of policy making has to be resolved.

Reproductive health policies must resolve the challenge of ordering priorities. These policies often compete against others that governments and agencies want to pursue. Legal drafting usually attempts precision and specification by fragmenting policies into particular provisions. Further, legislation and amendments to codified laws are often undertaken piecemeal, in response to concerns of the moment or individual preoccupations that rise to the surface of a governmental or legislative agenda. Legal provisions for instance on contraception may be separate from each other, so that it may be unclear whether prevention of implantation of a fertilized ovum is lawful contraception or unlawful abortion. Attention given to a new concern may not consider how one new legal provision fits within the context of existing laws, so that uncertainty of whether a new provision alters or is subject to prevailing provisions has to be resolved by judges. Uncertainty can be reduced, however, when legislation is based on a clearly articulated reproductive health policy

---

[1] In Indonesia, for instance, the Law on Population Development and Prosperous Family of 1992, lists 'control of the quantity of the people' as one of its objectives, in Article 3(2), and regulates access to contraceptives for the purpose of creating a 'small, happy, and prosperous family' (Article 14(1)).

es its intentions for integrating different services. Then it may be
for instance, that the policy to reduce resort to unsafe abortion applies to
ke post-coital or 'emergency contraception' lawful, even after fertilization
but before implantation. An integrated reproductive and sexual health policy
should also address both clinical and public health aspects of fertility, achieving individually drafted laws that fit into a coherent policy to protect and promote individuals' human rights to sexual expression and reproductive choice.

Reproductive health goals and values must be pursued with a realistic
assessment of how laws that are available to advance them are likely to operate in practice. For instance, to protect intended spouses against their partners'
HIV infection, several jurisdictions conditioned the grant of marriage licences
on couples' exchange of HIV test results. The effect in many cases was that
couples who knew of their HIV-positive status cohabited and started families
without marriage, or went to marry in other jurisdictions and returned home
as legally married couples. Further, sexual relations were more likely among
couples during prolonged engagements, and same-sex couples, legally pre-
cluded from marriage, were unaffected by this condition. False-positive test
results, more likely among low-risk individuals, were also sources of embarrassment and damaged relationships. Laws prohibiting marriage without
information exchange risked violation of the internationally protected human
right to marry and found a family,[2] and have been largely replaced by education, counselling, and voluntary testing provisions.[3] The policy to set legal
conditions for marriage did not discourage sexual relations between unmarried
couples to any significant extent, and has been almost universally abandoned
as ineffective, a human rights violation, and contrary to other policies to protect and encourage marriage and family life.

Countries have similarly set policies on abortion by reference to principles,
based on religious and other grounds, that favoured severe criminal condemnation. These policies have been widely applied in legal systems in which
women have had little if any influence. Evidence shows that policies to prohibit
all abortions, or to prevent medically conducted procedures except upon strict
medical grounds, result in widespread illegal and unskilled practice,[4] resulting
in women's death, infection, and impairment of future reproductive capacity.
Policies to liberalize restrictive abortion laws combined with policies for delivery of safe abortion services are almost invariably associated with reduction in
death, mutilation, and impairment of reproductive functions among women,
and not necessarily with an increase in rates of abortion.[5] Policies to reduce

---

[2] Universal Declaration of Human Rights (1948), Article 16.

[3] L. Gostin and Z. Lazzarini, *Human Rights and Public Health in the AIDS Pandemic* (New York: Oxford University Press, 1997), 21–3.

[4] M. F. Fathalla, *From Obstetrics and Gynecology to Women's Health: The Road Ahead* (New York and London: Parthenon, 1997), 239.

[5] Ibid.

numbers of both lawful and unlawful abortions can be pursued by promotion of voluntary birth control methods.

Policy to protect and advance reproductive health draws inspiration from various values and orderings of ethical priorities, but must take account of its anticipated consequences, balancing competing advantages over disadvantages. Some policies prioritize the value of protecting unborn human life over, for instance, the value of recognizing women as responsible decision-makers, but others conclude that the resulting costs of disrespectful and even inhumane treatment of women, and of causing maternal mortality by leaving women access only to unsafe illegal abortion, are excessive. This illustrates a type of challenge that reproductive health policy must resolve, namely balancing the conscientious pursuit of high but abstract principles against inadvertent harmful consequences, such as causing oppressive treatment of women and avoidable deaths. Principles that oppose oppressive treatment and avoidable death are reflected in international human rights treaties that countries legally commit themselves to implement through their domestic laws and practices.

2. *The Role of Law and of Lawyers*

It has been seen that law is an instrument by which states may regulate their affairs, and by which they may aim to give effect to the reproductive health policies that they find appropriate. The effect of law often depends on the respect it enjoys among those expected to obey it, since there are limits to the ability of non-military governments to enforce their will that the law be obeyed by coercive means. The habit of popular obedience to rules depends on their general acceptability. Laws may be based on custom followed in a community, but in modern times laws tend to be expressly enacted by politically composed legislatures. Their practice of law-making is generally seen to follow one of two models. The first is based on principles of virtue to which those governed by law are expected to conform, in order for society to achieve moral goals. The second is utilitarian or pragmatic, based on experience and practices that individuals are empowered or required to follow that are believed most likely to produce desired results.

Principle-based law may derive its provisions from a moral vision rooted in religion or, for instance, political philosophy. Some legal systems such as Islamic law give priority to sacred texts, and require that secular laws conform to authoritative interpretations. Practice-based or pragmatic law aims to achieve behaviours by public and private agencies and individuals that are considered to promote public good, or limit harmful consequences. Experience shows that laws based on moral principles may be enforced in ways that sometimes prove harmful in practice, and that pragmatic purposes may be advanced in ways that moral authorities sometimes consider to ignore or violate important values. Nevertheless, laws should be based on a sense of practical realities. When dealing with an adolescent girl's lawful access to contraception without her parents' consent, for instance, the highest court in the United Kingdom observed, in denying that there is a set legislated age of consent for medical and preventive health services, that 'If the law should impose . . . fixed limits where nature knows only a continuous process, the prize would be artificiality and a lack of realism in an area where the law must be sensitive to human development and social change.'[6]

Activities that affect a community's reproductive health have historically been regulated by moral or principle-based law. Sexual relations and human reproduction have been areas in which religious authorities have been accustomed to exercise moral influence. They may invoke the belief that human conception and birth are divinely regulated, and that such religious authorities themselves have been specially called to interpret and express truths that are divinely revealed to them. The emergence of a concept of reproductive health that is of secular origin, requiring implementation by pragmatic legal rules that measure the validity of such laws by their practical consequences, presents a special challenge to religious authorities. They are not accustomed to being held accountable to civil societies for the effects of pronouncements they make, since they believe what they pronounce to be divinely inspired and required. Their discomfort with and opposition to the formulation of the concept of reproductive health, as articulated in the Programme of Action of the United Nations International Conference on Population and Development, held in Cairo in 1994 (see Pt. I, Ch. 2, Sect. 2, and Ch. 6, Sect. 3.1), remains an obstacle to enactment of laws designed pragmatically to achieve reproductive health.

Nevertheless, democratic governments that are accountable to their electorates and that have endorsed the Cairo Programme bear responsibility to formulate and advance laws that serve their populations' reproductive health. Accordingly, laws must protect 'the right of men and women to be informed [about] and to have access to safe, effective, affordable and acceptable methods of family planning of their choice, as well as to other methods of their choice for regulation of fertility'.[7] The Cairo Programme protects access to such methods 'which are not against the law'. This provision respects the traditions embodied in law to which many countries endorsing the Cairo Programme adhere, and provides legislators and judges with means to exercise judgement on the relative weight to be given to moral or religious law that promotes spiritual values, and on secular law designed to achieve desired practical results.

---

[6] *Gillick v. West Norfolk and Wisbech Area Health Authority*, [1986] Appeal Cases 112 (House of Lords, England), Lord Scarman at 186.

[7] UN, *Population and Development*, i. *Programme of Action Adopted at the International Conference on Population and Development, Cairo, 5–13 September 1994* (New York: UN, Department for Economic and Social Information and Policy Analysis, ST/ESA/SER.A/149, 1994).

Epidemiological and social science research has shown that many traditional laws have harmful effects on women's reproductive health and wider interests.[8] Modern critiques of laws have arisen that are sometimes described as feminist, although not all representatives of women's interests describe themselves as such, and not all advocates of sensitivity to women's concerns are women. The practical damage done to women's health and status by moral or principle-based law, particularly on matters affecting human reproduction, has historically been overlooked or discounted, since institutions of moral authority such as religious institutions, legislatures, academic institutions, and professional associations have historically tended not to include women, and in many cases have deliberately excluded women. Accordingly, the law, as an instrument of government and the state, served purposes identified by men, and applied techniques that men considered appropriate but whose dysfunctions for women's lives and well-being men did not experience or appreciate.

Under conditions of equity between the sexes promoted by principles contained in national constitutions and national and/or international human rights law, all laws affecting reproductive health require review in order to assess their particular impact on women. Constitutional law is the central body of law that organizes principles by which government is conducted under the law, and that expresses the most significant or fundamental principles that governments that function under the rule of law are required to observe. International human rights laws express key principles that countries commit themselves to observe in their treatment of individuals, often drawn from principles expressed in nations' constitutional laws. Both constitutional and human rights laws recognize the equality of the sexes and individuals' entitlement to protect their lives and health, and reproductive health requires these laws to be observed.

The usual role of lawyers is to advise on the legality of proposed or past conduct, and to review legal options for the advancement of goals of those who seek their advice. There is an important contrast, which non-lawyers sometimes miss, between evasion of a law, which is illegal, and avoidance of a law. For instance, if a driver has little more than one hour to drive from town A to town B 70 kilometres away, and drives at 70 kilometres an hour on a regular road with a speed limit of 60 kilometres an hour, the driver has broken the legal speed limit but may hope to evade the consequences. If the towns are also joined by a motorway where the speed limit is 80 or more kilometres an hour, however, the driver will lawfully avoid the legal limit on the regular road by driving at 70 kilometres an hour on the motorway. Lawyers cannot advise legal evasion, because that is legal professional misconduct, but may advise

---

[8] See, for instance, Center for Reproductive Law and Policy (CRLP), *Reproductive Rights 2000: Moving Forward* (New York: CRLP, 2000), 38–44.

how restrictive laws can be lawfully avoided. For instance, when the Irish law prohibited abortion in the country, popular pressure led to an amendment to the national constitution to provide that women could lawfully travel elsewhere, notably to England, for legal procedures.[9] Similarly, when the English Court of Appeal held that the law in England prohibited a woman's use of her deceased husband's sperm to have his child posthumously, because she did not have his consent in writing to recover his sperm while he was unconscious, it also held that she could receive his sperm in order to be inseminated elsewhere, where his consent did not have to be evidenced in this form.[10] She was successfully inseminated in Belgium, and about six years later gave birth to his second child. Lawyers can sometimes propose how laws that cannot be evaded can lawfully be avoided.

3. *Legal Reform for Reproductive Health*

Laws are expressed in customs, codes, and legislated documents that fit within each country's traditions of legal development. Local lawyers and relevant legal literature need to be consulted to understand the particular laws and legal traditions of each country.[11] Some countries embody their law in comprehensive codes that contain all of the rights that governments, other agencies, and individuals may claim. Other countries set their law within a framework of custom that judges declare in individual cases, and into which particular enacted laws will fit. Yet other countries fit enacted laws within a framework of sacred law interpreted by religious authorities, which may declare an enacted law to be in violation of sacred principles, and accordingly inoperative.

Reproductive health law is not generally contained within a separate body of law. It describes laws that affect reproductive health, sometimes positively, such as where it facilitates education in sexual and reproductive health, and sometimes negatively, such as where it allows health care practitioners a right of conscientious objection to perform particular services without requiring them to refer patients who seek such services to other practitioners who do not have objections. Where all legal claims to rights are comprehensively codified, a section of the code may be prepared that will protect and promote reproductive health. Reproductive health rights will all be expressed within the detailed provisions of that section of the code, and any apparently inconsistent

---

[9] Thirteenth Amendment of the Constitution Act, 23 Dec. 1992.

[10] *R. v. Human Fertilisation and Embryology Authority, ex p. Blood*, [1997] 2 All ER 687 (Court of Appeal, England).

[11] See e.g. CRLP and International Federation of Women Lawyers (Kenya Chapter), *Women of the World: Laws and Policies Affecting their Reproductive Lives—Anglophone Africa* (New York: CRLP, 1997).

provisions in other parts of the code will be subordinate and subject to provisions contained in the reproductive health section. For instance, the Russian Federation has considered the enactment of a comprehensive law that would express the reproductive rights of citizens and the guarantees available to them for implementation of these rights.[12]

In contrast, many countries develop laws limited to advancing a particular goal in reproductive health care. For instance, in 1995 Guyana replaced its law that rendered abortion a serious criminal offence with a new law that gave priority to women's rights to avail themselves of safe abortion services.[13] In 1965, Guinea prohibited female genital cutting, often described as female genital mutilation (FGM), by including the practice within its Penal Code prohibition of castration.[14] In 1966, the Central African Republic issued an ordinance[15] prohibiting FGM in order to conform to the Universal Declaration of Human Rights, and Ghana enacted a law in 1994 explicitly prohibiting the practice of FGM.[16] Many other countries, in Africa and far beyond, have enacted specific laws for this purpose.[17] In 1990, the United Kingdom brought advanced reproductive technologies and research under the general control of the Human Fertilisation and Embryology Authority.[18] In 1996, the Second International Consultation on HIV/AIDS and Human Rights, organized by the Office of the United Nations High Commissioner for Human Rights and the Joint United Nations Programme on HIV/AIDS, laid out International Guidelines that states should embody in their legal codes or legislation for humane management of the HIV/AIDS pandemic (see Pt. III, Ch. 7).

Several countries in different regions of the world developing new constitutions have included provisions for the protection of reproductive rights. Article 40 of the 1991 Colombian Constitution, for example, protects the right to decide on the number and spacing of one's children. Other constitutions have more general provisions, such as on the right to liberty and security of the person, that have been applied to protect reproductive rights. For instance, in 1982 Canada adopted a Charter of Rights and Freedoms that included this right in general terms. In 1988, the Supreme Court of Canada found that the provisions of the Criminal Code that limited women's choice of abortion violated women's right to security of the person, and were therefore unconstitutional and inoperative.[19]

---

[12] Tabled by State Duma Deputy, N. V. Krivelskaya.
[13] Medical Termination of Pregnancy Act 1995, Act No. 7 of 1995.
[14] Penal Code of the Republic of Guinea (1965), Article 265.
[15] Central African Republic, Ordinance No. 66/16 of 22 Feb. 1966.
[16] Criminal Code (Amendment) Act, 1994, sec. 1
[17] See CRLP, *Reproductive Rights 2000: Moving Forward* (New York: CRLP, 2000), 41–2.
[18] Human Fertilisation and Embryology Act 1990, ch. 37.
[19] *R. v. Morgentaler* (1988), 44 Dominion Law Reports (4th) 385 (Supreme Court of Canada).

Less certain in their effects on reproductive health are constitutional amendments intended to protect human life from the moment of conception, such as have been introduced in the Irish[20] and Philippines[21] Constitutions and in several Latin American countries. Religions differ on when protected life comes to exist, but the Roman Catholic Church decided in 1869 that this is at the moment of conception, and encourages countries to adopt laws that give effect to this choice of time. These laws prioritize protection of unborn human life over lesser interests, but do not necessarily compel women to subordinate their interests in their own lives or the lives of their born children to the interests of their unborn children. Accordingly, where the lives of women or their dependent children would be endangered, for instance by successive pregnancies at short intervals, this constitutional provision would not necessarily limit legal recourse to abortion, even in countries that give special status to the Roman Catholic religion. For instance in Ireland, following an amendment to the national constitution by which the state guaranteed the right to life of the unborn child, with due regard to the equal right to life of the woman, the Supreme Court has held that abortion is legally allowed where it is probable that there is a real and substantial risk to the woman's life from continuation of pregnancy, including risk of suicide due to psychological imbalance.[22]

4. *The Evolution of Reproductive Health Law*

Contraception has detached sexual relations from reproduction, and the new reproductive technologies based on *in vitro* fertilization (IVF) have more recently separated reproduction from sexual relations, but the historical foundations of medical law were laid when sexual relations and human reproduction were unavoidably linked. Sexual activities were a special interest of moral and religious authorities, perhaps because they concern an inherent aspect of human nature and affect family creation and continuity. Religious leaders exercised strong influence over the law through judges and legislators who were respectful of their authority to make pronouncements concerning the mystery of human life. The law tended to condemn sexual conduct outside narrowly defined fidelity in religiously celebrated marriage, considering children conceived or born outside marriage as illegitimate. Under religious and moralistic influence, the early law addressing human reproduction and sexuality tended to be restrictive and censorious.

Both customary law declared by judges and legislation enacted by political assemblies were suspicious of human interventions in natural processes of

---

[20] Article 40.3.3, inserted by the Eighth Amendment to the Constitution Act, 1983.
[21] Article II, sec. 12.
[22] *Attorney General v. X.*, 1992 Irish Reports 1 (Supreme Court of Ireland), 55.

human reproduction, and condemned techniques of induced abortion, voluntary sterilization, and contraception that seemed to subvert or devalue the divine gift of conception and birth. The same vision served in later times to preserve reproductive choice by opposing laws that allowed involuntary sterilization. Early legislation on abortion, such as was enacted in 1803 in England, expressed the intention to protect women against interference in their pregnancies by unskilled and potentially harmful providers of abortion services. In time, the legislation came to be supported in defence of foetal and, later, embryonic life, with only guarded accommodation of medically indicated abortion when women's lives or permanent health were endangered by continuation of pregnancy. The criminal law in many countries punished induced abortion with its severest penalties short of execution, namely up to life imprisonment, and in time condemned women who sought abortions as well as those who performed them. Similarly, provision of information and of means by which women could prevent conception was condemned. In Canada, for instance, until 1969 the Criminal Code condemned supplying means and information of birth control under the heading of Crimes Against Morality.

4.1. *From morality to democracy*

The control of human reproduction and sexuality by penalties of the criminal law was supported by traditional political and religious institutions as a defence of marriage, the family, and moral values. For instance, voluntary sterilization remains a criminal offence in the laws of such religiously influenced countries as Argentina[23] and Poland.[24] An evolution in the relation between law and morality was triggered, however, in the English-speaking world and beyond, by publication in England in 1957 of the Report of the Committee on Homosexual Offences and Prostitution, known through the name of its chairman, Sir John (later Lord) Wolfenden, as the Wolfenden Committee Report. The Report observed that there must be an area of purely private morality and conscience, and that not every moral precept has to be embodied in law. The Report observed that, in a democratic society, 'there must remain a realm of private morality and immorality which is, in brief and crude terms, not the law's business'.[25] The Report favoured the moral neutrality

[23] Penal Code of Argentina, Law No. 11,719, text codified by Decree No. 3992, 21 Dec. 1984, Articles 90–2, as cited in CRLP and Estudo para la Defensa de los Derechos de la Mujer (DEMUS) *Women of the World: Laws and Policies Affecting their Reproductive Lives: Latin America and the Caribbean* (New York: CRLP, 1997), 24.
[24] Criminal Code of Poland, Article 156, as cited in M. Rutkiewicz, 'Towards a Human Rights-Based Contraceptive Policy: A Critique of Anti-Sterilization Law in Poland', *European J. of Health Law*, 8 (2001), 225–42.
[25] Home Office (UK), *Report of the [Wolfenden] Committee on Homosexual Offences and Prostitution* (London: Stationery Office, 1957) (Cmnd. 247), 24, para. 61.

of the law, and approached law as a pragmatic instrument concerned with practical outcomes that were not necessarily positively approved but that were acceptable within the limits of popular tolerance. The thrust of the Report was to change the foundations of criminal law relevant to sexual activity from a judgemental, moralistic basis to a pragmatic, tolerant, and democratic basis.

From the time of the Report, legislation was progressively liberalized in sexual and reproductive matters, including prostitution, homosexual relations between consenting adults in private, and abortion. For instance, the Abortion Act 1967 in Britain was followed by amendments in Canada's Criminal Code in 1969 that opened the way to lawful contraception and abortion, India's accommodating Termination of Pregnancy Act 1971 and, for instance, Zambia's similar Termination of Pregnancy Act 1974. In some countries, notably the USA, reform has come from higher courts[26] rather than from legislative assemblies. Three successive surveys of ten-year international trends in abortion legislation and court judgments since 1967, for 1967–77,[27] 1977–88,[28] and 1988–98[29] have shown a widespread, although not universal, evolution from moralistic laws towards laws concerned with protection and promotion of women's health and welfare.

4.2. *From crime and punishment to health and welfare*

There has been a movement of reproductive and sexual health law from a basis in criminal law enforcement of religious morality to a basis in individuals' interests in their own health and welfare. Laws have accordingly been progressively liberalized to allow advertisement and distribution of contraceptive means, access to contraceptive sterilization, and abortion. The movement was reinforced regarding infertility by use of means of medically assisted reproduction to overcome individuals' inabilities to conceive their own children, particularly through reproductive technologies. Committee reports from the 1980s, particularly in Australian states, the UK, Canada, and the USA,[30] noted how the assisted reproductive technologies challenged traditional and religious beliefs regarding the proper origins of human conception and life. Such beliefs were often prohibitive of some methods of achieving childbirth

---

[26] See *Griswold v. Connecticut* 381 United States Reporter 479 (1965) (Supreme Court of the United States) on contraception, and *Roe v. Wade*, 410 United States Reporter 113 (1973) (Supreme Court of the United States) on abortion.

[27] R. J. Cook and B. M. Dickens, 'A Decade of International Change in Abortion Law: 1967–1977', *American Journal of Public Health*, 68 (1978), 637–44.

[28] R. J. Cook and B. M. Dickens, 'International Developments in Abortion Law: 1977–1988', *American Journal of Public Health*, 78 (1988), 1305–11.

[29] R. J. Cook, B. M. Dickens, and L. E. Bliss, 'International Developments in Abortion Law: 1988–1998', *American Journal of Public Health*, 89 (1999), 579–86.

[30] S. McLean, *Law Reform and Human Reproduction* (Brookfield, Vt.: Dartmouth, 1992).

and conducting research to treat infertility that involved deliberate wastage of human embryos. The main effects of these committee reports, however, especially when their recommendations became embodied in legislation, were to accommodate many techniques available to provide infertile couples with children genetically related to both or at least one of them, and also to neither, and to regularize births of children artificially conceived on close analogy with children conceived naturally. Legal accommodation of medical interventions by which infertile and subfertile individuals could have the children they wanted came in many countries to parallel legal accommodation of medical interventions by which fertile individuals could prevent and overcome unplanned pregnancy, and space births according to their own choice and design.

4.3. *From health and welfare to human rights*

A further evolution in law on reproductive and sexual health is now apparent, moving the base from interests in health and welfare to a base in human rights principles. From 1981, for instance, the European Court of Human Rights has condemned national laws that prohibit sexual relationships between same-sex couples whose partners give competent, voluntary consent.[31] Human rights principles, such as respect for privacy and choice in family life, have afforded individuals protection against legislative interventions in their reproductive choices both to prevent unplanned pregnancy and childbirth and to use medical means to have children when they wish. In 1988, for instance, in the Supreme Court of Canada decision that held the restrictive Criminal Code provision on abortion unconstitutional and inoperative, the Chief Justice of Canada observed that: 'Forcing a woman, by threat of criminal sanction, to carry a foetus to term unless she meets certain criteria unrelated to her own priorities and aspirations, is a profound interference with a woman's body and thus a violation of security of the person.'[32]

Particularly significant in protection of reproductive choice by human rights principles and laws based on the Universal Declaration of Human Rights of 1948 have been documents and programmes coming from two UN conferences. The International Conference on Population and Development, held in Cairo in 1994, produced the Cairo Programme of Action, and the Fourth World Conference on Women, held in Beijing in 1995, produced the Beijing declaration and Platform for Action (see Pt. I, Ch. 6, Sect. 3). The Platform provides that:

The human rights of women include their right to have control over and decide freely and responsibly on matters related to their sexuality, including sexual and reproductive

---

[31] *Dudgeon v. United Kingdom* (1981) 4 EHRR 149.
[32] *R. v. Morgentaler* (see n. 19 above) at 402.

health, free of coercion, discrimination and violence. Equal relationships between women and men in matters of sexual relations and reproduction, including full respect for the integrity of the person, require mutual respect, consent and shared responsibility for sexual behaviour and its consequences.[33]

Human rights may be equally invoked to protect choice of resort to reproductive technologies to overcome infertility.[34] In the USA, the constitutional right of individual privacy that recognized a constitutional right to abortion[35] has been invoked to protect legal use of medically assisted reproduction.[36] Further, in England, a woman's right to use her husband's sperm recovered while he was unconscious and dying and without his prior consent given in conformity with the Human Fertilisation and Embryology Act 1990 was recognized, over the refusal of the Human Fertilisation and Embryology Authority, under principles of European Community law.[37]

The initial evolution, from addressing reproductive and sexual health issues through law on crime and punishment to applying the law on health and welfare, is incomplete internationally, and the further evolution to employ human rights law remains at its earliest stage. Moral visions exert a strong influence on legal systems, particularly those in which religious law is paramount, such as in Islamic legal systems. Many Islamic countries that have ratified the leading international human rights conventions have done so only subject to the reservation that shariah, Islamic religious law, not be compromised. This raises the question among international lawyers of the extent to which such countries are full members of the particular treaty regimes.[38] Nevertheless, the constitutions and many of the domestic laws of these countries recognize outcomes of married couples' reproductive choices, accommodate provisions of reproductive health programmes, and are compatible with human rights principles.

Accordingly, scope exists in many legal systems to move beyond criminal law prohibitions of choices in reproductive and sexual matters, to give effect to concepts of health, welfare, and individuals' enjoyment of their private and family lives. Further, widely endorsed and invoked principles of respect for human rights support health care providers' individual and professional initiatives to protect and serve the reproductive and sexual health and satisfaction of those who seek their services, and of all members of the communities to which service providers dedicate their professional lives. Movements in legal

---

[33] UN, Department of Public Information, *Platform for Action and Beijing Declaration: Fourth World Conference on Women, Beijing, China, 4–15 September 1995* (New York: UN, 1995).

[34] See Part I, Ch. 6, Sect. 4.3, for instance, on rights to the benefits of scientific progress.

[35] *Roe v. Wade* (see n. 26).

[36] J. A. Robertson, *Children of Choice: Freedom and the New Reproductive Technologies* (Princeton: Princeton University Press, 1994).

[37] *R. v. Human Fertilisation and Embryology Authority, ex p. Blood* (see n. 10).

[38] See *Reservations to the Genocide Convention*, Advisory Opinion, International Court of Justice Reports 1951, 15 (International Court of Justice).

systems in this direction occur at different paces, but movement in the reverse direction is an international anomaly.[39]

5. *Legal Principles Governing Reproductive Health Care*

The legal principles applicable to reproductive health that legal systems contain and express in their distinctive forms are relatively few, but are capable of applications that can maximize the protection and promotion of reproductive health.[40] Each legal system surrounds these core principles with refinements at different levels of detail and abstraction, developed in legislation or by judicial interpretation of customary or enacted law. The key principles that follow are widely found, however, as minimum basic principles that national legal systems contain to satisfy prevailing standards of justice through private and public accountability for reproductive health.

The key legal principles in the provision of services are:

- informed decision-making,
- free decision-making,
- privacy,
- confidentiality,
- competent delivery of services, and
- safety and efficacy of products.

Where a health care provider–patient relationship precedes a patient's request for reproductive health care, usually in the relationship between physician and patient, the provider may invoke a legally limited right of conscientious objection to performance of certain procedures, notably to voluntary sterilization and abortion, but is then obliged to refer the patient to a colleague who is known not to object (see below, Sect. 9).

Basic understanding of the law governing physicians comes from their treatment of patients, but many users of reproductive health services are not patients in the traditional sense. They may be described as 'patients' or as 'users', 'consumers' or, for instance, 'customers', but they are legally different. 'Patients' are people who are ill or who reasonably fear that they are at risk of becoming ill, and they seek therapeutic or preventive health care services. When their conditions are cured, adequately maintained, or otherwise secured, they no longer receive services. Chronically ill patients receive continuing

---

[39] In 1997, El Salvador amended its Penal Code to remove exceptions to its prohibition of abortion, which had formerly permitted abortion to save a woman's life or when pregnancy resulted from rape; see Decreto No. 1030, Articles 133–7 (1998).

[40] See generally, R. J. Cook and B. M. Dickens, *Considerations for Formulating Reproductive Health Laws* (Geneva: WHO, 2nd edn., 2000).

services, of course, for maintenance and prevention of deterioration of their conditions. However, while some recipients of reproductive health care are 'patients' in that traditional sense, such as pregnant women who want to maintain their own health and foetal health against risks, and those suffering from sexually transmitted diseases, many are not. Women seeking contraceptive services are usually healthy women who are sexually active or about to become so, and seek to limit the risks of unplanned pregnancy. This is a matter of lifestyle choice, sometimes called reproductive self-determination. While healthy and sexually active, furthermore, they may remain users of contraceptive services perhaps for decades, except for when they plan to build their families through spaced pregnancies.

The legal significance of the distinction between patients and other users of reproductive health services arises from the fact that, while physicians owe duties of care to their patients, they do not owe duties to other persons who seek their care. Physicians do not have to accept requests to take as patients anyone who asks. They can decline to undertake care for non-patients, provided that their choice is not based on a prohibited ground of discrimination such as race or HIV positivity,[41] but owe enforceable duties only to patients they have accepted as such, for instance to inform them of health care options. Physicians employed in hospitals and clinics may be legally bound to provide care for persons such facilities admit as patients, but facilities are not always obliged to accept applicants as patients, except in some cases of emergency. Nevertheless, the practice in this book is to describe all recipients of health care providers' services as 'patients', including both sick and healthy recipients, and those seeking protective services such as contraception, unless they are specifically identified not to be patients.

Physicians have a very limited privilege, the so-called 'therapeutic privilege', to moderate how they present information of therapeutic care options when explicit information may be countertherapeutic, for instance in compromising the patient's capacity to tolerate indicated care. The privilege cannot be lawfully used to manipulate or direct patient choice, but can be applied to maintain usual options of care when explicit detail of extraordinary risks of adverse outcomes would intimidate a sick patient who requires care. However, since the health of applicants for contraceptive services will not be prejudiced by forgoing such services, although their choice of conduct may be, there is no legal basis on which to withhold information of possible adverse effects of the treatment options available to them. Physicians have responsibilities to inform patients who have used reproductive health services of subsequently learned

---

[41] B. M. Dickens, 'Health Care Practitioners and HIV: Rights, Duties and Liabilities', in D. C. Jayasuriya (ed.), *HIV Law, Ethics and Human Rights* (New Delhi: UN Development Programme Regional Project on HIV and Development, 1995), 66–98, at 79–81.

risks associated with treatment they have received, particularly risks to reproductive functions, if the patients remain reasonably accessible to receive such information. Further, since failures in reproductive health care can affect the reproductive self-determination of patients' husbands, and the circumstances of the children they bear, in ways that legal systems recognize, physicians' protective responsibilities may apply to more than the patients who are direct recipients of their care.

Legal concerns in the provision of reproductive health care services include:

1. giving contraceptive and sterilization information and services;
2. giving antenatal, delivery and post-partum care, including access to emergency obstetrical services and perinatal care of newborns;
3. screening for, diagnosis, and treatment of obstetric and gynaecological morbidity, including reproductive tract infections (RTIs) and cervical and breast cancers;
4. screening for and diagnosis and treatment of sexually transmitted diseases (STDs) in both women and men;
5. rendering services for treating abortion complications, and when delivering legal, safe abortion services;
6. providing infertility services for women and men;
7. operating well-organized and dependable referral systems for complications requiring specialized care;
8. providing counselling and information on preventive care, health promotion, and access to treatment options;
9. eliminating induced hazards to reproductive health, such as female genital cutting or mutilation (FGM) and violence against women; and
10. being alert to the risk of HIV infection in patients and others, and non-discriminatory in responding to the risk.

6. *Decision-Making*

6.1. *Informed decision-making*

It has become conventional in many legal systems to express informed decision-making as 'informed consent'. This expression is inaccurate and often dysfunctional, however, because of its focus on a goal of inducing consent. It should be replaced by an expression such as informed decision-making or informed choice, in order to emphasize health service providers' duty to disclose information, rather than any purpose to obtain consent. The legal duty is to present information that is material to the choice that the medical patient and other users of family planning services have to make, in a form that they can understand and recall. The purpose is to equip them to exercise choice, and to review a choice that was previously made. Studies suggest that when female family planning users are able to exercise informed choice, family planning outcomes are enhanced and satisfaction and commitment to treatment are increased.[42]

Decisions both to accept recommended care and to decline it must be adequately informed. It has been recommended that '[w]henever a patient refuses a treatment, test, or procedure, a physician should document the informed refusal in the patient's medical record', including the reasons stated by the patient for refusal.[43] A patient receiving adequate information who declines a recommended option of reproductive health care must not be supposed to have done so because of a lack of understanding, or to be in need of any emphasis or amplification of information already adequately given. Overemphasis in support of a recommendation can be directive, and deny real choice. However, clinical judgement is required, since a physician has been held liable, for instance, for failing adequately to explain to a patient the significance of her decision to decline a pap smear test in several successive annual health checks when the prevailing advice was that women should receive the test at least once every three years.[44] Patients are clearly free to decline any test, but physicians and other providers responsible for the care of patients are required to react more actively to refusal of a pap smear test for a third or later year than to refusal for a first or second year after a test has been conducted and a negative result recorded.

Information that a health service provider is usually required to disclose will include:

- the patient's currently assessed reproductive health status regarding liability to unplanned pregnancy, STDs, conception and birth of a child affected by a reasonably foreseeable handicap, and infertility;
- reasonably accessible medical, social, and other means of response to the patient's condition and reproductive intentions, including the predictable success rates, side effects, and risks of each option;
- the implications for the patient's reproductive, sexual, and more general health and lifestyle of declining any of the options; and
- the provider's reasoned recommendation.

Underlying the duty to disclose is legal recognition that decisions on accepting or declining medical care are not themselves medical decisions. They are personal decisions that individuals make, in accordance with their own priorities

[42] Y. M. Kim, A. Kols, and S. Mucheke, 'Informed Choice and Decision-Making in Family Planning Counselling in Kenya', *Int. Family Planning Perspectives*, 24/1 (1998), 4–11.
[43] American College of Obstetricians and Gynecologists, Opinion of the Committee on Professional Liability, 'Informed Refusal', *Int. J. Gynecol. Obstet.* 74 (2001), 67–8 at 68.
[44] *Truman v. Thomas*, 611 Pacific Reporter 2d 902 (1980) (Supreme Court of California).

that have to be medically informed. The legal duty to supply adequate information for decision-making is not limited to the time of initiation of the provider–patient relationship, or of consideration of a new option for care. The legal duty to ensure that patients are duly informed is an ongoing duty that continues throughout the health care relationship.

Although a physician is not required periodically to repeat information previously given, the physician is required to address any new occasion that should reasonably cause him or her to question whether the patient would want to make a different decision than was previously made. The occasion to refresh or add to information may arise out of the patient's treatment, out of the physician's awareness of a new treatment option that may be more suited to the care or circumstances of the patient or, for instance, from statistical research or anecdotal data indicating that maintaining prevailing treatment may present a previously unrecognized risk. For example, when it was realized that sperm from men who had not been shown HIV negative at donation could be a source of HIV infection, practitioners who had used fresh sperm had to explain why they would no longer do so, but would use only screened, frozen sperm, unless a recipient accepted the risk, for instance, of her husband's fresh sperm.

There is no general legal duty to present new information to those who decided not to become patients when they declined previously offered care on the basis of information that was appropriate at the time it was given. It may be necessary to do so, however, if the person is an existing patient and the new information is relevant to care. Patients for whom providers have a continuing responsibility after they have completed a process of care may have to be given follow-up information of any material fact relevant to that care and the patient's continuing health that has become available after the patient's care has been completed. For instance, a physician has been held legally liable for failing to inform a patient that blood he had previously received by transfusion was later shown to have come from a pool that had been contaminated by a donor who had the AIDS virus, and that the recipient was unknowingly exposing his wife to infection.[45]

Relevant law on due disclosure is not specific to particular procedures, tests, or options. The law addresses such matters through provisions governing health care providers' competence to practise, and their continuing fitness where attendance at programmes of continuing education is a condition of holding a licence to practise that requires periodic renewal. Continuing education is of particular significance in areas of more intensive research. For instance, newly arising information on genetic causes of disease and on

[45] *Pittman Estate v. Bain* (1994), 112 Dominion Law Reports (4th) 257 (Ontario Court, General Division, Canada).

prevention and management of genetically derived pathologies should be available to patients in a timely fashion. Similarly, improved techniques and new outcome studies regarding reproductive technologies may present patients with fresh options, or, for instance, indicate the unsuitability for them of options that previously appeared appropriate.

General practitioners are expected to maintain general awareness of developments in the same way as other general practitioners, but specialists in a medical field are legally required to maintain the level of awareness of other specialists. They are not necessarily expected to monitor developments recorded in recent volumes of, for instance, general medical journals, but are expected to be familiar with literature in the journals of their specialty.[46]

Providers must exercise cautious judgement about incorporation into their practice of suddenly arising perceptions or fashions in treatment in advance of reliable data, in accordance with principles of evidence-based medicine, but should not delay application of findings based on sound evidence. If in doubt about adoption of new ideas or abandonment of possibly discredited practices, they should consult leaders within their field of specialty and available professional literature, particularly research findings published in their appropriate journals that have been peer reviewed.

Legal systems apply different levels at which health care providers should pitch the information they aim at patients. Some require a 'professional standard', according to which a provider is required to disclose information that would be disclosed by other, similarly situated providers in the same health care field.[47] Others require disclosure pitched at what a reasonable person in the general circumstances of the patient would consider material for the exercise of choice.[48]

Both levels require that providers relate the information they give to what they reasonably should know about those they treat, and to what they actually do know. That is, providers are required to present information based on a realistic sense of patients' lifestyles and reproductive intentions. They must have a sense of the probable sexual practices of their patients, and of probable sexual partners, and treat resulting knowledge and suppositions non-judgementally. They must also adjust the information they give to more specific knowledge they acquire about their patients, gained from questions that patients ask them in discussion, and for instance from medical or other examinations. They should not suppose that patients necessarily conform to a limited range of sexual practices, or to prevailing stereotypes. For instance, sexual

---

[46] *ter Neuzen v. Korn* (1995), 127 Dominion Law Reports (4th) 577 (Supreme Court of Canada).

[47] See *Sidaway v. Bethlem Royal Hospital Governors* [1985] Appeal Cases 871, [1985] 1 All ER 643 (House of Lords, England).

[48] See *Canterbury v. Spence* (1972) 464 Federal Reporter 2d 772 (US Court of Appeals, District of Columbia Circuit).

activity may not be confined to members of the other sex, and does not necessarily decline with advancing age or with loss or absence of a marital partner.

The legal duty to be non-judgemental can impose a strain or burden on providers' professionalism. As professionals, physicians may feel that they must act as social leaders and role-models in their communities, and express high moral standards, perhaps associated with religious teachings. Care of patients' needs may require, however, that they recognize and accommodate sexual practices that conventional religions find immoral and even unnatural. As health care professionals, however, they must restrain any instincts they may have for moral condemnation, and act non-judgementally to discharge their legal responsibilities to those whose medical treatment they undertake.

Providers are not usually required to disclose features about their own capacities to provide the care they offer, unless such features may compromise patients' safety or, for instance, create conflicts of interest (see below, Sect. 8.1). A provider who is undertaking a procedure for the first time without supervision need not so inform a patient, since the provider is legally obliged to maintain the standard of proficiency and care to which other, experienced providers are held. Similarly, an HIV-positive provider's confidentiality prohibits disclosure of that fact to prospective patients, unless there may be exposure to the provider's body fluids. Such providers may be limited, for instance, in conducting invasive surgery where they may cut themselves.[49]

6.2. *Free decision-making*

In addition to providers ensuring that patients are adequately informed for decision-making, they must be alert to how far those they treat are free to exercise independent choice. Many recipients of reproductive health services are never entirely free, because they are subject to factors in their social and family surroundings that are liable to influence their choices. Their hopes and fears, the well-being of those they care for and who depend on them, and, for instance, their material resources and their dreams for the future may limit the options among which they feel themselves free to choose, or may direct the choices they feel compelled to make.

Legal doctrine on free decision-making concerns patients' freedom from any bias introduced, consciously or unconsciously, by those to whom they turn for reproductive health advice or care. Providers' recommendations are liable to be influential and perhaps decisive, but recommendations must be made on the basis only of judgement addressed to patients' best interests, directed by their reproductive health status and their expression of their wishes, goals, and

---

[49] R. J. Cook and B. M. Dickens, 'Patient Care and the Health-Impaired Practitioner', *Int. J. Gynecol. Obstet.* 78 (2002), 171–7.

preferences. Those giving information of options must therefore take care not to be directive, and not to compel or unduly induce a particular decision, although they are entitled to make a recommendation in patients' interests. Patients' informed choices may not follow care-givers' recommendations nor appear to be in their medical interests. However, since health relates to physical, mental, and social well-being, providers must tolerate those they must inform to exercise choices according to their own assessments of their relevant circumstances and ranking of their physical, psychological, and social interests.

Providers must not permit patients' free decision-making to be distorted to favour providers' own material or other advantage, or mere convenience. For instance, a provider's recommendation or bias in favour of more expensive care when less expensive care would be equally appropriate may both compromise a patient's free decision-making, and constitute illegal and unethical conflict of interest on the part of the provider. A recommendation must be uninfluenced by personal advantage. A conflict of interest in possible performance of tests by laboratories of which providers are proprietors, for instance, should at least be disclosed to patients, with identification of alternative facilities.

Providers concerned that their approach to a patient or their style of practice may distort a patient's freedom of choice may consult their professional leaders or experienced colleagues who are able to offer an independent assessment. In clinical care of vulnerable patients, providers must exercise caution, for instance, in directing them towards forms of contraception on the basis of the providers' convenience or third-party payers' interests in economy, when alternative methods would be more suitable to patients' circumstances and better preserve their options for reproductive health.

How far providers should go to liberate patients from restrictions on choices that arise from the patients' social and family circumstances will depend on the features of each case. Providers are under no general legal duty to isolate or protect patients from the normal influences that affect their lives. They face legal liability only if they impose treatments on patients when it is obvious that recipients' resistance is being overborne by the insistence of third parties, such as partners, parents, or parents-in-law. Providers may be equally liable, for instance for negligence, for denying care that patients prefer because of knowledge of third parties' opposition.

The compromise of patients' freedom of decision-making that arises from their social vulnerability, poverty, or oppressive cultures presents providers with similar challenges. For instance, when a long-acting implantable contraceptive method, such as Norplant, is offered as an option to disadvantaged patients, they must be ensured adequately free choice with respect both to the initial implantation and to subsequent use and removal.

The introduction of untested medical methods of fertility control, or promotion, to inadequately informed patients, who then suffer injuries, may raise direct and indirect legal concerns. Direct legal liability is unlikely to be pressed when patients are not accustomed to bringing legal proceedings. However, investigators who allow themselves to appear as therapists, who fail to observe ethical guidelines and requirements of independent ethical review of research, for instance concerning patients' free participation in research, may face indirect legal liability. They may legally be exposed to sanctions in discipline proceedings by licensing authorities and by institutions with which they are associated, such as hospitals, universities, and professional bodies.

6.3. *The role of third parties*

6.3.1. *Partner authorization*

Health care providers must exercise great caution in supposing that their capacity to give sexual and reproductive health care to one partner in a marriage requires the authorization of the other. Unless recipients of their services explicitly approve consultation with spouses, disclosure of the request for or delivery of sexual or reproductive health care may violate a patient's confidentiality, and be illegal. Even where disclosure is a legal discretion it may still be unethical, exposing providers to professional disciplinary proceedings and sanctions.

It is widely recognized in law that mentally competent adults enjoy autonomy of choice in their medical and health care, that they do not require the consent of any third party, including a wife or husband, and are not subject to the veto of any third party, unless that third party has legal power to decline to pay the costs of such care. Providers who are advised by their own lawyers that partner consent is required, particularly in cases such as artificial insemination by sperm donor, should, of course, comply. Without such advice, however, providers may be in peril of legal violation if they suppose that such consent is required simply because it has been obtained in the past, or because it is customary in their community or facility to obtain it. Indeed, initiating discussions with spouses without patients' clear prior consent may constitute a serious legal breach of confidentiality. If a spouse needs to be informed of proposed care in order to cover the costs, disclosure is the responsibility of the proposed patient, not the health care provider, although providers may generalize information by reference, for instance, to gynaecological care, and not be specific. If providers render non-emergency care without prior arrangements for necessary fees to be met, they may be compromised in their legal capacity to seek payment from third parties, other than insurance agencies.

Young girls incapable of freely consenting to their marriage usually cannot be legally married simply on parental consent. Where such consent is a legally necessary condition of their marriage, because they are not of legal age for independent marriage, parental consent is not in itself a legally sufficient condition. Marriage requires both partners' free approval, and human rights are violated if individuals of any age are married against their will. However, parental consent to a legal minor's marriage makes the minor of adult status in the eyes of the law, and does not place him or (usually) her under the legal control of an older spouse. She can independently approve and disapprove medical procedures for herself, and make health care decisions for her child.

Husbands have no legally recognized cause of action against health care providers who treat their wives, on their wives' adequately informed and competent consent, without the husbands' authorization. Husbands' may have to be informed where health care services are payable only from family resources that husbands control, but husbands' legal duties are to provide their wives with medically necessary care that they have the means to provide. Health care providers asked to provide services that are not necessary to the preservation of patients' health, or that may be beyond the families' means to pay for, are entitled to seek assurances in advance that the services will be paid for. Nevertheless, such assurances sought from prospective patients do not justify any breach of their confidentiality by providers' discussions with spouses, unless they are authorized in advance by the prospective patients.

Providers may discuss with prospective patients whether delivery of services without their spouses' approval would provide the spouses with rights of divorce or other matrimonial remedies against such patients, for instance on grounds of cruelty or breach of a marriage contract between the parties or their families. A provider who is uncertain whether delivery of services to a patient that renders him or her liable to divorce would constitute professional misconduct, making the provider liable to sanctions by licensing authorities or by professional associations, should resolve the issue by discussions with relevant authorities or associations.

6.3.2. *Parental consent*

As children grow in intelligence, experience, and maturity, their ability grows comparably to discharge different functions and take responsibility for their decisions. The UN Convention on the Rights of the Child requires attention to 'the evolving capacities of the child'.[50] Although adolescents acquire full legal empowerment on the day they reach majority age, they have usually gained increasing legal rights earlier in their development. They may be empowered by legislation before majority age, for instance, to leave school and be employed, to buy tobacco or alcohol, to go unaccompanied to forms of entertainment, to vote, to drive motor vehicles, to consent to sexual activity, and to

---

[50] Article 5; see R. J. Cook and B. M. Dickens, 'Recognizing Adolescents' "Evolving Capacities" to Exercise Choice in Reproductive Healthcare', *Int. J. Gynecol. Obstet.* 70 (2000), 13–21.

marry. For many activities of adolescence, however, no chronological age is legislated.

In many countries there is no legally recognized age of consent to medical treatment, although health care providers are not uncommonly faced with literature that mistakenly states that there is. Such literature confuses law relevant to health care with legislation on the legal age of consent to sexual intercourse and, for instance, on the legal age of independent consent to marriage.

In health care law, there is generally no 'age of consent' but only a condition of consent, which is reached when a person, of whatever age, is capable of sufficient comprehension to give adequately informed consent. Where legislation sets an age of majority or medical consent, it usually affects only the point at which the governing legal presumption changes. At adult age, individuals are presumed capable to make health care decisions for themselves, unless evidence, such as of intellectual impairment, indicates that they are not. Legal minors or those below an age set for medical consent are presumed incapable, unless evidence of maturity and comprehension indicates that they are capable.

Providers who deny indicated sexual and reproductive health care to the mentally competent and mature adolescent children of families for whose care they have accepted responsibility, because the providers do not have consent of parents or other adult guardians and the adolescents refuse to have their parents or guardians informed, face legal liability for negligence and for abandonment. Further, where children of families for whose care providers are responsible are not clearly mentally competent or mature, but their parents or guardians have failed to exercise responsibility for their sexual or reproductive health and well-being, the children may lawfully seek and receive relevant health care services from providers independently. Providers who refuse such adolescent children's requests for services may bear some legal responsibility for predictable STDs, pregnancies, and other foreseeable consequences that requested services would prevent, particularly when the children are subject to sexual pressures against which they are not afforded the protection of their parents or guardians.

In some countries, legislation clearly states that medical services are not to be provided to legal minors without consent of parents or other adult guardians. Where such laws apply, there are usually parallel laws of equal effect that provide that parents or guardians are legally bound to provide their dependent children with medically indicated health care services, which include preventive health care services. Parents and guardians violate the law in refusing to authorize such services and to pay for them within their means. Health care providers have no legal responsibility to enforce or monitor parents' and guardians' duties owed to their dependants, although many countries have child welfare laws that require professionals who become aware of child abuse to notify police or child protection agencies. However, providers violate no right of parents or guardians by delivering services that they are legally entitled to make available on children's requests. This includes such sensitive services as contraceptive care and abortion.[51]

Outside comprehensively codified legal systems, the law on medical care of minors frequently provides additional powers of care that adult guardians may exercise, but does not exclude powers of decision-making about their care that mature minors can exercise independently. That is, the law empowers certain others to approve procedures, but does not disempower mature minors, who may effectively decline such care. They often remain subject, however, to the financial disability that they may not have the means to pay fees for services they request that are not covered by public or other funding. They may then remain dependent on payments by guardians, who usually expect to know the services for which they are required or asked to pay. Guardians' legal duties to pay for indicated services may entitle them to learn in advance what services minors have requested, compromising minors' confidentiality. A justification for providers informing parents or guardians of medical treatments undertaken or proposed for adolescent children may be that, since parents and guardians are legally responsible for the well-being of those under their care, they must know the medications and medical treatment their dependants receive. Providers will therefore have to discuss with legal minors who seek sexual and reproductive health care services which services will be given in confidence, and which services may be disclosed to parents or guardians. Disclosures to parents may preserve a level of confidentiality if generalized, and not indicating too much detail about origins of conditions or effects of treatments.

6.3.3. *Substitute decision-making*

Legislation on mentally impaired individuals that justifies their guardianship by competent other persons almost invariably affords those in charge of them the legal power to approve health care services that are indicated for their well-being, including appropriate sexual and reproductive health care services. The capacity of such individuals to give legally effective consent to sexual intercourse may be questionable, but experience shows that they may voluntarily engage in sexual behaviours with others that are not exploitive of them. It may be appropriate and consistent with their human rights, for instance to as much private life as possible, that they be allowed unchaperoned companionship with members of the other sex, and to give sexual expression to affection when protected against harmful consequences.

A legacy of the eugenics movement, including memories of the oppressive treatment of mentally impaired people under the Nazi administration, is the protective requirement that they not be subjected to contraceptive sterilization

---

[51] *Gillick v. West Norfolk and Wisbech Area Health Authority* (see n. 6).

procedures, except perhaps when judicially approved by decisions reached on a case-by-case basis.[52] Nevertheless, where sterility is a consequence of other treatment that is clearly for the therapeutic benefit of mentally impaired people, such as surgery for mentally impaired women who suffer cancer of the ovary or for mentally impaired men who suffer testicular cancer, treatment may be undertaken upon consent of those under whose care they are legally placed.

A number of judicial decisions have held that mental health legislation may not necessarily permit relatives of mentally impaired persons the legal power to consent to medical interventions on them, even when they are incapable of giving legal consent for themselves.[53] In such cases, only courts of law may authorize medical treatment, unless in cases of necessity to save life or permanent health. Where legislation or judicial decisions place such persons under the charge of others who are legally empowered to consent to their health care, consent may be given to protect or advance their sexual and reproductive health care, but legal power will usually be narrowly defined so as to permit only procedures that legal guardians are obliged to provide to meet dependent persons' needs. Power would not extend, for instance, to recruitment of dependent persons in research procedures not intended for their particular benefit.

It is a legal principle that mentally incompetent individuals' health care be governed by their competently formed wishes when they are known, for instance from their statements made and personalities shown at earlier times when they clearly had capacity. However, this principle cannot be observed when the individuals are not and perhaps have never been able to formulate or express wishes competently, or when no other persons are able to say reliably what their competent wishes were. The law then provides that such individuals be treated in ways that serve their best interests. That is, when treatment cannot be determined according to individuals' subjective wishes formed when they were competent, treatment must be determined according to the objective criterion of where each individual's best interests appear to lie. The role of family members or other guardians is to assist health care providers to reach an objective assessment of such best interests. The person's reactions to past experiences, his or her intellectual and emotional capacity, and, for instance, prospects of future institutional or domestic care may be described by those who know and are concerned for the person, in order to assist determination of what, if any, reproductive or sexual health care interventions will protect and advance his or her interests. Nevertheless, the eugenics legacy leaves doubts regarding the legality of irreversible, non-therapeutic surgical procedures, such as contraceptive sterilization, that are not judicially approved.

---

[52] See *Eve v. E.* [1986] 2 Supreme Court Reports 388 (Supreme Court of Canada).
[53] *Re F (A Mental Patient: Sterilisation)*, [1990] 2 Appeal Cases 1 (House of Lords, England).

7. Regulation of Information

7.1. Privacy

'Privacy' is sometimes considered an alternative expression to 'confidentiality', but a growing legal practice is to distinguish privacy from confidentiality and to determine the relationship between them.[54] Privacy consists in the right and power to control the information that others possess, and is almost invariably limited by the circumstances of everyday life. Individuals yield an aspect of their privacy, for instance, when they appear in public, and thereby permit others to observe them and to draw conclusions about them, such as their age, circumstances, and state of health.

Medical privacy is different, in that casual observers cannot draw accurate conclusions about individuals' health, particularly their reproductive health, from simple observation. Medical privacy is surrendered when patients tell providers how they feel, how they have behaved, how they propose to behave in sexual and other ways, and what they want providers to do for them, and particularly when they allow providers to examine them. The privacy they yield is particularly intimate and penetrating, because diagnosticians can learn information that patients themselves do not necessarily possess, may be unable to anticipate, or do not necessarily have the ability to understand. Privacy is critical to the functions of reproductive and sexual health clinics, because patients will feel unusually exposed and vulnerable to observation by strangers. If privacy is not ensured, patients may not return for care important to their own reproductive health and to the health of others, and potential patients may be deterred from going to them.

There are frequently legal provisions under which health care providers can obtain private information about individuals without their consent or even knowledge. Medical tests and reports that reduce privacy are sometimes involuntary, for instance under occupational health and safety laws, for immigration, and for school attendance. In some countries, men convicted, or only accused, of sexual assaults may be compelled to undergo HIV/AIDS testing for victims' health care. Health information may be compulsorily reportable, for instance to public health officers who monitor the prevalence of contagious or infectious diseases, including STDs. Publicly maintained registers of births will contain identifiable information of women who have given birth, and may include information of miscarriages, for instance after twenty weeks' gestation. Accordingly, by their own voluntary acts and direction of various laws, patients may find that their privacy is surrendered to health care providers.

---

[54] L. O. Gostin, *Public Health Law: Power, Duty, Restraint* (Berkeley, Calif.: University of California Press, 2000), 127.

Health care providers whose interactions with patients necessitate the compromise of privacy should minimize the extent to which this is required, consistently with their obligations to obtain information of patients' health and social histories relevant to their care, because an excess of disclosure may be legally indefensible. Compulsory acquisitions of information should be strictly limited to the purposes that justify the compulsion. All of those who receive information that compromises privacy, whether individuals volunteer that information freely or have no choice in the matter, are legally obliged to observe requirements of professional confidentiality.

7.2. *Confidentiality*

Confidentiality, the duty of providers and others who receive private medical information in the course of their employment to keep secret or private the information they gain about patients, is of critical concern regarding sexual and reproductive health. Sexual and reproductive matters are of particular sensitivity, and are not freely discussed in many families, communities, and cultures or between the sexes. Individuals who require and would benefit from sexual and reproductive health care may prefer to forgo it if they are not certain that their confidentiality will be strictly maintained. For instance, teenagers who are sexually active, or about to become so, may decide not to seek counselling from family physicians, school counsellors, or public clinics that would equip them to avoid STDs and pregnancy, for fear that their parents will be informed. Similarly, individuals inclined towards same-sex relationships may be fearful when those whose understanding they seek may make unauthorized or careless disclosures. To encourage individuals to seek information, a growing practice is to create 'hotlines' by which they can telephone anonymously for sexual and reproductive health advice, for instance concerning their risk of exposure to HIV infection. The fear that confidentiality will not be maintained deters many from seeking sexual and reproductive health services, and may literally cost lives, such as when women at risk of death from frequent or closely spaced pregnancy decline to seek information or means of birth control for fear of their husbands or in-laws being informed.

There are three predominant legal aspects of confidentiality, namely

- providers' duties to protect patients' information against unauthorized disclosures;
- patients' rights to know the information that their health care providers possess about them; and
- providers' duties to ensure that patients who authorize releases of their confidential health-related information to others exercise adequately informed and free choice.

Related concerns are legal provisions by which physicians have duties and discretions to release confidential information to others without their patients' knowledge, and when patients explicitly refuse consent.[55]

7.2.1. *Unauthorized disclosures*

Providers' protection of patients' information regarding sexual and reproductive health may have to go beyond the ordinary protection of family privacy, since the duty may concern information that individual partners in intimate relationships do not want to share even with each other. Treatment of STDs may require patients' disclosures, to providers, of sexual relationships outside marriage that would hurt patients to have disclosed to their partners. Health care providers face particular challenges to their legal duties and professional ethics when both partners in relationships are persons for whose care they are responsible, and infection in one partner endangers the other.

In some settings, wives may be fearful of serving their own interests in health and comfort, and the interests of children for whose care they are responsible, by negating the intentions of their husbands to father further children, particularly where existing children are all female. Accordingly, providers may have to be careful concerning the confidentiality of sterilization procedures and contraceptive care. The duty of confidentiality goes beyond care in conversation, since certain methods of provision of care may become apparent to husbands, in violation of wives' intentions to control the information their husbands acquire of wives' contraceptive practices. For instance, colourful containers of contraceptive pills may be difficult to conceal in simply furnished homes, and attendance for routine health checks may require explanation. Confidentiality of contraceptive care may be better secured by a long-acting injectable method, even when a less confidential alternative may be medically preferable.

Part of providers' duty of care owed to patients, arising through both legal contracts and the law of negligence, is to be vigilant to assure intended confidentiality. Counselling on methods of contraception, methods of sterilization, and, for instance, preventing spread of an STD, must be conducted in terms not only of the comfort and effectiveness of treatment options, but also of their confidentiality.

Infertility may damage the self-esteem of patients, and in some cultures be a legal ground for divorce. Further, a partner in a marriage may have psychological or other incentives to attribute the source of childlessness to the other partner. Practice shows that men may suppose their childlessness to be caused by their wives' inadequacy rather than by their own. While infertility is a

---

[55] B. M. Dickens and R. J. Cook, 'Law and Ethics in Conflict over Confidentiality?', *Int. J. Gynecol. Obstet.* 70 (2000), 385–91.

common concern to both partners in marriage for which they seek treatment, they may have adverse interests in information about the contribution the other makes to their failure to become parents.

Treatments to overcome childlessness that are acceptable to one partner may be unacceptable to the other, and options must be discussed, negotiated, and if possible agreed between partners. It may be illegal and unethical to initiate treatment resulting in birth within a marriage unless the treatment, such as use of donated sperm, receives the informed consent of both partners. Once agreement is reached and treatment is proposed, however, confidentiality of their joint care may be essential, for instance when the method, such as sperm donation, would deny the child legitimacy within the families of both partners, their community, and perhaps fellow adherents to their religious faith. The well-being of patients and the children intended to be reared in their families will turn not only on the clinical success of their reproductive health care, but also on its confidentiality.

7.2.2. *Disclosure to patients*

Patients' rights to know the information that their health care providers possess about them are widely recognized, but are subject to variations among different cultures. In some, it may be offensive to provide information damaging to patients' self-esteem without their request or careful preparation. For instance, adolescent patients have been harmed by sudden information, presented to them without counselling, as to the level of probability that any children they might later conceive would be at risk of inheriting a severe genetic disability.

An important legal distinction is that, while patients may have no right to demand the transfer into their possession of health care providers' records and correspondence about them, because such documents are the providers' legal property, patients are legally entitled to control the information about them that the documents contain. That is, the information is a separate legal interest or property from the documents and other materials in which it is contained. Accordingly, patients are entitled to information concerning themselves, and their requests cannot be rejected by providers claiming to have interests of their own in confidentiality of the documents and related materials. The right of confidentiality in their information belongs to the patients, who can direct providers to make it available to others, and to disclose it to themselves.

It does not follow, however, that patients legally entitled to information of their own health status are entitled as of right to take hold of and read the records, including notes and raw data that providers have made about them. Providers' legal duties are to make patients' information available to them in a form they can adequately understand, and in a way that will not result in their misunderstanding of their health circumstances and reproductive potential. Providers are not entitled to deny an appropriate interpretation of the information they possess, including information created by other health care providers. However, they should inquire what purposes patients intend to achieve by use of the information. They are then obliged to serve such purposes to the full extent of their information and ability. This may include giving a copy of a record to another physician a patient trusts to interpret it for the patient's purposes.

For example, where patients are fearful of venereal infection, they should be informed, when true, that their records show absence of infection. They may misunderstand a record that they read when it shows that they were tested to see whether or not they had been infected with named STDs. Patients may falsely focus on references in their records to particular diseases they fear, rather than on the negative results of tests. Negative results may not show that the risk is zero, but show a level that is below statistical significance, but enough to leave patients concerned. Providers must inform patients of the conditions by which they are found to be affected, counsel them on appropriate treatments, and recommend what care they consider best. However, providers must exercise their judgement concerning conditions that patients are found not to have, neither alarming patients concerning conditions their behaviour risked nor giving them a false sense of security against future risks. The legal duty is to give patients an adequate understanding, for their purposes, of information about their reproductive health, including both their present status and their potential future according to scenarios that patients indicate.

7.2.3. *Authorized disclosures*

Patients are entitled to require their health care providers to disclose to third parties, such as potential employers and insurance companies, the information that the providers possess about them. A precondition to compliance with such requests is that patients have some clear sense of what information providers possess about them. Whether or not patients have requested such disclosure to themselves (see 7.2.2 Disclosure to patients, above), providers have a legal duty to ensure that those who request a transmission of health information about themselves to third parties have an adequate opportunity to understand what information is then liable to be disclosed. This is an element of patients' adequately informed consent, although in law patients may be held to have voluntarily assumed the risk of disclosure of true but unfavourable information by requesting its disclosure to others without taking the opportunity to know the implications of their request.

Providers have to consider not only how to present truthful information in accordance with requests, but also whether patients have an adequate understanding of how requested disclosures may be of disadvantage to them, for instance by excluding them from personal, commercial, reproductive, or other opportunities. For instance, when an unmarried patient requests that her health records be provided to administrators of a school where she seeks employment, in order to show that she has no infection transmissible to children and for employment-related health insurance, she has to be told if the record will show her past pregnancy, and if the information should be limited to the purpose for which the request is made. Warning should also be given when patients request transfer of sensitive information to third parties who are under no legal duty or moral compulsion to treat it as confidential. Patients are entitled to insist on timely disclosure of records, but providers should offer an explanation when they fear that there is unawareness of unintended but likely negative effects of disclosure.

Providers' release of information in compliance with requests should be considered only within the scope of such requests, which they should interpret very conservatively. Accordingly, a response to a request concerning infection should not refer to past pregnancy. In case of uncertainty, providers should consult further with patients about the scope of requested disclosure, but should be aware that initiation of such consultation with patients in indiscreet ways may itself jeopardize confidentiality. For instance, providers should exercise great caution in leaving messages with third parties for patients to contact them, since this may inform the third parties that the patients are receiving care from these particular specialists, and expose the patients to unwelcome questioning or suspicion of why this is so. This is particularly important when clinic names refer to fertility, infertility, or venereal infection.

A request from patients with which providers are bound legally and ethically to comply fully and promptly is to transfer their records to other providers to whom the patients intend to transfer their care. Refusal cannot be based on, for instance, unpaid fees, since the records provide the new providers with information critical to the patients' right to care, and cannot be held as ransom for payment.

7.2.4. *Related concerns*

7.2.4.1. *Third-party interests*

It has been legally recognized that, while the duty of confidentiality is of great importance in the provider–patient relation, it is not the only duty, and it is not necessarily a duty that invariably outweighs all others. Further, there is latitude in how confidentiality serves the interests of patients. Although patients may not have authorized disclosures by explicit requests, it may be legally implied from their relationships that providers are free to make particular disclosures with the patients' implied consent. An obvious instance is when a physician decides to consult with a colleague about the significance of a finding in the patient's record. Further, when patients have voluntarily informed third parties that they are receiving care through particular providers, and such third parties approach the providers for assurances that the patients are not suffering from infection or other harmful health conditions from which the patients are in fact not suffering, the providers may so inform the third parties without having to obtain explicit authorization. If uncertain whether third parties have really been freely informed, however, providers should first consult the patients concerned.

Requests from third parties for health information about patients always present specialists with particular legal concerns. If they know that their patients have informed third parties, such as their husbands or wives, that they are under the specialists' care, and the information requested can be answered in a supportive or reassuring way, specialists may feel that they have consent to reply directly. Indeed, their failure to reply directly may be harmful, in that it may suggest that patients suffer from conditions that have negative implications. For instance, if a spouse inquires whether testing of a patient has shown that he or she suffers from an infection or malignancy, and testing has shown none to be present, the specialist may feel free to say so. Refusal to answer or a response that is not appropriately reassuring may be taken by the third party as evidence of the patient's ill-health. Further, a response that may reasonably give an impression that is both incorrect and disreputable or harmful to the patient may also in law be defamatory.

If providers are uncertain how replies may be understood, and when they know that patients have infections, malignancies, or other conditions the truthful disclosure of which may be a source of distress or disadvantage to them, providers are legally entitled to invoke the confidentiality of their professional relationships, to decline to answer. They may say that they are not free legally and/or ethically to disclose information arising from any professional relationship. Requesting parties may be advised to request such information from the patients themselves, or to ask the patients to request the providers to give answers to those making enquiries. Any patients who then authorize the release of information to third parties must be treated in accordance with the discussion above on authorized disclosures.

7.2.4.2. *Third-party peril*

A legal limitation of confidentiality that courts have recognized is that the duty of confidentiality ends where public peril begins.[56] In many countries, legislation requires health care providers who have become aware of patients' infections, by clinical diagnosis or otherwise, to so inform public health authorities. This is because of the legal limitation of individuals' rights to privacy (see above). However, reporting parties remain bound by duties of confidentiality outside the scope of their duty to report, and those who receive mandatory

---

[56] *Tarasoff v. Regents of the University of California*, 551 Pacific Reporter 2d 334 (1976) (Supreme Court of California) at 347.

reports are bound to treat the information they receive about individuals as confidential. Even when they are obliged to undertake contact-tracing, they cannot disclose the personal identities of persons about whom they have information. Some people who are contacted and warned that they have been exposed to risk of infection may recognize the source, but others may misidentify the person they believe is responsible.

A limitation of confidentiality may arise when reproductive health service providers acquire reasonable information in their professional capacity that those they are treating are placing identifiable third parties in preventable peril. This may be, for instance, because a patient may spread HIV infection or another STD to a partner through unprotected sexual intercourse. Providers may have legal duties to ensure such third parties' adequate protection, notably by ensuring that they are appropriately informed and counselled. Providers must be certain that their patients are aware of any risks they pose, and ask them what protections those at risk have. If assurances are given that seem adequate, in light, for instance, of patients' understanding, maturity, lifestyle, and demonstrated concern for the well-being of others at risk, providers will have discharged their legal responsibilities.

In case of uncertainty, providers may ask patients to return promptly with their partners for relevant counselling, or to have partners come alone or have the partners' own medical providers confirm that due counselling has been requested. Patients should be informed that, if partners' counselling is not assured, the providers are legally obliged, even without patients' consent, to inform their identified partners of the peril the providers have found to be present.

Providers must give those they are bound to warn information of the type of peril their patients present, without doing patients' confidentiality more than unavoidable damage. In hospital settings, for instance, providers have duties to protect staff such as waste disposal personnel and laundry workers against such injuries as may result from contaminated needles being left in bandages and bedding. They must give protection by general caution, education, and training, however, and not by disclosing that particular patients have, for instance, HIV infection or hepatitis. The danger to staff is not caused directly by patients, but by a provider's or institution's negligent safety strategy. Patients cannot legally invoke confidentiality to limit necessary disclosure of risks they themselves have refused or failed adequately to prevent. Where third parties at risk cannot reasonably be identified, providers discharge their legal duties by notifying appropriate public health or similar authorities that discharge policing functions for the community, whether or not reporting is mandatory under public health legislation.

In addition to holding providers bound to act appropriately to protect third parties against preventable serious harms that their patients appear likely to cause, courts have also held that providers who are not obliged so to act may be excused from legal liability if they exercise a discretion to act in reasonable protection of third parties. Whether they act protectively or not is an ethical rather than a legal matter (see Pt. I, Ch. 4). The legal doctrine of necessity may be invoked to excuse health care providers of legal liability when they take initiatives to protect others against their patients' tendencies to cause serious harm. However, while such initiatives may excuse health care providers from judicial sanctions, for instance for the breach of confidentiality they have committed, the initiatives are not justified in law. Professional licensing authorities and professional associations may consider the initiatives ethically improper and that they justify disciplinary sanctions. Further, lawyers may engage in professional misconduct if they assure or advise health care providers that they may behave in ways that are not legally justifiable, though excusable. Accordingly, the form of advice lawyers give will be that any proposed preventive initiatives are not legally justifiable, but that courts of law, as opposed perhaps to licensing authorities and professional associations, may find them excusable. Providers may consult with licensing authorities and professional associations before deciding whether to warn third parties whom they are not obliged to protect.

8. *Competent Delivery of Services and the Law of Negligence*

The law on competent delivery of services and negligence can have a distorting effect on health care practice, if providers believe that they have to treat patients in ways designed to defend themselves against risks of legal liability rather than in what they assess to be in the best interests of patients. Defending patients' health interests against real risks is good medicine, but undertaking 'defensive medicine' by use of procedures intended only to protect providers against fear of legal liability is not. In some countries, providers may decide, for instance, to turn to Caesarean delivery before properly assessing the safety to mother and child of natural delivery, and may feel bound to employ foetal monitors and induced delivery when no evidence of foetal distress is actually present. Providers' ongoing professional education should curb tendencies to practise harmful or wasteful variants of defensive medicine. In contrast, ensuring for instance that instruments used to treat a patient are adequately sterilized before use on another, for fear of transmission of contaminant agents that might cause, for instance, HIV infection, is a good form of defensive medicine, because its primary purpose is to defend patients. The growth of evidence-based medical practice, and courts' acceptance of empirically proven practice as setting the legal standard of care, should promote harmony between medical standards and legal standards of care that providers are required to satisfy.

In law, medical negligence is shown when four elements are all established by a complaining party.

1. A legal duty of care must be owed by a provider to the complaining party. The range of legal duties is set by each legal system; some finding legal duties owed, for instance, to patients' family members, unborn children, and even as yet unconceived children, where others do not. Much of lawyers' work lies in establishing legal duties owed to their clients, the complaining parties, by those they want to make liable to pay compensation to their clients. Other lawyers, whose clients have been sued, will work to deny that their clients, the defendants, owed such duties as a matter of law, or that any legally compensable wrong occurred.

2. Breach of the established legal duty of care must be shown, meaning that a provider failed to meet the legally determined standard of care (see next section, 1).

3. Damage must be shown, meaning a hardship or loss, perhaps of a future opportunity, that the law recognizes as an injury. For instance, courts usually recognize loss of future natural reproductive capacity as an injury. They have historically been reluctant to recognize parents' unplanned birth of a healthy child as a form of legal injury to them, but many courts are now considering this compensable to the extent of requiring negligent providers to pay the costs of confinement and inconvenience. Childrearing costs tend not to be included, but courts may allow recovery of these expenses where, for instance, a sterilization procedure that was negligently performed was sought because a family could not afford to rear a child.

4. Causation must be shown, meaning that the damage (see above) must be proven on a balance of probabilities to have been caused by the breach of duty of care (see above). Causation often requires evidence from expert witnesses (see section 2, below).

Central legal issues concerning competent delivery of sexual and reproductive health services are:

- the relation between legal and professional standards;
- standards for determining professional competence;
- delegated authority; and
- evidence for determining professional competency.

8.1. *Relation between legal and professional standards*

Courts are often inclined to defer to the standards of competence that health care professions require their members to observe, out of respect for the traditions of self-regulation that many societies maintain. However, many legal systems find that standards for delivery of services are matters of law as well as of professional discipline, because services are rendered under legal contracts whose terms, which are frequently implied rather than written, are to be interpreted as a matter of law, and enforced by courts of law. Even in the absence of contracts, courts also set standards of human conduct as a matter of social policy. If members of professions themselves could exclusively determine the standards of performance below which legal liability for negligence will arise, they might develop self-protective incentives to set standards modestly, at a lower level than would serve the public interest.

From their own expertise and experience, members of professions may develop practice standards or guidelines by which their credentialing authorities will measure providers' eligibility for specialist recognition, and by which their disciplinary authorities will determine the competence with which individual procedures were performed. The legal significance of such practice standards, where they exist, is that providers who fail to satisfy them are likely to be held in breach of their legal duty. Liability may arise because courts hold that providers, by contract or by imposition of the courts, undertake a duty of care, to perform according to that practice standard; that is, the courts can set the standard as the legal measure of providers' duty of care. Courts normally reserve the power, however, to find that, while breach of the professionally set standard creates legal liability, compliance with the standard does not necessarily satisfy legal standards. The courts ultimately set legal standards, as a matter of policy in the public interest, and may find that the standard of practice the profession has set is unacceptable to the wider community.

Professional standards of competence involve both professional skill and professional attitude, sometimes described as courtesy. Health care providers are required to be conscientious and sensitive not only in the skilful conduct of procedures, but also in demonstration of respect for their patients and colleagues. Unprofessional behaviour includes such matters as neglect of patients' modesty, such as by remaining in the room while patients undress or dress themselves, leaving them exposed to the sight of third parties while disrobed or under examination, smoking cigarettes while attending to them, and being distracted from care for them by attending to other personal or professional concerns. These insensitivities are difficult to regulate directly by law. Effective enforcement may be more readily achieved indirectly, through the legal power to impose professional discipline, including the disapproval of professional seniors and ineligibility for benefits such as promotions, due to the unsuitability of defaulting providers as role-models for junior colleagues.

The ethical component of professional competence may be heightened by reference to a wider literature than providers routinely consult, such as literature in bioethics (see Chapter 4). However, as part of the legal standard of care, providers will be expected to be familiar with their own specialist literature, which increasingly includes contributions from bioethics. Both specialists and general health care providers are legally obliged to keep up to date with developments in their field, which include ethical developments. For instance, providers of reproductive health care are expected to know about developments in emergency contraception, and that, where the offer of emergency contraception to rape victims is the professional standard of care, failure or refusal to offer it or to refer a victim to where she will receive it, constitutes abandonment, which is a professional disciplinary offence and legal negligence.[57] Providers of reproductive technologies are expected to be aware of controversies (whether or not regulated by law) and professional attitudes concerning such matters as not using fresh sperm nor donated sperm that has been preserved, until the donors are shown to have been HIV negative at the time of donation, commercial surrogate motherhood, sperm recovery from unconscious or dying men or recently deceased men, and induction of post-menopausal gestation.[58]

Many providers will recognize these latter concerns as controversial, but quite remote from their practice. More pressing are such issues as the prompt removal on request of contraceptive implants such as Norplant[59] and, for instance, husbands' opposition to services their wives would like to receive. Standards in the exercise of ethical judgement come under more strict legal scrutiny when providers have monetary or other personal incentives to behave in ways open to ethical question. Legal doctrine and health professional discipline address the possibility that providers will favour their own advantage, in dealings with patients who depend on them, by reference to principles on conflict of interest.[60] Some assessments are that such conflicts must always be avoided. In some countries, for instance, physicians are prohibited from owning interests in laboratories to which patients may be sent for testing of their samples. Often, however, a potential for conflict of interest can be satisfactorily resolved, ethically and legally, by disclosing the potential for conflict to a patient, and presenting the feasible option to seek services elsewhere where no such conflict exists.

The law tends to define conflict of interest widely, by reference to an external appearance of conflict, meaning a potential for conflict, not just the reality, so any possibility of conflict of interest has to be resolved. Whether resolution is through avoidance or due disclosure, a provider who does not achieve

[57] S. S. Smugar, B. J. Spina, and J. F. Merz, 'Informed Consent for Emergency Contraception: Variability in Hospital Care to Rape Victims', *Amer. J. Public Health*, 90 (2000), 1372–6.

[58] G. Serour and B. M. Dickens, 'Assisted Reproduction Developments in the Islamic World', *Int. J. Gynecol. Obstet.* 74 (2001), 187–93.

[59] E. Tolley and C. Naré, 'Access to Norplant Removal: An Issue of Informed Choice', *African J. of Reproductive Health*, 5 (2001), 90–9.

[60] R. G. Spece, D. S. Shimm, and A. E. Buchanan (eds.), *Conflicts of Interest in Clinical Practice and Research* (New York: Oxford University Press, 1996).

resolution will face legal and disciplinary liability for professional incompetence, often described as malpractice.

8.2. *Standards for determining professional competence*

In principle, each health care profession defines the services that its members profess themselves bound to deliver, and capable of delivering. Capability addresses both members' proficiency, including, for instance, dexterity and judgement in performance of professional acts, and the services the profession considers it ethical for its members to deliver. For instance, the American College of Obstetricians and Gynecologists has found that provision of emergency contraceptives is the standard of care for rape victims.[61] Professional ethics evolve over time, and practices unethical according to, for instance, the classical Hippocratic tradition, may now be considered ethical to be delivered by health care providers, and unethical for them to leave to patients themselves or to unskilled providers.[62] Equally, practices once considered ethical may cease to be so as professional perceptions evolve under such influences, for example, as respect for women's human rights. For instance, the practice of automatically consulting a woman's husband about her reproductive care is now dependent on her prior approval.

Legal systems differ on the extent to which they regulate health professions. The historical development of some systems has resulted in their tolerance of both qualified and unqualified health care practice. Protection of potential patients is achieved in these systems principally by precluding unqualified providers from passing themselves off as qualified. For instance, even when they hold recognized university-awarded doctorates, such as in psychology or pharmacology, those not qualified as physicians and licensed to practise medicine are not permitted to describe themselves simply as 'doctor' when offering health care. In general, the lay public is left considerable choice in purchase of services, under the principle of the marketplace *caveat emptor* ('let the purchaser beware').

More commonly, however, legal systems preclude the performance of medical acts from being offered or undertaken except by those who are academically qualified and professionally licensed to practise medicine within the jurisdiction. Legal systems also allow non-medically qualified personnel, such as medical students, to perform acts under medical supervision and may allow

---

[61] American College of Obstetricians and Gynecologists (ACOG), *Practice Bulletin, Criminal Management Guidelines for Obstetrician-Gynecologists No. 25 (Emergency Oral Contraception)* (Washington, DC: ACOG, 2001).

[62] WHO/International Federation of Gynecology and Obstetrics (FIGO) Task Force, *Abortion: A Professional Responsibility for Obstetricians and Gynecologists. Report of the WHO/FIGO Task Force, Campinas (Brazil) Workshop, 2–5 March 1997* (London: FIGO, 1997).

for instance nurses to conduct some abortion procedures initiated by physicians, in recognition of medically directed team practice (see below, Sect. 8.3). Some laws permit licensed nurses and, for instance, paramedical personnel to perform limited medical acts without medical supervision. Unqualified individuals are also allowed to treat themselves in minor ways, and to give similarly superficial ('band-aid') domestic care to family members such as dependent children. Further, under laws on medical necessity, emergency care may be given by anyone who honestly believes another to be in immediate grave peril and who then, in the absence of access to anyone better able, takes reasonable initiatives for rescue.

Some overlap exists between qualified and unqualified health care practice concerning services that do not require skills developed through supervised training, but that depend on sensitivity and judgement in human interactions and familiarity with reliable literature relevant to the services in question. For instance, counselling concerning wise goals in sexual and reproductive health care may be undertaken not only by qualified health care professionals, but also by schoolteachers, ministers of religion, and, for instance, social workers. The availability in some countries of contraceptive pills without prescription, like the availability of condoms, justifies non-physicians advising on their use. Similarly, as countries increasingly approve access without prescription to emergency contraception ('over the counter' availability), pharmacists and their staff may provide advice on use of these means.[63]

Unqualified individuals who legally offer services related to health care risk legal liability through recklessness in what they do, but are not held to a professional standard unless they hold themselves out as having skills beyond those ordinarily expected of non-professionals. They do not attract greater legal liability simply for having offered advice for a lengthy period of time, since their claim of experience is not necessarily a claim to expertise.

Qualified health care professionals claiming to act as such will legally be held to a professional standard of competence. General practitioners in their discipline, such as medicine and nursing, will be expected to maintain the standard of practice of other general practitioners, while those holding or claiming specialist status will be held to the standards that prevail within the specialty. An important element of professionalism, in both general and specialized practise, is to recognize the limits of one's skills and the need to make timely referral of patients to other, appropriate providers who are able to offer patients the care they need.

Although it is common to speak of 'the' professional standard of care, courts often recognize that the standard includes a range of practices that are

---

[63] See R. J. Cook, B. M. Dickens, C. Ngwena, and M. I. Plata, 'The Legal Status of Emergency Contraception', *Int. J. Gynecol. Obstet.* 75 (2001), 185–91.

acceptable to satisfy the standard. The law acknowledges that standards evolve, and that at each end of the central body of practice there will be practices that are either somewhat dated or innovative. A respected minority of the profession may maintain earlier practices that are not discredited but that mainstream providers no longer follow. Similarly, a respected minority may find newer practices that are not in the mainstream to be preferable, and incorporate them in their practice not as research but as routine care. The legal concept of standard professional practice therefore covers a spectrum, from reputable but largely abandoned care, through mainstream practice, to newly established practice that may in time become mainstream.

Outside the range of standard practice, however, will be antiquated, discredited care, and unproven treatment still at the stage of experimentation. For example, the use of general anaesthesia for early abortion was once common, but such procedures are now undertaken with no more than local anaesthesia, often on an outpatient basis. The continuing use of general anaesthesia for early termination of pregnancy warrants assessment by the profession, not only because of its drain on professional and funding resources, but particularly because of unnecessary risks posed to patients. Adequately informed patients may be willing to take the risks if they consider general anaesthesia preferable for them. The performance of abortion without available anaesthesia, which has been interpreted as introducing a punitive or deterrent component to the procedure, requires professional assessment on grounds of patients' comfort, dignity, and free and informed choice. Withholding of available anaesthesia raises both professional ethical and legal concerns.

Before patients are offered reproductive health care, providers may be expected to identify the need for assessments that do not fall within the field of obstetrics and gynaecology. Providers who lack the capacity, for instance, to undertake genetic diagnosis, prognosis, and counselling are required to advise patients regarding the services that appropriate, reasonably accessible geneticists offer, access to such specialists, and the implications of patients proceeding with their reproductive intentions in the absence of such services. This applies both to patients who intend to have children when they are unaware that the children could be at risk of harmful genetic inheritance, and patients seeking contraception or sterilization because they fear their children's harmful genetic inheritance when, with due counselling and care, the harm to born children could be avoided or overcome, such as by pre-implantation genetic diagnosis.

8.3. *Delegated authority*

It has long been recognized in law that medical care often involves team work, and that providers frequently act following obtaining patients' consent for treatment by delegating tasks to those they supervise. This is the basis on which many medical functions discharged by nurses and other health care professionals are legally justified, and on which medical students undertake medical acts and health care practice before they are qualified. Team work and delegation are frequently essential in reproductive health care, and accommodated in law. Where the law reserves certain practices only to licensed physicians, or creates immunities from legal liability only for such physicians, the law recognizes that physicians may act along extended lines of authority. Further, delegation may be general, to a form of care to be rendered to whichever patient is eligible to receive it, rather than specific to the care of a particular patient, such as when nurses act under medically directed standing orders.

For instance in Britain, when the Abortion Act 1967 amended the law, it maintained the previous criminal liability for performing abortion, but created a new immunity for acting in specified, more liberal circumstances. However, the immunity was expressed to protect only 'a registered medical practitioner'. Nurses later objected to their conduct of prostaglandin-induced abortion procedures, which were developed after 1967 and considered superior to many surgical procedures that were previously indicated. The Royal College of Nursing feared that nurses instrumental in performing prostaglandin-induced abortions were not protected by the immunity from criminal liability legislated in the 1967 Act. In these procedures, doctors inserted catheters for drug administration, but nurses administered the drugs and managed the subsequent expulsion of uterine contents, so initiating and completing the abortion. However, the highest court interpreted the power of a registered medical practitioner to perform an abortion under protection of the Act to include procedures performed by delegation of authority. Accordingly, nurses and others acting under delegated medical authority were held to enjoy the same immunity as delegating physicians.[64]

When physicians delegate authority to others, they remain obliged to conduct appropriate supervision, and are legally liable if their supervision falls below the legally regulated standard. Further, under many legal systems, even when physicians' supervision satisfies the legal standard, they will be held vicariously liable (that is, liable without any personal fault) to patients, and others to whom legal duties are owed, if they are injured by activities performed by those to whom authority to act has been delegated. Physicians should therefore ensure that their insurance protection or self-protection plan membership covers legal liability that arises when they are not at personal fault. They may also want to enquire whether those to whom they delegate functions, such as nurses, can indemnify them for any vicarious legal liability they incur, such as by having their own insurance.

---

[64] *Royal College of Nursing of the United Kingdom v. Department of Health and Social Security*, [1981] 1 All ER 545 (House of Lords, England).

8.4. *Evidence for determining professional competency*

Competency standards are determined by both courts of law and professional disciplinary tribunals. Providers are liable to be called on to answer for their clinical, institutional, and economic practices before such tribunals. They are also liable to serve as expert witnesses to assist courts and tribunals in the identification and measurement of competency standards by which all members of the profession are bound. The credentials that constitute expertise will usually be set by courts and tribunals themselves, usually paying respect not only to the academic and professional qualifications possessed by those offered as expert witnesses but also to the recognition they have achieved and the leadership they have provided within their own profession.

However expert providers may be, they may feel reluctant to testify to professional standards of competency at hearings where fellow providers are defendants facing penalties. A so-called conspiracy of silence may develop within a profession that compromises parties' ability to acquire expert witnesses necessary for the due administration of justice. In the face of this, courts of law assessing patients' claims for compensation may hear only insubstantial evidence. Courts will allow the parties to present evidence from expert authorities on specialized matters that are beyond the courts' or lay juries' own capacities to judge, particularly regarding whether the care delivered satisfied professional standards of competency, concerning proficiency of performance and/or ethical sensitivity. Those appearing as expert witnesses should always remember, however, that they are not acting as advocates for the parties that engage them and pay them fees for their attendance before the court or other tribunal. Their only allegiance is to the integrity of their professional knowledge and to their assessment of the facts placed before them. They damage their credibility and professional standing by deliberately attempting to aid the case of the party that calls them, or to weaken the other party's case. As experts and professionals, they have no personal or professional interest in the outcome of the case, but are present only as distinterested expert witnesses to assist the court or tribunal.

Where courts of law are asked by public prosecutors to impose criminal penalties for wrongdoing and negligence, the prosecutor will usually be required to present compelling evidence that the defendant provider's proven behaviour fell short of the professional standard by presenting expert evidence of what that standard requires. In professional disciplinary tribunals, the representative of the profession will be expected similarly to demonstrate the standards it claims were violated. Standards must be strictly proven as facts, which prosecuting authorities in criminal cases usually must establish beyond reasonable doubt, and which in disciplinary cases must be established by clear and convincing evidence.

8.5. *Sexual misconduct*

Non-consensual sexual intercourse with patients is obviously a serious criminal offence and a compensable wrong committed against them, but the concern of competent delivery of health care services extends far beyond this self-evident truth. Many licensing authorities and professional associations consider consensual sexual behaviour with patients to be professional misconduct, even though no crime has been committed. This is because such conduct may constitute an exploitation or abuse of the professional's authority and the patient's dependency and vulnerability, of which the professional takes advantage for personal gratification. Further, behaviour with sexual aspects falling far short of sexual intercourse may be held to constitute professional misconduct.[65] It may also be a ground for legal action, for instance in legal systems that recognize the deliberate or even the negligent infliction of emotional damage, or any breach of fiduciary duty,[66] to justify compensation. Health care providers' abuse of their power over patients for their personal sexual or other gratification usually persuades courts that a remedy for breach of at least civil (meaning non-criminal) law should be available. Some courts recognize abuse of power as a wrong in itself, and others may find breach of a fiduciary duty to act conscientiously to be compensable.

Conduct that has been considered sexual abuse of patients and professional misconduct typically involves male providers and female patients, suggesting a need of more female reproductive health workers, perhaps to make women patients feel more secure when treated by male colleagues. Instances also exist of the reverse, and of health providers' improper sexual behaviour with patients of their own sex. Further, misconduct has been found when health care providers have engaged in sexual behaviours with their patients' spouses and other partners, such as in forming relationships with patients' partners when knowing of sexual or other difficulties between them. Beyond conduct that unmistakably exploits patients' sexual, emotional, or other vulnerability, conduct that humiliates, disparages, or embarrasses patients on grounds of sex may be considered sexual misconduct. This includes making unwarranted observations about a patient's sexual performance or attractiveness, whether of a negative or affirmative nature, and making sexual jokes. Such jokes need not make the patient the object of ridicule, but may be misjudged attempts to make her or him feel comfortable, or to distract attention from an occasion of embarrassment. Misconduct also includes having patients undress or dress in

[65] See, for instance, College of Physicians and Surgeons of Ontario, *Final Report of the Independent Task Force on Sexual Abuse of Patients* (Toronto: College PSO, 1991).
[66] In *Norberg v. Wynrib* (1992), 92 Dominion Law Reports (4th) 449, for instance, the Supreme Court of Canada upheld a $50,000 award to a patient when her physician made her agreement to sexual intercourse a condition of writing a prescription for a drug to which she was addicted.

the presence or sight of the health care providers, providers' colleagues, or other service recipients.

Health care providers in the field of sexual and reproductive health are legally expected to exercise a high level of caution and self-awareness concerning liability to suspicion of sexual misconduct, because of the unusually intimate, sensitive, and sexually related examinations they may conduct, the types of histories they may request from patients and the types of treatments they may administer and monitor. It may be expected that, when possible in any reasonable way, their practice would allow physical examinations of patients to be conducted by providers of the same sex, and that, particularly when male providers are examining females, and perhaps also when they are consulting with females, they will remain in the sight of female colleagues, within the limits of patients' confidentiality. Alternatively, patients may be required or invited to have a family member such as a mother or sister, or a friend, accompany them and be easily accessible, again subject to requirements of confidentiality.

A common feature of health care providers' sexual abuse of patients has been that the patients feel embarrassed and ashamed, and sometimes inclined to blame themselves, so that they do not present complaints immediately, or at all. A response by some licensing authorities is to require licence holders who become aware of other providers' sexual misconduct to report the circumstances to the authorities, so that proper investigations and appropriate disciplinary proceedings can be initiated, and particularly so that patients who have suffered abuse can be offered appropriate counselling, care, and rehabilitation. When sexual abuse is broadly defined to include sexually sensitive discourtesies, professional colleagues may become aware of abuses that patients themselves do not recognize.

A policy of 'zero tolerance' of sexual misconduct may be considered to justify sanctions against providers who fail to report the misconduct of others. The legal power that licensing authorities possess usually includes imposition of such sanctions as withdrawal or suspension of licensure for professional misconduct that is not itself an offence when committed by persons outside the profession, such as making sexual jokes or gratuitous comments on sexual attractiveness. Voluntary professional associations' legal powers to investigate and discipline members usually arise as a term, often implied, of the contractual relationship created by payment of membership fees. Under either statutory licensing or contractual legal power, professional authorities and associations can offer the public assurances that their policy with regard to providers' sexual misconduct is strict and uncompromising.

A limitation or dysfunction of a zero tolerance policy is that it may not distinguish between abuse of patients and the attraction and affection that may genuinely arise, without exploitation, between a provider of care and a recipient that, in other circumstances, might be accepted to include a sexual expression, and evolve through courtship into marriage. Professional institutions' interventions to regulate members may appear an unjustified intervention in patients' lives and choices, and even a denial of patients' rights. Nevertheless, some authorities hold the view that patients' choices can never be made freely in such unequal relationships that involve emotional dependency. Even rejecting this uncompromising approach, however, providers are expected to recognize when their interest in patients transcends professionalism and is becoming personal, and to terminate the professional relationship and its emotional aspects, such as by advising and facilitating transfer of care to other providers, before allowing any sexual or intimate expression of affection. Providers who are uncertain about the propriety of a relationship they anticipate and favour should be able to consult professional colleagues, authorities, and associations, and professional seniors and peers, without suspicions of professional misconduct arising.

9. *Conscientious Objection*

By specific laws governing reproductive health services or general laws concerning human rights, sometimes embodied in countries' constitutional laws, many legal systems protect health care providers from legal obligations to perform procedures to which they have conscientious objections.[67] In most legal systems, this right of protected conscience covers only conscience based on adherence to a religious faith, but some laws on freedom of political, philosophical, or other expression may accommodate a right of non-participation in professional practice to which individuals object on grounds of more general conscience. In the field of reproductive health, most conscientious objection is raised to participation in abortion procedures and contraceptive sterilization, but it could be relevant for instance to legally available commercial surrogate motherhood, and prenatal sex-identification for possible sex-based abortion.

Laws on conscientious objection are normally inapplicable when patients are in emergency circumstances, such as when their lives or permanent health are at risk. This does not violate the conscience of providers in many cases involving abortion or sterilization, because of the ethical and religious principle of 'double effect'.[68] This provides, in its simple form, that an action that is good in itself, such as preserving endangered human life, may be performed

[67] See B. M. Dickens and R. J. Cook, 'The Scope and Limits of Conscientious Objection', *Int. J. Gynecol. Obstet.* 71 (2000), 71–7.
[68] J. Boyle, 'Toward Understanding the Principle of Double Effect', *Ethics*, 90 (1980), 527–38.

despite the fact that the objective can be achieved only by causing an unavoidable harmful effect. The action itself must be either good or morally indifferent, the good effect must not arise by inherently wrongful means, and there must be proportionate justification for allowing the harmful effect to occur. It does not matter that the harmful effect is anticipated, provided that it is not intended. For instance, an ectopic or tubal pregnancy that endangers a woman's life can be removed without the procedure being regarded as a procedure to perform an abortion, and a man's testicular cancer can be treated by removal of the testicles without the procedure being regarded as a sterilization, although its effect is to leave him sterile.

The legal burden of proving that a conscientious objection is raised in good faith usually falls on the person claiming relief from an otherwise legally binding duty to act. This burden is sometimes discharged adequately by the claimant making a solemn declaration of religious or other conscience. The scope of relief from a duty on grounds of conscience is normally interpreted narrowly. Health care professionals who object, for instance, to performing abortions may be exempted from conducting such procedures and perhaps from preparing patients for immediate performance of abortion procedures, but not from providing more general care, including for post-operative recovery and changing dressings. Further, only those who otherwise would be required to perform services directly on patients for the purposes to which they object can invoke grounds of conscience to obtain exemption. Hospital staff cannot refuse such functions as delivery of patients' meals, arrangement and replacement of their bedding, preparing operating rooms, and booking of appointments, on the ground of conscientious objection to the medical service the patient is intended to receive. It has been legally held, for instance, that a physician's secretary has no conscientious right to refuse to type an abortion referral letter.[69]

Institutions and clinics as such, even when established by religiously or otherwise committed agencies, cannot invoke conscientious objection, although they are often entitled to distinguish the services they offer from those unavailable to patients. When a hospital presents itself to the public or is publicly funded in whole or in part as a facility on which members of the public can rely for lawful and medically indicated health services, it cannot endanger the lives or health of those induced to rely on its delivery of care by refusing an indicated service. The duty of such facilities is to employ adequate staff to provide competent delivery of services to which some staff members may object on grounds of conscience, or to have standing arrangements under which patients are safely and conveniently referred to alternative facilities where such services are available.

---

[69] *Janaway v. Salford Area Health Authority*, [1989] Appeal Cases 537 (House of Lords, England).

In many countries, public hospitals are governmental facilities, and litigation brought against them may be resisted on grounds of their legal entitlement to governmental immunity. Senior administrators who refuse to allow medically indicated treatments to be delivered in such public facilities on the basis of their personal conscience may be liable to ethical disciplinary proceedings by professional licensing authorities, however, if they are licenced health care professionals. Further, immunities that protect government facilities before national courts may render the state itself liable before international human rights tribunals for breaches of individuals' human rights (see Pt. I, Ch. 6).

Providers who invoke conscience to refuse to perform services on patients entitled to receive them are usually legally obliged to refer their patients to other appropriate providers, within their own facility or conveniently accessible elsewhere, who will provide the service. Under some religious doctrines, it may constitute a wrong not only to perform a prohibited procedure but to have complicity in its performance through referral. Legal systems often afford priority to patients' rights of access to lawfully available therapeutic and preventive health care procedures over providers' personal conscientious objection. They interpret providers' conscientious exemption to apply only to actual performance of procedures, but not to justify refusal of appropriate referral. Failure or refusal of due referral may be found to constitute legal negligence or abandonment of patients.[70]

In contrast, except in circumstances of emergency, providers are usually free not to accept applicants for their care as patients. That is, not every person has a legal right to become a patient of a chosen or accessible provider. Physicians and others may decline to accept persons who request services from them, on grounds among others of conscience, and in that case bear no legal duty to refer applicants elsewhere. However, they may be in breach of human rights laws if their claim of conscience amounts to discrimination against persons seeking their services on such grounds as their religion, marital status, sexual orientation,[71] or HIV-positive status.[72]

Further, licensing authorities and professional associations, in their definition of professional ethical responsibilities, may require that more be done to assist applicants for services than is required by the general law. Authorities and associations may review the practice of providers who invoke conscience to decline to perform procedures in public facilities but who participate in such

---

[70] *Zimmer v. Ringrose* (1981), 124 Dominion Law Reports (3rd) 215 (Alberta Court of Appeal, Canada).

[71] *Korn v. Potter* (1996), 134 Dominion Law Reports (4th) 437 (British Columbia Supreme Court, Canada); *McBain v. Victoria* (2000), 3 Commonwealth Human Rights Law Digest 153 (Federal Court of Australia).

[72] See Gostin and Lazzarini, *Human Rights and Public Health*, at 52–4, 75–8; and *Bragdon v. Abbott* (1998), 524 United States Reporter 624 (Supreme Court of the United States).

procedures in private practice. Since the duty of proving conscience usually falls on such providers, performance in private practice of procedures refused in public facilities will compromise their ability to discharge this duty.

Related issues include whether a medical or other health care student with a conscientious objection to a reproductive health procedure such as abortion can refuse instruction and examination in performance of skills relevant to the procedure without forfeiting the right of qualification. Another is whether medical schools run by institutions with religious or other objections to certain health care procedures can decline to give instruction in relevant skills without forfeiting the right to accreditation, and to licensure of their graduates. Since the right of conscientious objection does not apply where patients' lives or permanent health are at risk, it appears that providers who may conscientiously object to performance of procedures in routine cases must nevertheless be capable of performing them in emergency, and be appropriately trained and qualified for this purpose. Further, although they may be entitled to object on grounds of conscience to initiate abortion procedures, practitioners must be capable to treat patients for instance to remove a dead embryo or foetus, and to provide indicated care when an abortion process has already started, whether spontaneously or not, and has become inevitable, and in cases of incomplete abortion.

Similarly, medical schools responsible for training graduates to serve needs of the public, including in conditions of emergency, may be required to instruct students in procedures they might properly refuse to initiate in routine cases. It has been seen that, under religious teaching on the principle of double effect, procedures that achieve pregnancy termination only indirectly, such as treatment of ectopic pregnancy, and procedures to treat incomplete abortion, are not prohibited, and licensing authorities should require appropriate health care professionals to be competent in their performance.

10. *Safety and Efficacy of Products*

The law of product liability is not a direct concern to many physicians, including obstetricians and gynaecologists as such, although any who develop new pharmaceutical products or design new devices will become involved in such concerns as they move towards introduction and marketing. Providers proposing to develop new drugs or devices will be bound by relevant legal requirements to conduct research with human participants to establish safety and efficacy. The most immediate legal significance of drug and device safety is that reproductive health service providers are required, as part of their continuing competence to practise, to be aware of improvements in products available to patients, and of data and relevant anecdotal evidence of products failing to meet levels of efficacy and safety they were formerly believed to meet. Further, such health care providers are expected to offer their patients the safest and most effective means of care of which patients can reasonably avail themselves, whether under public funding of services or private means, including under private health care insurance policies or organizations.

Legal systems approach product safety through principles either of liability based on proven fault, or alternatively of so-called strict or no-fault liability.[73] The latter requires the manufacturer of a product to become in effect the guarantor of its safety for the purpose for which it is designed and marketed. Whether liability is based on principles of fault or not, deficiencies leading to liability for products may arise from inadequate design, inadequate manufacture, for instance with defective materials or deviating from the specified design, or inadequate instruction or warning concerning proper use and limitations of the product.

The significance of this law for providers who are not researchers, designers, manufacturers, or retailers of a product concerns their liability for recommending a specific product for a patient. Even if they select and supply a product such as an interuterine device and charge a patient for it separately from services for the individual's care, they will not be considered to have become retailers of the product, but to be undertaking a professional service rather than a sale of goods transaction. When they employ devices for the purposes for which they are designed, and in accordance with the manufacturers' instructions, they can claim legal indemnity from the manufacturers if they incur legal liability for injuries to patients that follow from such use. Whether others can be found legally liable for negligence when they supply devices or drugs for the purposes for which their marketing and promotion are approved is a matter on which laws vary.

Providers accept responsibility for any accidental or deliberate uses they make of products that differ from their approved purposes or methods of use, for instance, dosage levels for drugs. Although professional practice may allow so-called off-label uses of drugs, when they are prescribed for purposes that depart from the conditions or dosage levels for which they have been tested and approved, such practice provides no legal defence for off-label use that results in harm.

Physicians are required under legal provisions on competence to pay regard to the information they receive from manufacturers of drugs and devices concerning contra-indications to their use, and should make adverse incident reports to manufacturers concerning harmful outcomes of which manufacturers have not warned them. Physicians must apply the information they

---

[73] On US law, for instance, see D. Owen, 'Products Liability Law Restated', *South Carolina Law Review*, 49 (1998), 237–92.

receive from manufacturers with appropriate professional skill and judgement, and be alert to information in the literature they should read, as part of their professional responsibility, of scientific criticism of manufacturers' trade information. They may also be required, for instance, to inspect devices and the packaging of drugs they supply to patients directly, in order to ensure that there are no defects apparent upon competent inspection that would render them unfit for use, such as passage of expiry dates for effectiveness of drugs.

Of particular concern are practices of providers and institutions, often driven by the needs of economy or pressure of scarcity, to reuse devices advertised by the manufacturer and/or marketed by a retailer as being for single use only. As a matter of experience, many single-use devices are known to be safe for a number of reuses, subject perhaps to effective sterilization. Manufacturers may refrain from promoting the devices as fit for repeated use or reuse after sterilization, not simply to increase sales from single use, but to avoid legal liability in testing and in, for instance, specifying safe techniques of sterilization and a number of reuses after which devices should be discarded. Providers and institutions bear legal liability for the harmful consequences that follow reuse.

Liability may be limited if providers offer patients the option to have first use or subsequent use of a single-use device, perhaps adding the cost of the former to charges for services. Liability arising from subsequent use may be due to the transmission of infection following defective sterilization, associated perhaps with use of diluted solvents or error in sterilization procedures, or due to mechanical misfunction of the device resulting from fatigue of its materials or from damage caused by sterilizing solvents. Even when patients give adequately informed consent for reuse of single use devices, and accept the irreducible minimum risks of their misfunction, they are not legally held to accept risks of providers' negligent handling or inspection of devices.

11. *Criminal Law*

It has been observed above that the general evolution in reproductive and sexual health law has been from control by criminal law and punishment to accommodation in laws on health and welfare, and on human rights (see above, Sect. 4). This is true with regard to contraception, sterilization, abortion, and, for instance, same-sex relationships. Nevertheless, a role remains for criminal law, the purpose of which is to protect individuals against harms they may suffer individually but the danger of which is primarily regarded as threatening to the well-being of the society at large. For instance, incest has long been a crime in many countries, and though it is sometimes described as a victimless crime, there have been no strong moves towards decriminalization. Rape is a grave wrong to the victim who suffers it, but society in general is outraged when the person and integrity of any one of its members is so violated, and when any one of its members commits this outrage against another person. The victim's private remedy against the assailant, such as to sue for monetary compensation for personal injury, is considered insufficient to satisfy society's need of protection and deterrence. Enforcement of criminal law and punishment must be ensured for the public sense of justice to be satisfied.[74]

Society's first reaction to recognition of wrongful conduct is to punish it as a crime, and this instinct remains alive. New crimes are regularly created, and often remain on statute books after the harm at which they were directed has abated. The social sense of harm may abate by the successful deterrence or prevention of conduct considered harmful or, for instance, by development of social tolerance. The landmark UK report of the Wolfenden Committee on prostitution and homosexuality, in 1957,[75] both recorded shifts in social tolerance and opened thinking further, leading particularly to decriminalization of homosexual acts between consenting adults in private in the Sexual Offences Act, 1967.[76] Shifts can also be towards intolerance of customary practices a society finds no longer acceptable, such as in Ghana in 1994 when female genital cutting (mutilation) was criminalized.[77] When immigrant populations made this practice newly apparent in the UK, it was criminalized there too, in 1985.[78]

Reproductive developments offer a rich field for criminal law control, particularly with the advent of new technologies and their applications that arouse initial and sometimes enduring hostility. In the UK, for instance, arranging commercial surrogate motherhood agreements was criminalized in 1985,[79] extending the criminal prohibitions many countries have against commerce in human sperm and ova. The Human Fertilisation and Embryology Act 1990[80] is more regulatory than purely prohibitory, since it establishes the Human Fertilisation and Embryology Authority as a licensing agency for reproductive technologies, and applies criminal punishments for acts that lack or violate licences. The Act prohibits some practices, such as placing non-human live embryos and gametes in women, and its punishment for prohibited and unlicensed practices can be severe, including up to ten years' imprisonment. Several countries have proposed severe punishment for such practices as attempted human reproductive cloning, and have introduced criminal laws

---

[74] *Bodhisatwa Goutam v. Subhra Chakraborty* (1996) 1 SCC 490 (Supreme Court of India).
[75] Home Office (UK) (see n. 25).   [76] UK Statutes 1967, ch. 60.
[77] Criminal Code (Amendment) Act, 1994 (Ghana); published in *International Digest of Health Legislation*, 47 (1996), 30–1.
[78] Prohibition of Female Circumcision Act 1985 (UK), Statutes 1985, ch. 38.
[79] Surrogacy Arrangements Act 1985 (UK). Statutes 1985, ch. 49.
[80] Statutes 1990, ch. 37.

against prenatal sex diagnosis for purposes of sex-based abortion, such as in India.[81]

The Indian legislation has been so ineffective in practice that judges in the Supreme Court of India have required governmental efforts to apply it adequately.[82] This shows that judicial action may be taken in addition to legislative action to apply the existing criminal law against sexual and reproductive conduct considered socially harmful. For instance, the historical concept of maim, which no one can lawfully consent to suffer, might be applied, in the absence of prohibitive legislation, to condemn at least the more invasive forms of female genital cutting. In this spirit in 1998, the Supreme Court of Canada extended the law of assault to reverse two lower courts, and a long-standing body of legal understanding, to find a man convictable of aggravated assault for having consensual sexual intercourse with two women.[83] He knew that he had tested HIV positive, but denied any infectious disease when one woman asked him before unprotected intercourse, and did not disclose his infection to the other who did not ask him in the same circumstances. At trial, neither woman had tested HIV positive, but the Supreme Court held that his lie to one woman and non-disclosure to the other could have negated their consent to intercourse. The Court held that the risk of HIV/AIDS is qualitatively different from that of other sexually transmitted infections and pregnancy, and that exposing uninformed partners to that risk is within the scope of criminal prohibition.

Many applications of criminal law to reproductive and sexual conduct appear defensible, although legislators sometimes show an unreflective disposition to hurry to criminalize practices they find new and threatening. A significant critique of criminalization is that it may suppress development of ethical sensitivity and reflection. If risk of ethical error seems too grave to tolerate, such as regarding, for instance, 'mercy killing' of disabled people, criminal prohibition may be justified and preferable. In the case of other ethically challenging issues, however, criminal law leaves little accommodation of conscientious objection, and compromises rational argument for objective assessment of proper reaction to matters on which reasonable people may differ. It may also blur legitimate distinctions, for instance between prenatal sex diagnosis that perpetuates devaluation of girl children, and sex-selection that is used in later pregnancies to balance family composition, and between reproductive and therapeutic cloning. Criminal law may be invoked to reinforce ethical objection, but may also be implemented as an act of political power at the cost or impoverishment of ethical reflection and discussion. The

---

[81] Prenatal Diagnostic Techniques (Regulation and Prevention of Misuse) Act 1994.
[82] S. Ghoshal, 'A Year when Judges Took Action for India's Health', *Lancet*, 359 (2002), 53.
[83] *R. v. Cuerrier* (1998), 127 Can. Criminal Cases (3d) 1 (Supreme Court of Canada).

Wolfenden Committee considered that not everything that is unethical or immoral need be made criminal. The Committee considered that: 'Unless a deliberate attempt is to be made by society, acting through the agency of the law, to equate the sphere of crime with that of sin, there must remain a realm of private morality and immorality which is, in brief and crude terms, not the law's business.'[84]

---

[84] Home Office (UK) (see n. 25), para. 61, 24.

6

Human Rights Principles

1. *Overview*

Human rights are expressed in national constitutions and laws and in regional and international conventions. They are tools that direct government agencies, individuals, and institutions towards the appropriate shaping of their own policies and practices, and equip them with the principles and language to urge improvements in the policies and practices of others. Many individuals and groups find human rights empowering because they provide means by which they can legitimately assert their interests. Governmental agencies can employ human rights to advance social justice among the people they lead and serve, and individuals and groups can employ human rights to require governmental agencies to observe the standards of conduct to which they have committed themselves.

Enduring challenges in advancing human rights are the lack of understanding of how to invoke human rights to prevent wrongs and, when wrongs have occurred, how to remedy them through the application of human rights. The application of human rights in the health care context remains particularly challenging because there is little, although growing, experience of their application at the national and international levels. In addition, those who are unfamiliar with the language of rights may characterize human rights as an alien intrusion on national sovereignty. Nevertheless, most states have national constitutions that claim to embody the key principles of respect for human rights, and many states have subscribed to regional and international treaties that specify the human rights they protect.

The protection and promotion of rights relating to reproductive and sexual health have gained momentum in recent years, due in large part to the 1994 United Nations (UN) Conference on Population and Development, held in Cairo, and the 1995 Fourth UN World Conference on Women, held in Beijing. These two conferences led to the recognition that the protection of reproductive and sexual health is a matter of social justice, and that the realization of such health can be addressed through the improved application of human rights contained in existing national constitutions and regional and international human rights treaties. The Programme of Action[1] resulting from the 1994 Cairo Conference, and the Declaration and Platform for Action[2] resulting from the 1995 Beijing Conference, were strengthened in subsequent five-year reviews in 1999[3] and 2000[4] respectively.

The movement towards fostering compliance with reproductive and sexual health rights has been enhanced through work by the UN,[5] national and international non-governmental organizations[6] and professional medical associations,[7] and through academic initiatives. These efforts have been reinforced by, for example, research into women's perspectives on the exercise of their reproductive rights,[8] and research into the challenges of protecting reproductive rights in different regions.[9] These activities will be referred to collectively as 'the Cairo process'.

[1] UN, *Population and Development*, i. *Programme of Action adopted at the International Conference on Population and Development, Cairo, 5–13 September 1994* (New York: United Nations, Department for Economic and Social Information and Policy Analysis, ST/ESA/SER.A/149, 1994) (hereinafter Cairo Programme).

[2] UN, Department of Public Information, *Platform for Action and Beijing Declaration. Fourth World Conference on Women, Beijing, China, 4–15 September 1995* (New York: UN, 1995) (hereinafter Beijing Platform).

[3] UN, General Assembly, *Report of the Ad Hoc Committee of the Whole of the Twenty-First Special Session of the General Assembly: Overall Review and Appraisal of the Implementation of the Programme of Action of the International Conference on Population and Development*, A/S-21/5/Add.1 (New York: UN, 1999).

[4] UN, General Assembly, *Report of the Ad Hoc Committee of the Whole of the Twenty-Third Special Session of the General Assembly: Further Actions and Initiatives to Implement the Beijing Declaration and the Platform for Action*, A/S-23/10/Rev.1) (New York: UN, 2000).

[5] UN Population Fund (UNFPA), *Ensuring Reproductive Rights and Implementing Sexual and Reproductive Health Programmes including Women's Empowerment, Male Involvement and Human Rights* (New York: UNFPA, 1998).

[6] Development Alternatives with Women for a New Era (DAWN), *Implementing ICPD: Moving Forward in the Eye of the Storm* (Suva, Fiji: DAWN, 1999); Health, Empowerment, Rights and Accountability (HERA), *Confounding the Critics: Cairo Five Years on* (New York: HERA, 1998); International Planned Parenthood Federation (IPPF), *Charter on Sexual and Reproductive Rights and Guidelines* (London: IPPF, 1996); Women's Environment and Development Organization (WEDO), *Risks, Rights and Reforms: A Fifty Country Survey Assessing Government Actions Five Years After the International Conference on Population and Development* (New York: WEDO, 1999).

[7] See, for instance, Commonwealth Medical Association, *A Woman's Right to Health, Including Sexual and Reproductive Health* (London: Commonwealth Medical Association, 1996); R. J. Cook and B. M. Dickens, 'The FIGO Study Group on Women's Sexual and Reproductive Rights', *Int. J. Gynecol. Obstet.* 67 (1999), 55–61.

[8] R. P. Petchesky and K. Judd (eds.), *Negotiating Reproductive Rights: Women's Perspectives across Countries and Cultures* (London and New York: Zed Books, 1998).

[9] Center for Reproductive Law and Policy (CRLP) and Estudo para la Defensa de los Derechos de la Mujer (DEMUS), *Women of the World: Laws and Policies Affecting their Reproductive Lives: Latin America and the Caribbean* (New York: CRLP, 1997); CRLP and International Federation of Women Lawyers—Kenya Chapter, *Women of the World: Laws and Policies Affecting their Reproductive Lives: Anglophone Africa* (New York: CRLP, 1997). See also references at Women's Human Rights Resources website at: www.law-lib.utoronto.ca/diana, last accessed 9 May 2002.

Human rights, whether found in national constitutions and laws or regional or international human rights treaties, are a means through which laws and policies that foster respect for reproductive self-determination can be enhanced, and norms and practices that inhibit reproductive self-determination can be addressed.[10] The Cairo Programme explains that:

reproductive rights embrace certain human rights that are already recognized in national laws, international human rights documents, and other consensus documents. These rights rest on the recognition of the basic right of all couples and individuals to decide freely and responsibly the number, spacing and timing of their children, and to have the information and means to do so; and the right to attain the highest standard of sexual and reproductive health. It also includes their right to make decisions concerning reproduction free of discrimination, coercion and violence, as expressed in human rights documents. (para. 7.3)

This chapter explains how different human rights have been and might be applied to protect different interests in reproductive and sexual health. It is recognized that the content and meaning of rights evolve as they are applied in different countries to different reproductive and sexual health concerns. Often, common patterns emerge among different countries in how rights are most effectively applied, but those patterns are also subject to refinement and change as understandings about the nature of reproductive and sexual health problems evolve.

2. *Sources and Nature of Human Rights*

Human rights are rooted in historic, prestigious, and authoritatively endorsed national constitutions and laws, and international treaties and documents. Older constitutions tend to protect only the more classical civil and political rights, while more modern constitutions, such as the South African Constitution of 1996, also protect economic, social, and cultural rights, including the right to health. Given the increasing interdependence of rights, courts in countries with constitutions that protect only civil and political rights are beginning to import notions of health into the meaning of civil and political rights. For example, state neglect of an individual's basic health needs has been interpreted as a denial of the right to security of the person, and the right to non-discrimination has been applied to ensure equitable access to health care. Courts and human rights commissions in countries with constitutions that also protect economic, social, and cultural rights are beginning to outline what is required by these rights in local contexts.

---

[10] For legal developments on reproductive rights, see *Annual Review of Population Law* website: http://www.law.harvard.edu/programs/annualreview, last accessed 30 Apr. 2002.

The Preamble to the 1948 Universal Declaration of Human Rights added substance to the United Nations Charter, which in 1945 observed that a purpose of the newly created organization is 'to reaffirm faith in fundamental human rights, in the dignity and worth of the human person, [and] in the equal rights of men and women'. The Universal Declaration discloses its origins in principle-based natural law or deontological orientations to ethics (see Pt. I, Ch. 4, Sect. 4.1), opening with the observations that:

Whereas recognition of the inherent dignity and of the equal and inalienable rights of all members of the human family is the foundation of freedom, justice and peace in the world,

Whereas disregard and contempt for human rights have resulted in barbarous acts which have outraged the conscience of mankind . . . [and]

Whereas it is essential . . . that human rights should be protected by the rule of law . . .

The General Assembly [of the United Nations] . . . proclaims this Universal Declaration of Human Rights as a common standard of achievement for all peoples and all nations, to the end that every individual and every organ of society . . . shall strive . . . by progressive measures, national and international, to secure their universal and effective recognition and observance . . .

The Declaration thereby constitutes an international ethic that every country should seek to achieve and maintain through its law.

Countries now commit themselves under the Universal Declaration and international law, particularly through various international human rights conventions to which they voluntarily adhere, to respect and give effect to standards of governmental conduct expressed in these conventions that have their origins in ethical values. That is, human rights are rooted in ethics, and should be given effect through law, legal procedures, and voluntary conduct at both national and international levels. Policies that governments apply, through legal power or other means, that violate human rights are unethical. Many countries' own courts have condemned national policies, laws, and practices that violate human rights, and increasingly countries submit their policies and laws to the scrutiny of international human rights tribunals and periodically to that of international human rights treaty monitoring bodies.

The provisions of human rights law relevant to reproductive and sexual health, and procedures to implement such rights, are elaborated below. Perhaps the greatest potential effects of ethical analysis are prospective and preventive. Those responsible for planning and implementing health policies can measure their provisions and monitor their effects according to the human rights provisions that are a modern legal expression of ethical values. An increasingly detailed body of judicial decisions reached by both domestic and international tribunals, and of standards set by domestic and international human rights monitoring bodies, indicates the ethical criteria of acceptable reproductive and sexual health policy, law, and practice. Perhaps the most critical concern that judicial decisions address is the content and meaning of the human rights in issue.

Human rights were reinvigorated after 1948 by a revival of a natural law philosophy, seen as an orientation of modern bioethics. The discussion of ethics, addressed above in Chapter 4, distinguishes between negative and positive ethical rights, and the same distinction is relevant to the legal nature of human rights. In the same way as in ethics negative rights can be described as 'rights to be left alone', negative human rights entitle individuals to behave as they consider right, without subjection to regulation or control by governmental agencies. In contrast, positive human rights depend on governmental or other accommodation and provision beyond an individual's own resources. The existence of rights depends on duties. Negative rights depend on the duty of governmental and other restraint from intervention in their exercise. Positive rights depend on the duty of governmental or other intervention by affirmative acts to facilitate the enjoyment of rights. In many circumstances, the negative and positive aspects of rights coincide, because of legislation that empowers individual initiative and requires governmental action. Where legislation has supported oppressive power of government, however, recognition of individuals' negative reproductive and sexual rights requires the repeal of laws through which governments could lawfully intervene in their exercise. Accordingly, respect for a newly recognized negative right requires positive legislative action, or an authoritative judicial ruling holding an offensive law inoperative. Once taken, however, this action would limit any future governmental intervention in individuals' exercise of such rights.

The promotion of negative human rights by exclusion of governmental action is challenging where there has been a tradition of strong, authoritarian governmental intervention, inspired by the defence, for instance, of perceived moral values or military or economic interests. More challenging, however, may be promotion of positive human rights, because they may depend on a government's financial resources and the political will to allocate them to the service of such rights. The challenge is even greater regarding positive human rights to reproductive and sexual health care, since these have been recognized only in relatively recent years. These rights remain opposed by powerful forces of traditional religion, which once set the agenda of public and private morality and continue to exert political influence on many governments. The right to reproductive choice as a negative right has been successfully asserted in many countries by judicial decisions restricting governmental intervention. However, the right to such choice has not been as successfully advanced as a positive right, since courts are less willing and able to direct governmental discretion on resource allocation.

In almost every country of the world, individuals with the resources to purchase or otherwise obtain contraceptive means for themselves enjoy the human right to decide on the number and spacing of their children as a negative right. However, in many countries, those who cannot afford to purchase contraceptive means do not enjoy this human right, because the means by which they can exercise this right are inaccessible to them. Their governments do not implement the right as a positive right by provision of contraceptive means, and judicial tribunals do not require that they should as a matter of law. Where courts do not characterize human rights as positive rights, they are of little if any practical avail to people disadvantaged by poverty, ignorance, and powerlessness, who in many countries have marginal or minority racial or ethnic status. The challenge for the twenty-first century is to secure all human rights as negative rights, and to advance those that depend on the allocation of governmental resources as positive rights.

Human rights treaties, designed to give legal force to the Universal Declaration of Human Rights, include the International Covenant on Civil and Political Rights (the Political Covenant),[11] the International Covenant on Economic, Social and Cultural Rights (the Economic Covenant)[12] and regional treaties such as the European Convention on Human Rights (the European Convention),[13] the American Convention on Human Rights (the American Convention),[14] and the African Charter on Human and Peoples' Rights (the African Charter).[15] In addition, several international treaties are directed to the relief of injustices individuals may suffer on account of an innate characteristic. These treaties include the International Convention on the Elimination of All Forms of Racial Discrimination (the Race Convention)[16] and the Convention on the Rights of the Child (the Children's Convention).[17] Most directly relevant, however, is the Convention on the Elimination of All Forms of Discrimination against Women (the Women's Convention),[18] which explicitly addresses human rights regarding family planning services, care and

[11] UN, *International Covenant on Economic, Social and Cultural Rights* (New York: UN, 1996), GA Res. 2200 (XXI), 21 UN GAOR Supp. (No. 16) at 52, UN Doc.A/6316 (hereinafter *Economic Covenant*).
[12] Ibid. at 49.
[13] UN, *European Convention on Human Rights*, United Nations Treaty Series, 213 (New York: UN, 1959), 221.
[14] Organization of American States, *American Convention on Human Rights*, Organization of American States Treaty Series, 1 (1969) 1.
[15] Organization of African Unity, *African Charter on Human and Peoples' Rights* (Addis Abbaba: OAU, 1981), Doc. CAB/Leg/67/3/Rev. 5.
[16] UN, *International Convention on the Elimination of All Forms of Racial Discrimination* (New York: UN, 1965).
[17] UN, *Convention on the Rights of the Child* (New York: UN, 1989), GA Res. 44/25, annex, 44 UN GAOR Suppl. (No. 49) at 167, UN Doc. A/44/49 (1989), entered into force 2 Sept. 1990, 1577 UNTS 3.
[18] UN, *Convention on the Elimination of All Forms of Discrimination against Women* (New York: UN, 1979), 34 UN GAOR Suppl. (No. 21) (A/34/46) at 193, UN Doc. A/Res/34/180 (hereinafter Women's Convention).

nutrition during pregnancy, information, and, for instance, education to decide the number and spacing of one's children.

These leading international human rights treaties establish committees whose functions are to monitor states' compliance with the obligations states have accepted. The Women's Convention establishes the Committee on the Elimination of Discrimination against Women (CEDAW) to monitor whether states have brought their laws, policies, and practices into compliance with the Women's Convention. Similarly, the Political Covenant establishes the Human Rights Committee (HRC), the Economic Covenant establishes the Committee on Economic, Social and Cultural Rights (CESCR), the Children's Convention establishes the Committee on the Rights of the Child (CRC) and, for example, the International Convention on the Elimination of All Forms of Racial Discrimination establishes the Committee on the Elimination of Racial Discrimination (CERD).

These committees meet once or twice or three times a year. Committees consider the reports of member states on what the states have done to bring their laws, policies, and practices into compliance with treaty obligations. Once committee members have considered and discussed reports through dialogues with representatives of reporting states, committees will issue Concluding Observations on reports.[19] To assist countries in discharge of their reporting obligations, the committees have developed useful General Comments or General Recommendations on specific treaty articles that explain the content and meaning of the specific rights. Some committees have the ability to hear complaints from individuals or groups from consenting countries, or to undertake inquiries into alleged violations in consenting countries (see Pt. I, Ch. 7). The opinions that the committees form in response to these complaints or inquiries also add to the content and meaning of rights, by showing how rights or a group of rights are applied to particular facts.

3. *Rights Relating to Reproductive and Sexual Health*

3.1. *Evolution of reproductive rights*

Control of women's reproduction and sexuality has a history that reaches back into antiquity. Over the centuries, governments have used criminal laws as a primary instrument to express and control morality, particularly through the prohibition of birth control and abortion or through penalizing and stigmatizing certain forms of sexual behaviour. Gradually, however, with the spread of democratic government, a realization has emerged of the harmful effects on

---

[19] UN, *Manual on Human Rights Reporting* (Geneva: UN, 1997).

the health and welfare of individuals caused by the punitive control of reproduction and sexuality. This has fostered an approach to laws and policies
designed to promote individuals' interests in their health and welfare. A more
recent approach challenges patriarchal laws by advocating increased access to
reproductive and sexual health services as a matter of human rights and social
justice.

The three approaches, from criminalization, through the promotion of
health and welfare, to an emphasis on human rights and justice, exist in many
countries, and are not necessarily mutually exclusive. The tendency to use
criminal law to punish and stigmatize disapproved behaviour remains, but is
waning because of an increased understanding that this approach is often dysfunctional. Many countries have used a health and welfare rationale to legalize
and, in some cases, provide or subsidize reproductive and sexual health services. An increasing number of countries have reformed laws and policies to
facilitate the provision of reproductive and sexual health services because of
a growing recognition of the importance of respecting the human rights of
women in general, and reproductive and sexual health rights in particular.

The Cairo process introduced a new focus on meeting the reproductive
health needs and preferences of individual women and men, rather than, as in
the past, on achieving demographic or population-based targets. Key to this
new approach is the empowerment of women within their families and communities and the protection of their human rights, particularly those relevant
to their reproductive and sexual health. The challenge ahead is to turn the
political commitments made by governments in Cairo and Beijing into legally
enforceable duties to respect reproductive rights. There is a growing awareness
that national and international interactions to develop favourable practices
and norms need to continue over time, and not end with court decisions or the
approval of international documents. That is, the Cairo and Beijing commitments need to be seen as a dynamic, ongoing law-making and implementation
process through which non-binding commitments become politically, socially,
and legally binding.

Empirical evidence that demonstrates the dysfunctions of many doctrinally
based criminal laws has contributed to the modern movement in reproductive
health away from reliance on concepts of crime and punishment, in favour of
the promotion of health and welfare. During the decade of the 1990s, for
instance, abortion law reform has been achieved in many countries.[20] Reforms
have, however, been frustrated by religious and moral opposition in some
countries, and some attempts to restrict the availability of legal abortion have
been successful. In addition, some national constitutions have been amended

---

[20] R. J. Cook, B. M. Dickens, and L. E. Bliss, 'International Developments in Abortion Law
from 1988 to 1998', *American J. of Public Health*, 89 (1999), 579–86.

to claim to protect life from the moment of conception, in attempts to restrict reproductive choices. Efforts to institute sex education in schools have been challenged in most regions of the world, and barriers to the provision of reproductive and sexual health information and services persist.

Defending and articulating a woman's right to personal choice and freedom in her decisions concerning her body and her reproductive options are important aspects of what has emerged as a movement to define and protect women's reproductive rights. Recognition of the importance of women's self-determination to their health and well-being is growing. It is increasingly unacceptable, for instance, for a husband to dominate his wife by the use or threat of violence, or to force her into unwanted sex or to continue an unwanted pregnancy. Violence against commercial sex workers, who are vulnerable to abuse because their activities are often outside the protection of the law, is no longer tolerable. Equally unacceptable is state enforcement of positive and negative population policies at the expense of individual human rights to reproductive choice.

Understanding of the multiple dimensions of reproductive and sexual health has been developed through research undertaken in a variety of different disciplines, including empirical disciplines in health and social sciences, and normative disciplines such as law and bioethics. This research has informed our understanding of the causes and human consequences of reproductive and sexual ill-health, and thus how human rights might be applied to prevent and remedy some of the causes of ill-health. The protection of reproductive rights has evolved over time as individuals have found the courage to step forward to address, and in some cases remedy, the abuses of rights they or others have suffered. Protective spheres for the advancement of vital interests relating to reproductive and sexual health have emerged out of these individual and collective struggles. These spheres are known collectively as reproductive rights.

3.2. *Duties to implement reproductive rights*

A person's interest or need becomes a right in so far as a duty binds another to respect that interest. The binding force that creates a duty can be either legal or moral, and thus a right itself may be legal, moral, or both. The challenge ahead is to apply legal, moral, or other authority to create duties that require the protection and promotion of rights relating to reproductive and sexual health.

The CEDAW General Recommendation on Women and Health explains the legal duties that obligate states that are parties to the Women's Convention to respect rights by not obstructing their exercise, to protect rights by taking positive action against third-party violators, and to fulfil rights by employing governmental means to afford individuals the full benefit of their human rights (see Pt. III, Ch. 6, Sect. 2). This Recommendation addresses obligations to advance human rights to women's health in the following ways:

> The obligation to *respect* rights requires States Parties to refrain from obstructing action taken by women in pursuit of their health goals. States Parties should report on how public and private health care providers meet their duties to respect women's rights to have access to health care (para. 14) . . . The obligation to *protect* rights relating to women's health requires States Parties, their agents and officials to take action to prevent and impose sanctions for violations of rights by private persons and organizations (para. 15) . . . The duty to *fulfil* rights places an obligation on States Parties to take appropriate legislative, judicial, administrative and budgetary, economic and other measures to the maximum extent of their available resources to ensure that women realize their rights to health care (para. 17).

The General Recommendation explains that studies that show high rates of maternal mortality and morbidity within particular states, and that show a large number of couples who would like to limit their family size but lack access to any form of contraception, provide important indications to states of their possible breaches of duties to ensure women's access to health care. The Recommendation also emphasizes the importance of states addressing in their respective reports to CEDAW the steps they have taken to deal with preventable conditions, such as HIV/AIDS.

3.3. *Restrictions and limitations of rights*

Under international human rights law, restrictions of some rights are permissible if such restrictions are necessary to achieve overriding objectives such as public health, the rights of others, commonly agreed morality, public order, the general welfare in a democratic society, and national security. There are some rights, such as the right to life, the right to be free from torture, and the right to freedom of conscience and religion, that are absolute and cannot be limited in any circumstances, even in times of emergency. Other rights can be restricted for legitimate reasons, provided that:

- the restriction is imposed in accordance with the law;
- the restriction is based on a legitimate interest, as defined in the provisions guaranteeing the right, such as the preservation of public health or the rights of others;
- the restriction is proportionate to that interest; and
- the restriction constitutes the least intrusive and least restrictive measure available effectively to achieve that interest.[21]

---

[21] UN, *HIV/AIDS and Human Rights: International Guidelines* (Geneva: UN, 1998), at 42, for summary see Pt. III, Ch. 7. Limburg Principles on the Implementation of the International Covenant on Economic, Social and Cultural Rights, *Human Rights Quarterly*, 9 (1987), 122–35, paras. 46–56.

For example, the right of confidentiality of a patient who is HIV positive can be restricted in the situation where the right of another specifically identified individual is at imminent risk of harm. If it has been established that the HIV-positive patient refuses to inform his or her partner, and it is strictly necessary for the purpose of preserving the health of that identified person, the law and codes of medical ethics then allow for protective disclosure of this otherwise confidential information. Limited disclosure is for the legitimate reason of preserving the life or health of an identifiable person.

4. *The Application of Human Rights to Reproductive and Sexual Health*

Interests relating to reproductive and sexual health may be protected through specific human rights. Rights that can be most relevantly invoked, and how rights are shown to have been violated, depend on the particular facts of an alleged violation and on the underlying causes of reproductive or sexual ill-health.[22] The rights addressed below are not exhaustive, but indicative of rights that may be developed to advance reproductive interests.

Rights are interactive, in that each depends to a greater or lesser degree on the observance of others. The following discussion shows ways in which specific rights may be applied to protect reproductive and sexual health. It also addresses how national laws and international standards such as those contained in the Cairo Programme, the Beijing Platform, and CEDAW General Recommendations have been used and can be further used to develop criteria by which to measure compliance with these rights.

Most countries have committed themselves to respect individuals' human dignity and physical integrity through their own national constitutions and other laws, and their membership in regional and international human rights conventions. The separate human rights that contribute to reproductive and sexual health can be clustered around reproductive and sexual health interests relating to:

- life, survival, security, and sexuality;
- reproductive self-determination and free choice of maternity;
- health and the benefits of scientific progress;
- non-discrimination and due respect for difference; and
- information, education, and decision-making.

These interests can be categorized differently, depending on the issues at stake and people's perceptions of those issues. Health, for instance, has been seen as

---

[22] CRLP, *An Unfulfilled Human Right: Family Planning in Guatemala* (New York: CRLP, 2000); D. D. Dora and D. D. da Silveira (eds.), *Direitos Humanos, Etica e Direitos Reprodutivos* (Human Rights, Ethics, and Reproductive Rights) (Porto Alegre, Brazil: Themis, 1998).

a component of the right to security of the person as well as a right standing on its own, often called the right to health. The clustering of specific human rights around reproductive and sexual health interests is fluid and can be arranged in different ways. The right to education, for example, is relevant both to the advancement of health and to facilitate decision-making. Separately expressed rights are not insulated from others, but interact dynamically with and inform other rights.

The purpose of clustering is to show how different human rights can be cumulatively and interactively applied to advance interests in reproductive and sexual health. The purpose is not to suggest that there is any single 'correct' approach to categorizing reproductive and sexual health interests or to clustering human rights around them. As human rights are applied more vigorously to reproductive and sexual health needs, different ways of applying human rights to serve those needs will emerge.

4.1. *Rights relating to life, survival, security, and sexuality*

Rights relating to life, survival, security, and sexuality are increasingly applied to require a state to eliminate barriers to the basic services necessary for the reproductive and sexual health of its residents. These rights include the right to life and survival, the right to liberty and security of the person, and the right to be free from torture and from inhuman and degrading treatment. Notions of health are illuminating the content and meaning of these rights at the national level, particularly in national courts, and at the regional and international levels.

In some countries, these rights have been applied to require governments to provide services necessary to protect reproductive and sexual health. Effective application of these rights is needed in order to require governments to take the steps necessary to ensure, for example, that women can go through pregnancy and childbirth safely, to protect the confidentiality of patients seeking reproductive health services,[23] to ensure respect for human rights of people living with HIV/AIDS,[24] to reduce violence against women, including female genital cutting or mutilation,[25] and trafficking in women.[26]

Where a denial of rights, especially those rights that relate to personal integrity and liberty, has been established, a court might consider how this

---

[23] *Insurralde, Mirta, T. 148 PS. 357/428*, Corte Suprema de la Provincia de Sante Fe, Argentina, 1 Aug. 1998 (court found that a doctor was not liable for breaching patient confidentiality by reporting an adolescent girl to the authorities for seeking treatment for complications resulting from an allegedly illegal abortion), reported in B. M. Dickens and R. J. Cook, 'Law and Ethics in Conflict over Confidentiality?', *Int. J. Gynecol. Obstet.* 70 (2000), 385–91.

[24] UN, *HIV/AIDS and Human Rights*.

[25] A. Rahman and N. Toubia (eds.), *Female Genital Mutilation: A Guide to Laws and Policies Worldwide* (London: Zed Books, 2000).

[26] Asian Women's Fund, *Proceedings of the 1998 Regional Conference on Trafficking in Women* (Tokyo: Asian Women's Fund, 1999).

denial has disrupted an individual's life plan, and order remedies that take account of that disruption. The Inter-American Court of Human Rights, in finding violations of the right to personal liberty, the right to humane treatment, and the right to a fair trial for the unlawful detention and torture of a woman,[27] ordered reparations that take account of that disruption to her life plan.[28] The Court explained that:

It is obvious that the violations committed against the victim in the instant Case prevented her from achieving her goals for personal and professional growth, goals that would have been feasible under normal circumstances. Those violations caused irreparable damage to her life, forcing her to interrupt her studies and to take up life in a foreign country far from the context in which her life had been evolving, in a state of solitude, poverty, and severe physical and psychological distress. Obviously this combination of circumstances, directly attributable to the violations that this Court examined, has seriously and probably irreparably altered the life of Mrs Loayza-Tamayo, and has prevented her from achieving the personal, family and professional goals that she had reasonably set for herself.[29]

As a result of this decision, it would seem reasonable where denial of rights relating to reproductive and sexual health disrupts the life plan of an individual, and where that life plan is both reasonable and attainable in practice, the Inter-American Court will order reparations that reasonably accommodate that disruption.

4.1.1. *The right to life and survival*

The Political Covenant, Article 6(1), states: 'Every human being has the inherent right to life. This right shall be protected by law. No one shall be arbitrarily deprived of his life.'

Historically, this right generally has been applied only to prohibit governments from imposing capital punishment in an arbitrary way. However, judicial tribunals are beginning to apply the right to life to matters relating to health by addressing the positive nature of the right, and by providing a context of health and human dignity to the right to life. For example, the Human Rights Committee (HRC) has explained that 'the expression "inherent right to life" cannot be properly understood in a restrictive manner, and the protection of this right requires that States adopt positive measures'.[30] When explaining what positive measures might be adopted, HRC gave, as an example, measures necessary to reduce infant mortality and to increase life expectancy. HRC has

---

[27] *Loayza Tamayo v. Peru*, Inter-American Court of Human Rights, Judgment of 17 Sept. 1997 (ser. C.), No. 33 (1977).

[28] *Loayza Tamayo v. Peru*, Inter-American Court of Human Rights, Sentence on reparations, 27 Nov. 1998 (ser. C), No. 42 I.6.

[29] Ibid., para. 152.

[30] UN, 'Human Rights Committee General Comment 6, Article 6 (Right to Life), 1982', *International Human Rights Instruments* (New York: UN, 1996), HRI/Gen/1/Rev. 2, 6–7, para. 5.

specified through its General Comment on Equality between Men and Women that states are now required to provide data on 'pregnancy and childbirth-related deaths of women' (see Pt. III, Ch. 6, Sect. 4, para. 10).

The Inter-American Court of Human Rights held the government of Guatemala responsible for the treatment of street children resulting, in some cases, in the loss of life. In explaining the positive obligations to protect life, the Court explained that:

The right to life is a fundamental human right, and the exercise of this right is essential for the exercise of all other human rights. If it is not respected, all rights lack meaning. Owing to the fundamental nature of the right to life, restrictive approaches to it are inadmissible. In essence, the fundamental right to life includes, not only the right of every human being not to be deprived of his life arbitrarily, but also the right that he will not be prevented from having access to the conditions that guarantee a dignified existence. States have the obligation to guarantee the creation of the conditions required in order that violations to this basic right do not occur and, in particular, the duty to prevent its agents from violating it.[31]

Where a state neglects to provide the means necessary to prevent women from dying from pregnancy and childbirth, they are failing in their obligation to ensure 'access to the conditions that guarantee a dignified existence'.

4.1.1.1. *Essential obstetric care*

The right to life is the most obvious right that could be applied to protect women at risk of dying in childbirth, due to lack of essential or emergency obstetric care. For example, the Supreme Court of India decided that the right to life contained in the Indian Constitution[32] was breached when various government hospitals denied an individual emergency treatment for serious head injuries.[33] The Court explained that the state cannot use financial constraints to ignore its constitutional obligation to provide adequate medical services to preserve human life, and even detailed which measures the state might take to comply. While this decision addressed emergency medical care to treat head injuries, the reasoning could be applied to require governments to provide essential obstetric services where they are not sufficiently available.

The European Commission of Human Rights considered a complaint alleging a state's violation of the right to life of a woman who had died in childbirth.[34] The Commission held that the complaint was inadmissible on technical grounds. However, the Commission took the opportunity to emphasize that

[31] *Villagran Morales et al. v. Guatemala*, Series C, No. 63, 19 Nov. 1999, para. 144.
[32] Article 21 of the Indian Constitution, on the Protection of Life and Personal Liberty, reads: 'No person shall be deprived of his life or personal liberty except according to procedure established by law.'
[33] *Paschim Banga Khet Mazdoor Samity v. State of West Bengal* (1996) 4 SCC 37, digested in *Commonwealth Human Rights Law Digest*, 2 (1998), 109 (Supreme Court of India).
[34] *Tavares v. France* (1991), Eur. Comm. HR, Application No. 16593/90, (09/12/91 unpublished) (European Commission of Human Rights).

the right to life in the European Convention[35] has to be interpreted not only to require states to take steps to prevent intentional killing, but also to take measures necessary to protect life against unintentional loss. The European Commission had earlier considered a claim that a governmental vaccination programme that resulted in damage and death to babies was a violation of the right to life.[36] The Commission found that appropriate and adequate measures to protect life had been taken in this case. The Commission explained, however, that had the state not shown that such measures had been taken, the state would have been found in breach of its duty under human rights law to safeguard life and health. This shows that states are bound to explain and justify their efforts to protect their citizens' lives and health.

Given the magnitude of the estimated 1,400 maternal deaths worldwide each day, it is remarkable that so few legal proceedings have made their way into national courts to require governments to take appropriate measures to identify the causes of maternal mortality, and take measures necessary to prevent further maternal deaths. This inaction is due in part to members of communities in which maternal mortality is high not understanding how governmental neglect of the conditions in which women bear pregnancies and give birth violates their right to life.

Effective protection of the right to life requires that positive measures be taken that are necessary to ensure, as the Cairo programme requires, 'access to appropriate health-care services that will enable women to go safely through pregnancy and childbirth and provide couples with the best chance of having a healthy infant'.[37] Positive measures might include that progressive steps are taken to ensure that, at an increasing rate, births are assisted by skilled attendants, as required by the Cairo and Beijing processes. Where such measures have not been taken, states need to be encouraged to take steps to ensure compliance with their treaty obligations to protect and promote pregnant women's right to life (see Pt. I, Ch. 7, Sect. 3.4. on Performance Standards).

4.1.1.2. *Anti-retroviral and associated treatment*

The Supreme Court of Venezuela recognized the interrelationship between the rights to life[38] and to health[39] contained in the Venezuelan Constitution when

---

[35] European Convention, Article 2, reads: 'Everyone's right to life shall be protected by law. No one shall be deprived of his life intentionally save in the execution of a sentence of a court of law following his conviction of a crime for which this penalty is provided by law.'

[36] *X v. United Kingdom* (1978), Application No. 7154, Decision 12 July 1978, Decision & Reports 14: 31–5, June 1979 (European Commission of Human Rights).

[37] Cairo Programme, para. 7.2.

[38] Article 58 of the 1961 Venezuelan Constitution reads: 'The right to life is inviolable . . .'.

[39] Article 76 of the 1961 Venezuelan Constitution reads: 'Everyone shall have the right to protection of his health. The authorities shall oversee the maintenance of public health and shall provide the means of prevention and attention for those who lack them. Everyone is obliged to submit to health measures established by law, within the limits imposed by respect for the human person.'

ruling in favour of a claim for HIV treatment.[40] In underscoring the positive nature of the right to life, the Court required the Ministry of Health to:

- provide the medicines prescribed by government doctors;
- cover the cost of HIV blood tests in order for patients to obtain the necessary anti-retroviral treatments and treatments for opportunistic infections;
- develop the policies and programmes necessary for affected patients' treatment and assistance; and
- make the reallocation of the budget necessary to carry out the decision of the Court.

While the successful claim was brought on behalf of 172 individuals living with HIV, the Court applied the decision to all people who are HIV positive in Venezuela.

Similar judgments by the Supreme Court of Mexico,[41] and the Constitutional Court of South Africa,[42] have ordered the governments to provide necessary treatment to Mexicans with HIV/AIDS, and to pregnant women with HIV/AIDS in South Africa respectively. The Inter-American Commission on Human Rights agreed to hear the claims that Chile[43] and El Salvador[44] are in breach of their duties under the American Convention on Human Rights for not providing necessary medications for all of their residents with HIV/AIDS. Pending the consideration of these claims, the Inter-American Commission required the governments of Chile and El Salvador to continue to provide prevailing access to such medications as a precautionary measure.

As a result of these decisions, it is now timely to explore how additional claims might be brought on behalf of those who are at increased risk of death because of governmental failure to provide reproductive and sexual health services. Those at such risk include women needing life-saving obstetric care or life-saving treatment for incomplete abortions, as well as individuals needing life-saving treatment for conditions relating to HIV/AIDS. Such claims would certainly be feasible under the codified laws in civil law countries, given the

[40] *Cruz Bermudez, et al. v. Ministerio de Sanidad y Asistencia Social (MSAS)*, Case No. 15789 (1999) http://www.csj.gov.ve, last accessed 13 June 2000 (Supreme Court of Venezuela); M. Torres, 'The Human Right to Health, National Courts, and Access to HIV/AIDS Treatment: A Case from Venezuela', *Chicago J. International Law*, 3 (2002), 105–14.

[41] *Jose Luis Castro Ramiriez* (1997), Amparo Appeal No. 2231 (Supreme Court of Mexico).

[42] *Minister of Health v. Treatment Action Campaign* (2002), Case CCT 8/02 (Constitutional Court of South Africa) (Report pending, judgment available at http://www.concourt.gov.za/date 2002.html)

[43] *Juan Pablo et al. v. Chile*, Annual Report of the Inter-American Commission on Human Rights, *OEA/Ser./L/V/II.114, doc. 5 rev. (2001)*, online: http://www.cidh.org/annualrep/2001eng/chap.3a.htm#C, last accessed: 10 May 2002.

[44] *Jorge Odir Miranda Cortez v. El Salvador*, Report No. 29/01, Case 12.249, 7 Mar. 2001 (Inter-American Commission on Human Rights).

Venezuelan Supreme Court decision, and, in light of the Supreme Court of India's judgment, they would be credible in most Commonwealth countries that apply the common law system of customary and enacted laws. Governmental health administrations might be wise to plan their resource allocations and programmes in anticipation of judicial sympathy with the courts in Venezuela and India. Moreover, health administrators will be called on to explain in a variety of forums, including courts of law and of public opinion, the adequacy of their responses to their obligations to reduce maternal mortality, and mortality related, for instance, to HIV/AIDS.

4.1.2. *The right to liberty and security of the person*

The Political Covenant, Article 9(1), states: 'Everyone has the right to liberty and security of person . . . No one shall be deprived of his liberty except on such grounds and in accordance with such procedures as are established by law.'

The right to liberty and security of the person is one of the strongest defences of individual integrity in the reproductive and sexual health care context. The right is being applied beyond its historical prohibition of arbitrary arrest or detention, to require governments to provide health services when the lack of services jeopardizes liberty and particularly health security of the person. The Inter-American Commission of Human Rights has recognized a right to the satisfaction of basic health needs as part of a right to personal security in observing that:

The essence of the legal obligation incurred by any government . . . is to strive to attain the economic and social aspirations of its people by following an order that assigns priority to the basic needs of health, nutrition and education. The priority of the 'right to survival' and 'basic needs' is a natural consequence of the right to personal security.[45]

If governments and agencies to which they delegate responsibility to administer health services fail to provide conditions necessary to protect reproductive and sexual health, they might be held responsible for the denial of the right to liberty and security of the person.

4.1.2.1. *Unsafe abortion*

Unsafe abortion is the second largest cause of maternal mortality in some countries, such as Colombia.[46] Where unsafe abortion is a major cause of maternal death, it may be possible to apply the right to liberty and security to

---

[45] Inter-American Commission of Human Rights, *1980–1981 Annual Report*, 125, cited in *1989–1990 Annual Report*, 187.

[46] Ministerio de Salud, DANE, Presidencia de la República, DNP, OPS, UNFPA, UNICEF, PROFAMILIA, 'Por Qué se Mueren las Mujeres en Colombia?' (Why do Mothers Die in Colombia?), *Revista PROFAMILIA*, 14/28 (1996), 14–28.

require governments to improve services for treatment of unsafe abortion, and to change restrictive laws to ensure access to contraceptive and abortion services. Experience consistently shows that stronger enforcement of restrictive laws is ineffective and almost invariably dysfunctional in forcing women, who are disrespectfully characterized as criminals, into even less safe practices. It is widely recognized that restrictive abortion laws do not reduce the number of abortions but only their safety, and may actually increase the number by denying women access to counselling that may present acceptable alternatives to abortion and reduce repeat abortions.

The right to liberty and security has been applied by national courts in abortion cases to protect a woman's freedom to decide if, when, and how often to bear children. In Canada, for instance, the Supreme Court held that a restrictive criminal abortion provision violated a woman's right to security of the person.[47] Several constitutional courts, including those of France,[48] Italy,[49] and the Netherlands,[50] have found that liberal abortion laws are consistent with women's right to liberty. Even laws expressed only prohibitively usually have an implied exception that allows lawful abortion when a woman's life or enduring health is in danger. However, the punitive context of the law deters women from seeking medical treatment, and doctors from proposing it, where the public at large and medical practitioners in particular are not informed that restrictively worded laws have an implied exception that allows lawful abortion for preservation of life and health. The tragedy is that many women risk and lose their lives undertaking unsafe procedures when the existing law would permit their abortions to be performed legally and safely.

4.1.2.2. *Female genital cutting (FGC)*

Female genital cutting (FGC), also described as mutilation or circumcision, affects many human rights, but it centrally implicates rights to liberty and security of the person. This is obviously so when applied to young girls, but the principle can be applied equally regarding adolescent and older women who, for family and cultural reasons, find their future impaired without submitting to such procedures. FGC can be classified into increasing degrees of invasiveness (see Pt. II, Ch. 2), but even a minor form implicates the rights to liberty and security when conducted on a young girl incapable of providing her own

---

[47] *R. v. Morgentaler* (1988), 44 DLR (4th) 385 (Supreme Court of Canada).

[48] *Judgment of Jan. 15, 1975*, Conseil Constitutionnel, 1975 Recueil Dalloz-Sirey [D.S. Jur.] 529, Journal Officiel, 16 Jan. 1975 (Constitutional Council, France).

[49] *Judgment No. 108/81 of 25 June 1981*, 57 Raccolta Ufficiale della Corte Costituzionale 823, 1981 (Constitutional Court of Italy).

[50] *Juristenvereiniging Pro Vita v. De Staat der Nederlanden (Ministerie van Welzijn, Volksgezondheid en Cultuur)* (1990) Nederlandse Jurisprudentie, No. 43, 1990, entry 707, as summarized in *European Law Digest*, 19/5 (1991), 179–80 and reported in the *Annual Review of Population Law*, 17 (1990), 29 (The Court, The Hague).

consent due to immature age and family and communal pressure. Beyond violations to girls' liberty, there are often dangers to their security from un-hygienic and unskilled practice. The lifelong effects of the procedure can also implicate rights to found a family, since the effect of procedures can limit child-bearing capacity.

Adolescent and older women may feel pressures to accept FGC where it is an expectation in their community that they be treated, and a condition of their marriage. The Children's Convention obliges States Parties to 'take all effective and appropriate measures with a view to abolishing traditional practices prejudicial to the health of the child' (Article 24(3)). The Women's Convention obliges States Parties to protect women against harmful practices, but also to reform the cultures in which traditional expectations oppress women and endanger their health (Articles 5(*a*) and 12). Moreover, CEDAW through its General Recommendation on Female Circumcision requires States Parties to 'take effective and appropriate measures with a view to eradicating the practice of female circumcision'.[51] Accordingly, while the right to resist FGC is a negative right in so far as capable women are free to resist such genital cutting, it is better regarded as a positive right. That is, states have affirmative duties to prevent the practice by prohibiting health professional involvement, and unskilled practice, and also educating communities to aban-don the practice.

It may be claimed that the liberty rights of mature women entitle them to consent to the procedure, and to ask health professionals to perform it safely. However, the Political Covenant provides that liberty not be denied 'except on such grounds and in accordance with such procedures as are established by law'. Beyond laws that would define the more invasive types of FGC as unlaw-ful maiming, an increasing number of countries have enacted laws to prohibit the practice by people in general and physicians and other health care practi-tioners in particular.[52] Some laws may, however, permit re-infibulation follow-ing childbirth, although some medical associations on human rights grounds consider this also to be professional misconduct.

4.1.2.3. *Confidentiality*

Women's liberty and security require clinic policies and laws that ensure their care and confidentiality. Under the Women's Convention, CEDAW has made a General Recommendation reiterating the importance of confidentiality. The Recommendation observes that, although lack of confidentiality affects both men and women to a certain degree, 'it may deter women from seeking advice

---

[51] United Nations, 'CEDAW General Recommendation 14 on Female Circumcision, 1990', in UN, 'Human Rights Committee Comment', 108–9.
[52] Rahman and Toubia (eds.), *Female Genital Mutilation*.

and treatment and thereby adversely affect their health and well-being. Women will be less willing, for that reason [unreliable confidentiality], to seek medical care for diseases of the genital tract, for contraception or for incomplete abortion and in cases where they have suffered sexual or physical violence' (see Pt. III, Ch. 6, Sect. 2, para. 12(*d*)).

Given this clear explanation of the impact of failures to respect confidentiality, health care administrators and providers can appreciate that lack of respect for confidentiality can deter women from seeking treatment particularly for conditions resulting from stigmatizing situations such as violence, or conditions such as vesico-vaginal fistulae (VVF), incomplete abortion, or sexually transmitted infections (STIs). As a result, failure adequately to respect confidentiality offends a woman's right to security of her person and possibly her right to health.

The right to liberty and security of the person can be applied to require that states take positive measures to ensure protection of confidentiality in the delivery of reproductive health services to women who are at particular risk. They include women, especially adolescent girls, presenting with stigmatizing conditions, such as unmarried or extra-marital pregnancy, or incomplete abortion. Sometimes, adolescents hesitate to seek reproductive health services because they fear that their confidentiality might be breached.[53] They fear, perhaps incorrectly, that information about their sexual behaviour, which they have to give for appropriate health care, will be disclosed to their parents, parents of their partners, teachers, and others. As a result, special care and attention need to be given to informing adolescents in the community through positive assurances that their confidentiality will be protected, and to training health personnel appropriately. Clinics may have to withhold information not only of what treatment their patients have received, but also of who their patients are, although some disclosure of identity may be required for billing purposes. Clinics may have to ensure that their own names do not disclose their services, such as that they treat only pregnant patients or those with STIs.

There are exceptions to the rule of confidentiality. Disclosure is permitted under most codes of medical ethics where it can be shown that there is an immediate or future risk to the health and life of others. The Supreme Court of India upheld a disclosure by a hospital of the HIV-positive status of a man who was planning to marry a particular woman.[54] The Court explained that the Code of Medical Ethics, developed by the Indian Medical Council, does permit disclosure in very limited circumstances, such as where there is an imminent risk to an identifiable person (see Pt. I, Ch. 5, Sect. 7.2.3).

---

[53] C. A. Ford, S. G. Millstein, B. L. Halpern-Felsher, and C. E. Irwin, 'Influence of Physician Confidentiality Assurances on Adolescents' Willingness to Disclose Information and Seek Future Health Care', *Journal of the American Medical Association*, 278 (1997), 1029–34.

[54] *Mr. X v. Hosptial Z* (1998) 8 SCC 296 (Supreme Court of India).

4.1.2.4. *Compulsory diagnostic testing*

Both women and men may be subject to involuntary diagnostic testing by invasive and non-invasive means. Non-invasive testing may be conducted without consent on tissue samples, such as blood, hair, and urine, that become available for other purposes. Whether or not testable material is acquired in violation of an individual's security of the person, its non-consensual testing violates liberty of the person. Women are as liable as men to have, for instance, urine and hair samples tested for drug use and other forensic purposes, but women alone are liable to have HIV testing of samples given in prenatal care or recovered at childbirth. A critical human rights objection to involuntary HIV testing is that a positive result may expose patients to immense discrimination, in access to health services and in many other aspects of their lives, including, for instance, employment and housing, and not be compensated by appropriate provision of medical care.

Contrasts are often drawn between voluntary or consensual testing (including tests to which individuals agree and which they may take the initiative to request), compulsory testing, which is undertaken without individuals' approval and even over their objections, and mandatory testing. Mandatory testing is undertaken when testing is made a condition of individuals undertaking acts that they want to undertake but are not compelled to undertake. For instance, athletic competitors may be subject to tissue tests for use of banned drugs, but can choose not to compete, in the same way as drivers may be subject to spot testing of breath for alcohol use, but a person is not obliged to drive. A human rights violation and social dysfunction may arise, however, when women who attend clinics for prenatal care are subject to mandatory HIV testing, since they can deny the test only to the prejudice of their and their child's prenatal health monitoring. Similarly, when childbirth centres make HIV testing of, for instance, cord blood a condition of their care, such mandatory testing can be avoided only by a rejection of the safety to mother and child that their facilities afford.

There is, however, an alternative argument that favours mandatory testing based on the human right to security of the person. The care required for a child born to an HIV-positive mother can promote the health and very survival of the child, but can be available only if the mother's HIV-positive status is determined. That is, the human rights of the child can be served only by compromise of the mother's liberty interest in rejecting testing. Since parents owe their children legal duties of care and protection, this denial of the mother's liberty may come within the exception to Article 9(1) of the Political Covenant, in constituting a ground and procedure established by law. Further, in health care settings where universal precautions cannot be maintained against the risk of health care providers' exposure to HIV infection, the protection of providers who treat pregnant women, women in labour, and newborn children may require that they identify HIV-positive women. In these circumstances, the human right to security of providers may be in conflict with the liberty rights of pregnant women. Social advantage suggests that the interests of providers may prevail, but only on the condition that HIV-positive women and their children enjoy security against discrimination on grounds of disability.

An approach to accommodating the right to security of the health care providers and the right to liberty of the pregnant woman is suggested by the United States Centers for Disease Control Revised Recommendations for HIV Screening of Pregnant Women. They recommend testing of all pregnant patients, but respect the right of the patient to refuse testing. The Recommendations state that '[a]ll health-care providers should recommend HIV testing to all pregnant patients, pointing out the substantial benefit of knowledge of HIV status for the health of women and their infants. HIV screening should be a routine part of prenatal care for all women.'[55] These Recommendations go on to explain that:

Although HIV testing is recommended, women should be allowed to refuse testing. Women should not be tested without their knowledge. Women who refuse testing should not be coerced into testing, denied care for themselves or their infants, or threatened with loss of custody of their infants or other negative consequences. Discussing and addressing reasons for refusal (e.g. lack of awareness of risk or fear of the disease, partner violence, potential stigma, or discrimination) could promote health education and trust-building and allow some women to accept testing at a later date.[56]

These Recommendations, however, presuppose the availability of effective interventions in the form of highly active combination anti-retrovirals, and recommend that information be given on their availability before testing.

The contrast between HIV testing and HIV screening is important to public health services. Testing is individual and identified, but screening is often of tissue samples that are anonymously derived from a population group, whether supplied deliberately for this purpose or left over from other purposes. Screening of the prevalence of HIV infection among representative members of a population group, such as pregnant women or mothers of newborn children, is not the same as testing individuals to determine their HIV status. When prevalence screening studies are conducted on anonymous left-over tissue samples, no individual's liberty interests are involved, and individuals' consent is not necessarily required. Consent may be required if all members of the population studied may become negatively stigmatized, but proper care in how results are publicized should reduce this risk and the need for consent. The

[55] United States Centers for Disease Control, 'Revised Guidelines for HIV Counseling, Testing and Referral and Revised Recommendations for HIV Screening of Pregnant Women', *Morbidity and Mortality Weekly Report*, 50 (RR-19) (2001), 1–85 at 75.
[56] Ibid.

benefit of screening studies is that they can identify health deficits or risks in particular communities or population groups, so that remedial services and supplies can be appropriately made available to them. That is, such studies can serve individuals' security interests.

4.1.3. *The right to be free from inhuman and degrading treatment*

The Political Covenant, Article 7, states: 'No one shall be subjected to torture or to cruel, inhuman or degrading treatment or punishment. In particular, no one shall be subjected without his free consent to medical or scientific experimentation.'

The traditional application of the right to be free from torture and from cruel, inhuman, and degrading treatment was only to ensure that prisoners are treated in humane ways. Courts and human rights tribunals are now moving beyond this, however, to ensure that the inherent dignity of women is respected, protected, and fulfilled. To ensure that 'no one shall be subjected without his free consent to medical or scientific experimentation', important work has been done to protect free and informed decision-making in the context of biomedical research in human reproduction.[57] Examples, explored below, show how tribunals are adding content to this right by importing understanding of sexual and reproductive health and well-being into determination of what is considered to be inhuman and degrading treatment.

4.1.3.1. *Rape and the subsequent denial of justice*

Human rights tribunals are beginning to apply the right to be free from torture and inhuman and degrading treatment to hold states accountable for the rape of women by governmental officers, and applying the right to a fair trial where subsequent recourse to judicial protection has been neglected or abused.

The Inter-American Commission found Mexico responsible for the illegal detention and interrogation by Mexican military officers of three sisters, Ana (20 years old), Beatriz (18 years old), and Cecilia (16 years old), and their mother, Delia Gonzalez Perez, in violation of their right to their liberty and personal security under the American Convention on Human Rights.[58] They also found Mexico responsible for the raping by Mexican military officers of the three sisters in violation of their right to their physical and moral integrity, and in the case of Cecilia, her right to protection as a child under the American Convention, and their right not to be subjected to torture under the American Convention and the Inter-American Convention to Prevent and Punish Torture.[59] They also found that the rapes violated their rights to respect of their

[57] See the World Medical Association, Declaration of Helsinki, in Pt III, Ch. 2.

[58] *Ana, Beatriz and Cecilia Gonzalez Perez v. Mexico*, Report No. 53/01, Case 11. 565, 4 April 2001, para. 27.

[59] OAS Treaty Series, No. 67.

privacy and recognition of their dignity.[60] The Commission's decision against
Mexico is consistent with its findings in the Report on the Situation of Human
Rights in Haiti under the Raoul Cedras Administration. The Commission
determined that rape and abuse of Haitian women were violations of their
right to be free from torture and inhuman and degrading treatment, and of
their right to liberty and security of the person.[61]

Consistently with the Inter-American Commission, the European Court of
Human Rights has found that the rape and ill-treatment of a 17-year-old
woman of Kurdish ethnicity by Turkish government security forces while she
was in detention constituted torture and inhuman and degrading treatment.[62]
The Committee against Torture, the committee established to monitor state
compliance with the Convention against Torture and other Cruel and Inhuman
or Degrading Treatment or Punishment[63] is increasingly vigilant about the
application of this Convention where there are frequent allegations of using
rape and other forms of sexual violence as forms of torture and ill-treatment.[64]

The Inter-American Commission on Human Rights settled a case against
the government of Peru for the rape of a young woman by a doctor employed
by the state public health system and her subsequent denial of justice by the
courts.[65] In the Settlement, the government acknowledged the wrong done to
the young woman and agreed to take appropriate steps to resolve her case and
prevent the occurrence of similar cases. The government agreed to inform
the Peruvian Medical Association about the doctor's violation of the young
woman's integrity so that the Association may proceed with appropriate professional sanctions against him. Peru also agreed to pay for the victim's rehabilitation in the form of housing, land, social assistance, health care associated
with the rape, and the means by which she could start a small micro-business.

4.1.3.2. *Denial of abortion services (including following rape)*

The Human Rights Committee addressed the inhuman and degrading nature
of maternal death from unskilled abortion in considering a report submitted
by the government of Peru under the Political Covenant. When examining

---

[60] Para. 52.

[61] Inter-American Commission on Human Rights, *Report of the Situation of Human Rights in Haiti* (Washington, DC: IACHR, 1995), OEA/Ser.L/V/II.88/Doc 10 at 93–7.

[62] *Aydin v. Turkey*, 25 EHRR 251 (1997) (European Court of Human Rights).

[63] UN, *Convention against Torture and Other Cruel and Inhuman or Degrading Treatment or Punishment* (New York: UN, 1984), GA Res. 39/46, annex, 39 UN GAOR Supp. (No. 51) at 197, UN Doc. A/39/51, entered into force 26 June 1987.

[64] UN, Committee against Torture, *Conclusions and Recommendations on Indonesia* (New York: UN, 2001), CAT/C/XXVII/Concl. 3 at para. 7(f); C. Benninger-Budel, *Violence against Women: 10 Reports/Year 2000* (Geneva: World Organization Against Torture, 2000).

[65] *Marina Machaca v. Peru*, Friendly Settlement of 6 Mar. 2000, Inter-American Commission Case 12.041 reported in S. Tuesta, *The Search for Justice* (Lima: Movimiento Manuela Ramos, 2000), 43–8.

what the country had done to bring its laws, policies, and practices into compliance with the Covenant, the Committee addressed the human rights of women, including the rights denied them by Peru's restrictive criminal abortion law. In its Concluding Observations, the Committee expressed its concern 'that abortion gives rise to a criminal penalty even if a woman is pregnant as a result of rape and that clandestine abortions are the main cause of maternal mortality' in Peru.[66] The Committee found that the restrictions of the criminal law subjected women to inhuman treatment. Moreover, the Committee explained that this aspect of the criminal law was possibly incompatible with the rights of men and women to enjoyment of other rights set forth in the Covenant. The Committee said this would include women's right to life, since men could request medical care of a life- or health-endangering condition without fear that they or their care-providers would face criminal investigation and prosecution.

The Committee recommended that 'necessary legal measures should be taken to ensure compliance with the obligations to respect and guarantee the rights recognised in the Covenant' (para. 19). Moreover, the Committee explained that the 'provisions of the Civil and Penal Codes [of Peru] should be revised in light of the obligations laid down in the Covenant', particularly the right of women to equal enjoyment of the rights under the Covenant (para. 22). The requirement that a country conform to human rights standards, if necessary by amending national laws, shows that governments can be expected to comply with the duties their countries have assumed to protect rights relating to reproductive and sexual health.

A state is responsible, at a minimum, to require its health care providers and facilities to ensure women's reasonable access to safe abortion and related health services, as its law permits. Moreover, where a national law that strictly penalizes abortion is shown to result in inhuman treatment of women and undue maternal mortality, the state can be obliged to consider legal reform so that its law complies with human rights standards for women's health and dignity. A new national policy could be expressed in law that more adequately balances limitations on abortion with women's several rights relating to safe and humane access to health services necessary to protect their lives and dignity, to their security in health and to be free from inhuman and degrading treatment.

4.1.3.3. *Involuntary sterilization*

The Inter-American Commission on Human Rights has recently settled a case against the government of Peru, brought on behalf of an indigent woman

---

[66] UN, Human Rights Committee, *Concluding Observations on Peru* (New York: UN, 1996), UN Doc. CCPR/C/79/Add. 72 at para. 15.

who was sterilized against her will, which procedure ultimately caused her death.[67] Peru accepted that the then government had committed violations of the right to humane treatment, the right to life, and the right to equal protection of the law, and of the obligation to respect rights without discrimination for reasons of sex, social origin, economic status, birth, or any other social condition variously protected by the American Convention on Human Rights, the Additional Protocol to this Convention in the Area of Economic, Social and Cultural Rights, the Inter-American Convention on the Prevention, Punishment and Eradication of Violence against Women, and the Convention on the Elimination of All Forms of Discrimination against Women.

4.1.3.4. *Denial of adequate medical treatment*

Decisions of human rights courts and tribunals are beginning to import notions of health into the content and meaning of the right to be free from inhuman and degrading treatment. That is, courts are increasingly requiring states to ensure that health services are provided when their denial would be inhuman and degrading. The Human Rights Committee has held that denying a prison inmate adequate medical treatment for his mental condition constitutes inhuman treatment and a denial of respect for the right to liberty and inherent dignity of his person.[68] The European Court of Human Rights has held that a governmental deportation of a person at an advanced stage of terminal AIDS back to his own country, where he would have no hope of receiving appropriate care, would constitute inhuman treatment.[69]

Accordingly, a state might be held bound to ensure provision of appropriate treatment for AIDS patients, essential obstetric care, and treatment for obstetric fistulae or unsafe abortion, because lack of such provision could constitute inhuman treatment and denial of respect for the inherent dignity of women. Care could provide for a woman's access to medically indicated treatment, which may include services to treat a high-risk pregnancy, and to terminate pregnancy safely where her life or continuing health, including mental health and social well-being, are at risk.

4.1.3.5. *Sexuality*

As has been explained in Chapter 2, human sexuality serves more than the purpose of reproduction. It enhances human bonding, spousal or partner attraction, intimacy, affection and fidelity, and social stability, thereby maximizing

---

[67] *Maria Mamérita Mestanza Chávez v. Peru*, Case 12.191, Decision on Admissibility, 3 Oct. 2000 (Inter-American Commission on Human Rights), settlement 14 Oct. 2002.

[68] *Williams v. Jamaica*, Comm. No. 609/1995, UN Doc. CCPR/C/61/D/609/1995, 17 Nov. 1997 (UN Human Rights Committee).

[69] *D v. United Kingdom* (1997), 24 EHRR 423 (European Court of Human Rights). Contrast *Karara v. Finland* (1998), European Commission on Human Rights, Application No. 40900/98, 29 May 1998, available at http: //hudoc.echr.coe.int/hudoc

human development and security. Rights relating to sexuality include the right to liberty and security of the person, the right to private and family life, the right to health, and the right to non-discrimination on grounds of sexual orientation.[70] To date, the courts have generally addressed the issue of sexuality as a negative right, under the right to private life. That is, criminalizing private sexual conduct between consenting adults of the same sex is a violation of the right to private life[71] (see below, Sect. 4.2.1), and also the right to non-discrimination on grounds of sexual orientation[72] (see below, Sect. 4.4.6). Some courts have found, however, that particularly exploitive, degrading, or violent sexual practices, such as incest and sado-masochism, are unlawful, even though there might be some degree of consent to such acts.[73]

The reason for addressing sexuality primarily under the right to be free from inhuman and degrading treatment is that sexuality is inherent in being human, and prohibition of private expressions of sexuality denies individuals' rights of being fully human. Courts have yet to apply the right to be free from inhuman and degrading treatment in a comprehensive way, but recent work in sexuality might enrich their means to do so.[74] It has been observed that 'Sex refers to the sum of biological characteristics that define the spectrum of humans as females and males.'[75] This observation is derived from biology, which characterizes animal and plant life by reference to sex. Lower animals have sex only for purposes of reproduction. In contrast, human sexuality and sexual behaviour are manifest when reproduction is not possible, or not intended, and after pregnancy has been achieved. Sexuality is a distinctively human characteristic, since

Sexuality refers to a core dimension of being human which includes sex, gender, sexual and gender identity, sexual orientation, eroticism, emotional attachment/love, and

[70] J. D. Wilets, 'International Human Rights Law and Sexual Orientation', *Hastings Int. and Comparative L. Rev.* 18 (1994), 1–120; International Gay and Lesbian Association (ILGA)—Europe Region, *Equality for Lesbians and Gay Men: A Relevant Issue in the EU Accession Process* (Brussels: IGLA—Europe, 2001).

[71] *Dudgeon v. United Kingdom* (1981), 4 EHRR 149 (European Court of Human Rights); *Norris v. Ireland* (1988) 13 EHRR 186 (European Court of Human Rights); *Modinos v. Cyprus* (1993) 16 EHRR 485 (European Court of Human Rights); *Toonen v. Australia* UN GAOR, Human Rights Committee, 15th Sess., Case 488/1992, UN Doc CCPR/C/D/488/1992, Apr. 1994 (UN Human Rights Committee).

[72] *Toonen v. Australia* (see n. 71).

[73] *R. v. Brown*, [1993] 2 All ER 75 (House of Lords, England).

[74] See, generally, *Symposium Issue on Sexuality, Reproductive Health Matters*, 6/12 (1998); S. T. Fried, *Annotated Bibliography: Sexuality and Human Rights* (New York: International Women's Health Coalition, 2002), available at www.iwhc.org, last accessed 9 May 2002.

[75] Pan American Health Organization WHO, *Promotion of Sexual Health: Recommendations for Action—Proceedings of a Regional Consultation Convened by PAHO/WHO in Collaboration with the World Association for Sexology, Antigua Guatemala, Guatemala, May 19–22, 2000* (Washington, DC: PAHO, 2001), available in English at http://www.paho.org/English/HCP/HCA/PromotionSexualHealth.pdf, and in Spanish at http://www.paho.org/Spanish/HCP/HCA/salud_sexual.pdf, last accessed 14 Apr. 2002.

reproduction. It is experienced or expressed in thoughts, fantasies, desires, beliefs, attitudes, values, activities, practices, roles, relationships. Sexuality is a result of the interplay of biological, psychological, socio-economic, cultural, ethical and religious/ spiritual factors. While sexuality can include all of these aspects, not all of these dimensions need to be experienced or expressed. However, in sum our sexuality is experienced and expressed in all that we are, what we feel, think and do.[76]

Further it has been observed that:

Sexual health is the experience of the ongoing process of physical, psychological, and socio-cultural well being related to sexuality. Sexual health is evidenced in the free and responsible expressions of sexual capabilities that foster harmonious personal and social wellness, enriching individual and social life. It is not merely the absence of dysfunction, disease and/or infirmity. For sexual health to be maintained it is necessary that the sexual rights of all people be recognized and upheld.[77]

Accordingly, denying or obstructing means of achieving sexual health, that is, 'well being related to sexuality', may constitute treatment that is inhuman in negating individuals' human character and dignity.

4.2. *Rights relating to reproductive self-determination and free choice of maternity*

Rights relating to reproductive self-determination and free choice of maternity have been developed through interrelated rights, including the right to decide the number and spacing of one's children, the right to private and family life, the right to marry and to found a family, and rights requiring maternity protection. The exercise of these rights needs to be examined in the contexts in which individuals live, whether it be the family, community, or cultural contexts. Some community and cultural norms, and laws governing family formation, relations, and dissolution offend women's rights and make it difficult for them to exercise their reproductive rights.[78]

4.2.1. *The right to decide the number and spacing of one's children and the right to private and family life*

The Women's Convention, Article 16(1), states:

States Parties shall take all appropriate measures to eliminate discrimination against women in all matters relating to marriage and family relations and in particular shall ensure, on a basis of equality of men and women . . .

---

[76] Ibid.   [77] Ibid.
[78] United Nations Special Rapporteur on Violence Against Women, *Cultural Practices in the Family that are Violent toward Women* (New York: UN, 2002), E/CN/.4/2002/83; United Nations Special Rapporteur on Violence against Women, *Violence against Women in the Family* (New York: UN, 1999), E/CN/.4/1999/68.

(*e*) The same rights to decide freely and responsibly on the number and spacing of their children and to have access to the information, education and means to enable them to exercise these rights . . .

The Political Covenant, Article 17(1), states: 'No one shall be subjected to arbitrary or unlawful interference with his privacy, family, home or correspondence . . .'.

The right to decide the number and spacing of one's children and the right to private and family life are protected by various international and regional human rights treaties and by various national constitutions. For example, the 1998 Constitution of Ecuador provides that: 'The State shall guarantee the right of persons to decide on the number of children they want to conceive, adopt, maintain and educate. It is the obligation of the State to inform, educate and provide means that contribute to the exercise of this right.'[79] The right to decide on the number and spacing of one's children is not specifically protected in the more historical constitutions, but the right to private and family life is usually applied by national courts to protect an individual's right to reproductive self-determination.

The implementation of such rights, however formulated, reduces state power to compel individuals to account to governmental officers for their reproductive choices, and to compel individuals to employ their reproductive capacities in compliance with governmental preferences. Free choice of maternity is increasingly recognized as an attribute of private and family life, in order that individuals may propose whether, when, and how often to have children, without governmental control, accountability, or coercion. The common approach now is that choices on reproductive practice and health, including maternity, are private decisions between consenting partners, not democratic or governmental decisions. Accordingly, women may in principle protect their health in reproduction by determining whether and when to plan pregnancy.

Governments may propose to influence reproductive choices through incentives and moderate disincentives, but cannot apply compulsion or coercive means, such as by punishments or inflictions of harm to individuals' enjoyment of their lives.

4.2.1.1. *Denial of contraceptive sterilization*

It has been argued that the denial of voluntary sterilization for contraceptive purposes violates the right to private life.[80] Some countries, such as

[79] Article 39, the Constitution of the Republic of Ecuador, 11 Aug. 1998.
[80] M. Rutkiewicz, 'Towards a Human Rights-Based Contraceptive Policy: A Critique of Anti-Sterilization Law in Poland', *European J. of Health Law*, 8 (2001), 225–42.

Argentina[81] and Poland,[82] prohibit sterilization for contraceptive purposes. Such restrictive laws can have the effect of denying individuals their right to private life, including their right to decide the number and spacing of their children. Prohibiting voluntary sterilization for contraceptive purposes would be particularly burdensome for individuals for whom this is the only feasible contraceptive method.

4.2.1.2. *Choice of termination of unintended pregnancy*

The issue of choice of termination of unplanned or health-endangering pregnancy remains problematic in many countries. Governmental agents such as police officers have powers of inquiry and investigation where criminal abortion is suspected that may prevail over human rights of privacy. Women are often deterred from seeking health care when they know that governmental officers, including police officers, could gain access to their health care information. The deterrent effect on women is especially strong when others' knowledge of their pregnancy, or possible pregnancy, risks their exposure to discrimination or disadvantage. They may fear, for instance, loss of personal and family reputation where pregnancy outside marriage is stigmatized, and subjection to personal violence, which in some cultures, notwithstanding prohibitive law, may go so far as to accommodate or only lightly punish a so-called 'honour killing'. Further, a premature end to a pregnancy of which those bound or disposed to notify police officers are aware may expose a woman, and perhaps others close to her, to investigation on suspicion of unlawfully inducing abortion.

4.2.1.3. *Putative father's veto*

Courts respecting women's choices on pregnancy and childbirth have relied on rights to private life to prevent potential fathers, whether married or unmarried, from forcing women to bear children against their will. The European Commission has held that a husband could not veto his wife's lawful abortion and force her to endure pregnancy against her will.[83] This decision gives priority to a wife's right of decision with respect to childbearing over a husband's right to family life in the birth of his child. Husbands' rights do not include the right even to be consulted about abortion, because wives' rights of confidentiality and privacy prevail. This reasoning supports the argument that a state

[81] Penal Code of Argentina, Law No. 11,719, text codified by Decree No. 3992, 21 Dec. 1984, Articles 90–2, as cited in CRLP and Estudo para la Defensa de los Derechos de la Mujer (DEMUS), *Women of the World: Laws and Policies Affecting their Reproductive Lives: Latin America and the Caribbean* (New York: CRLP, 1997), 24.
[82] Polish Criminal Code 1997, Article 156, sec. 1, as cited in Rutkiewicz, 'Towards a Human-Rights Based Policy'.
[83] *Paton v. United Kingdom* (1980), 3 EHRR 408 (European Commission on Human Rights).

can have no greater interest in the birth of a child than a husband or biological father. As a result, the state has little if any power to prevent women's choice about whether and when to have a child, or women's full exercise of their right to private and family life.[84] A state is free to manifest its professed commitment to prenatal life in positive ways that are consistent with women's privacy rights, such as by provision of prenatal care and nutritional supplements for pregnant women.

A study of maternal mortality in Nepal indicates how the right of women to privacy is not sufficiently protected by prevailing practices regarding decisions to seek health care. The Nepalese study demonstrates that the husband is the most frequent decision-maker in whether to seek hospital maternity care,[85] and that delay in seeking care is a contributing factor to maternal deaths. The husband alone made the decision to seek care in 42.5 per cent of all families that sought hospital care, and the husband and family of the husband together made the decision in 39.1 per cent of the cases. In only 11.5 per cent of cases did maternal family members make the decision. The Nepalese experience suggests that a great deal of effort is needed to educate husbands and wives and their families on the importance of seeking maternity care promptly, and the importance of respecting the woman's decision to seek care promptly when she feels in need of assistance.

4.2.1.4. *Same sex intimacy*

The right to private life has been applied numerous times by the European Court of Human Rights, and in one case before the UN Human Rights Committee, to void laws criminalizing homosexual conduct between consenting male adults.[86] The Human Rights Committee explained that 'it is undisputed that adult consensual sexual activity in private is covered by the concept of "privacy"',[87] and that the instigator of the case 'is actually and currently affected by the continued existence' of laws prohibiting same sex intimacy between consenting adults.[88]

The Committee specifically rejected the contention that laws prohibiting same-sex intimacy can be justified on public health grounds by explaining that:

criminalization of homosexual practices cannot be considered a reasonable means or proportionate measure to achieve the aim of preventing the spread of HIV/AIDS. The Government of Australia observes that statutes criminalizing homosexual activity tend to impede public health programmes 'by driving underground many of the people at risk of infection'. Criminalization of homosexual activity thus would appear to run

---

[84] R. J. Cook, 'International Protection of Women's Reproductive Rights', *New York University Journal of International Law and Politics*, 24 (1992), 645–727 at 706.

[85] Family Health Division, Dept. of Health Services, Ministry of Health, Nepal, *Maternal Mortality and Morbidity Study* (Kathmandu: Ministry of Health, 1998), at p. ii.

[86] *Toonen v. Australia* (see n. 71).   [87] Ibid., para. 8.2.   [88] Ibid.

counter to the implementation of effective education programmes in respect of HIV/ AIDS prevention. Secondly, the Committee notes that no link has been shown between the continued criminalization of homosexual activity and the effective control of the spread of the HIV/AIDS virus.[89]

The Committee also explained that its members cannot accept that 'moral issues are exclusively a matter of domestic concern, as this would open the door to withdrawing from the Committee's scrutiny a potentially large number of statutes interfering with privacy'.[90]

4.2.2. *The right to marry and to found a family*

The Political Covenant, Article 23, states:

1. The family is the natural and fundamental group unit of society and is entitled to protection by society and the State.
2. The right of men and women of marriageable age to marry and to found a family shall be recognised.
3. No marriage shall be entered into without the free and full consent of the intending spouses.
4. States Parties to the present Covenant shall take appropriate steps to ensure equality of rights and responsibilities of spouses as to marriage, during marriage and at its dissolution. In the case of dissolution, provision shall be made for the necessary protection of any children.

The obligations of states to protect the family are found in many human rights treaties (see Pt. III, Ch. 4). Wording similar to that of Article 23(1) of the Political Covenant is found in Article 18 of the African Charter, requiring protection of the family. The exact wording of Article 23(1) is repeated in Article 17(1) of the American Convention. Article 23(2) is slightly revised in Article 17(2) of the American Convention, to read: 'The right of men and women of marriageable age to marry and to raise a family shall be recognized . . .'.

Article 10(1) of the Economic Covenant stresses the importance of states ensuring protection and assistance for the 'establishment' of the family and for 'the care and education of dependent children'. It reads: 'The widest possible protection and assistance should be accorded to the family, which is the natural and fundamental group unit of society, particularly for its establishment and while it is responsible for the care and education of dependent children. Marriage must be entered into with the free consent of the intending spouses.'

The Women's Convention stresses the importance of equal rights within the family. Article 16 reads:

(1) States Parties shall take all appropriate measures to eliminate discrimination against women in all matters relating to marriage and family relations and in particular shall ensure, on a basis of equality of men and women:

---

[89] Ibid., para. 8.5.   [90] Ibid., para. 8.6.

180   *Medical, Ethical, and Legal Principles*

    (*a*) The same right to enter into marriage;
    (*b*) The same right to choose a spouse and to enter into marriage only with their free and full consent;
    (*c*) The same rights and responsibilities during marriage and at its dissolution . . .

(2) The betrothal and marriage of a child shall have no legal effect, and all necessary action, including legislation, shall be taken to specify a minimum age for marriage and to make the registration of marriages in an official registry compulsory.

The right to marry and found a family is not always absolute, and may be circumscribed by, for example, laws against incestuous unions and particularly on legal minimum ages of marriage. Laws setting a legal minimum age of marriage, if implemented, can help to ensure that young women are of sufficient age and maturity to be able voluntarily to consent to marriage, and to avoid the physical health risks of premature childbearing and the mental health consequences of early marriage.

Research shows that, while many countries have set a legal minimum age of marriage, governments generally do not provide the resources or the leadership for their effective implementation.[91] They could do this, for instance, through a requirement of marriage licensing dependent on submission of evidence of age, such as dated certificates of birth. This is relevant to the case, for instance, in India, where marriage registration is not legally required.[92] In its Concluding Observations on the report of the government of India, submitted under the Political Covenant, the Human Rights Committee explained that:

While acknowledging measures taken to outlaw child marriages (Child Marriage Restraint Act) [this 1929 Act sets the minimum age of marriage at 18 for girls and 21 for boys], . . . the Committee remains gravely concerned that legislative measures are not sufficient and that measures designed to change the attitudes which allow such practices [child marriages] should be taken . . . The Committee therefore recommends that the Government take further measures to overcome these problems. . . .[93]

The Committee's concern about child marriages entered 'without free and full consent of the intending spouses' is underscored by a study in Rajasthan, India, which explained that:

Even today, mass child marriage ceremonies arranged by parents, where hundreds of boys and girls wed each other, are very common. The mean age at marriage for women (16.1 years) is among the lowest in the country. Once the girl goes to her marital home, it is her duty to beget a child as soon as she can. . . . Forcing early

    [91] UNICEF, *Early Marriage: Child Spouses* (Florence: UNICEF Innocenti Research Centre, 2001), 4–5.
    [92] J. Sagade, 'Socio-Legal and Human Rights Dimensions of Child Marriage in India', doctoral thesis, Faculty of Law, University of Toronto, 2002, 117–18.
    [93] UN, Human Rights Committee, *Concluding Observations on India* (New York: UN, 1997), UN Doc. CCPR/C/79/Add.81, at para. 16.

pregnancies and motherhood on teenage girls under the banner of social custom and family is tragic.[94]

The tragedy of child marriages is not unique to Rajasthan. CEDAW expressed similar concerns in its Concluding Observations on the report of Nepal in noting that:

traditional customs and practices detrimental to women and girls, such as child marriage, dowry, polygamy, deuki (a tradition of dedicating girls to a god or goddess, who become 'temple prostitutes', which persists, despite the prohibition of the practice by the Children's Act), badi (the ethnic practice of forcing young girls to become prostitutes) and discriminatory practices that derive from the caste system are still prevalent.[95]

4.2.2.1. *'The family is entitled to protection by society and the State'*

There is significant scope for the right to marry and to found a family to be applied to advance women's reproductive integrity and safe motherhood, because this right imposes positive obligations on the state to protect the right. State authorities can be liable for not providing vulnerable women and girls with effective protection against the acts of private individuals that jeopardize the integrity of family life, such as by requiring daughters to be surrendered to them in payment of debts, as has been known in some regions of the world.[96] Courts of law are, of course, public authorities, and obliged to apply and develop the law consistently with national constitutions and human rights treaties binding their states. Where state officials do not constrain those who arrange marriages of children under the legal age of marriage, or against the will of one of the parties to the marriage, the government would be accountable for the violation of such individuals' right to enter into marriage with their free and full consent.

The human right to family life is seriously jeopardized by neglect of the needs of women to receive reproductive, including maternity, care when they are at risk of maternal death or disability. In addition, the rights to family life of children and fathers are prejudiced due to the harmful impact of mothers' deaths on the potential of surviving infants, children, and other family members to lead healthy lives. Children of women who die following childbirth are 'three to ten times more likely to die within two years than those with both

---

[94] V. Pendse, 'Maternal Deaths in an Indian Hospital: A Decade of (No) Change?', *Safe Motherhood Initiatives: Critical Issues. Reproductive Health Matters*, special edition (1999), 119–26.

[95] UN, Committee on the Elimination of Discrimination against Women, *Concluding Observations on Nepal* (New York: UN, 1999), UN Doc. CEDAW/C/1999/L.2/Add.5, at para. 37.

[96] A. Armstrong, 'Consent and Compensation: The Sexual Abuse of Girls in Zimbabwe', in W. Ncube (ed.), *Law, Culture, Tradition and Children's Rights in Eastern and Southern Africa* (Aldershot: Ashgate, 1998), 129–49.

living parents'.[97] Preservation of maternal health and prevention of maternal death are so central to the enjoyment of family life that they are part of the human rights entitlements not only of women but also of children and husbands.

4.2.2.2. *Marriageable age*

The right to marry and to found a family available to persons of 'marriageable age' may be applied to achieve the desirable result of adolescent girls marrying later, giving them more choice over the age at which they have children. The expression 'marriageable age' in Article 23(2) of the Political Covenant needs to be interpreted in light of the Children's Convention. Article 1 of that Convention explains that 'a child means every human being below the age of eighteen unless, under the law applicable to the child, majority is attained earlier'.

National family laws have traditionally set ages at which adolescents could marry without parental consent, and even over parental objection. This age often coincided with the general age of majority (traditionally 21 but now commonly 18). A lower age was also set at which adolescents could marry provided that their parents consented, or 'emancipated' them. In addition, laws often had an exception allowing an underage girl to marry if she was pregnant, in order that her child would be legitimate at birth.

An objection to parental consent laws is that they protect marriages the parents arrange. Daughters may accept the arrangements as an act of obedience to their parents rather than of emotional commitment to their husbands and to raising their own children. Accordingly, the better view may be that the reference in legal provisions to 'marriageable age' not be taken to refer to the minimum age of marriage with parental consent, but to the age of marriageability without the legal requirement of emancipation by parents.

This view is reinforced by the health advantages, for both mothers and children, of marriages not being undertaken before adolescent girls have achieved sufficient physical maturity to bear pregnancy and deliver safely, and the emotional and intellectual maturity for self-care, child-care, and resort to necessary assistance. Physical maturity can be approximately related to a chronological age, but this age may not be as reliably related to emotional and intellectual maturity.

4.2.2.3. *Health and social effects of child marriage*

The Human Rights Committee and other treaty monitoring bodies could benefit significantly from the work of women's health specialists in adding

[97] A. Starrs, *The Safe Motherhood Action Agenda: Priorities for the Next Decade. Report on the Safe Motherhood Technical Consultation, Colombo, Sri Lanka, 18–23 October 1997* (New York: Family Care International, 1998), 16.

content and meaning to an understanding of 'marriageable age'. For example, a serious health dysfunction of early marriage and childbearing is younger girls' vulnerability to suffer different forms of obstetric fistulae. A fistula is a maternal disability arising from obstructed labour that has been reported particularly in Africa and Asia.[98] It has been explained that:

an obstetric fistula is a hole which forms in the vaginal wall communicating into the bladder (vesico-vaginal fistula—VVF) or the rectum (recto-vaginal fistula—RVF) or both (recto-vesico-vaginal fistula RVVF), as a result of prolonged and obstructed labour . . . The immediate consequences of such damage are urinary incontinence, faecal incontinence if the rectum is affected, and excoriation of the vulva from the constantly leaking urine and faeces. Secondary amenorrhoea is a frequently associated problem. Women who have survived prolonged obstructed labour may also suffer from local nerve damage which results in difficulty in walking, including foot drop.[99]

The social stigma resulting from obstetric fistulae can be devastating to those who cannot obtain prompt surgical repair. It has been explained that:

The social consequences of these physical disabilities are severe. Most victims of obstructed labour in which the fistula subsequently occurred will also have given birth to a stillborn baby. In some areas, a high percentage of fistulae occur during the first pregnancy. Women who live in cultures where childlessness is unacceptable will therefore suffer from this fact alone. As long as they are incontinent of urine they are also likely to be abandoned by their husbands on whom they are financially dependent, and will probably be ostracised by society.[100]

Moreover, in many situations, 'social isolation compounds the woman's own belief that she is a disgrace and has brought shame on her family. Women with VVF often work alone, eat alone, use their own plates and utensils to eat and are not allowed to cook for anyone else. In some cases they must live on the streets and beg.'[101]

The denial of the right to enjoy marriage and to found a family that failure to prevent and remedy this condition causes is obvious from the history of women who suffer it. States need to ensure that adolescent girls are of sufficient physical maturity for marriage and childbearing. Once adolescent girls are married, states need to ensure that they obtain the necessary health care to survive pregnancy and delivery. In the event of complications, such as obstetric fistulae, states are obliged to ensure that women quickly obtain necessary surgical treatment in order that they may create and enjoy their families.

[98] WHO, *Obstetric Fistulae: A Review of Available Information* (Geneva: WHO, 1991), WHO/MCH/MSM/91.5.
[99] Ibid. at 3.   [100] Ibid.
[101] M. Bangser, B. Gumodoka, and Z. Berege, 'A Comprehensive Approach to Vesico-Vaginal Fistula: A Project in Mwanza, Tanzania', *Reproductive Health Matters* (1999), 157–65 at 158.

4.2.2.4. *Free and full consent*

The burden falls on those employing state authority, whether by enacting legislation or by taking executive or judicial action, to ensure that entry into marriage relationships conforms to human rights standards concerning voluntary choice to marry.

The Committee on Economic, Social and Cultural Rights (CESCR), in its Concluding Observations on the report from Suriname, recommended that 'the laws permitting persons to marry without the acknowledgement or consent of the partner be abolished'.[102] In its Concluding Observations on the report of Cameroon, CESCR also deplored 'the lack of progress made by the Government in combating . . . the forced early marriage of girls'.[103]

Significantly, the National Court of Justice of Papua New Guinea decided in favour of a girl who wanted to continue her education and find a job, over her family's opposition, instead of being married involuntarily.[104] In so doing, the Court declared unconstitutional the 'head pay' custom of providing young women for marriage or other employment in victims' families as part of legitimate compensation for causing accidental deaths.

The Court's judgment is consistent with CEDAW's General Recommendation on Equality in Marriage and Family Relations.[105] This Recommendation makes the following observation on Article 16(1)(*a*) and (*b*) of the Women's Convention:

A woman's right to choose a spouse and enter freely into marriage is central to her life and to her dignity and equality as a human being. An examination of States parties' reports discloses that there are countries which, on the basis of custom, religious beliefs or the ethnic origins of particular groups of people, permit forced marriages or remarriages. Other countries allow a woman's marriage to be arranged for payment or preferment and in others women's poverty forces them to marry foreign nationals for financial security. Subject to reasonable restrictions based for example on a woman's youth or consanguinity with her partner, a woman's right to choose when, if, and whom she will marry must be protected and enforced at law.

This Recommendation has been echoed in HRC's General Comment 28, on Equality of Rights between Men and Women, which explains that:

States are required to treat men and women equally in regard to marriage in accordance with article 23. . . . Men and women have the right to enter into marriage only with

---

[102] UN, Committee on Economic, Social and Cultural Rights, *Concluding Observations on Suriname* (New York: UN, 1995), UN Doc. E/C 12/1995/6, para. 16.

[103] UN, Committee on Economic, Social and Cultural Rights, *Concluding Observations on Cameroon* (New York: UN, 1999), UN Doc. E/C.12/1/Add. 40, para. 14.

[104] *Re Miriam Willingal* (10 Feb. 1997), MP No. 289 of 1996 (unreported), digested in *Commonwealth Human Rights Law Digest* 2 (1998) 57 (National Court of Justice, Papua New Guinea).

[105] UN, Committee on the Elimination of Discrimination against Women, 'General Recommendation 21, Equality in Marriage and Family Relations', *International Human Rights Instruments*, 173.

their free and full consent, and States have an obligation to protect the enjoyment of this right on an equal basis. Many factors may prevent women from being able to make the decision to marry freely. One factor relates to the minimum age for marriage. That age should be set by the State on the basis of equal criteria for men and women. These criteria should ensure women's capacity to make an informed and uncoerced decision. A second factor in some States may be that either by statutory or customary law a guardian, who is generally male, consents to the marriage instead of the woman herself, thereby preventing women from exercising a free choice. (see Pt. III, Ch. 6, Sect. 4, para. 23)

4.2.3. *The right to maternity protection*

The Economic Covenant, Article 10(2), states: 'Special protection should be accorded to mothers during a reasonable period before and after childbirth . . .'.

The exact wording of Article 10(2) of the Economic Covenant, above, is also found in Article 27(1) of the 1992 Constitution of Ghana. Other examples of national constitutional rights relating to family life that require the protection of motherhood include Article 10 of the 1980 Constitution of the Arab Republic of Egypt, which provides that '[t]he State shall guarantee the protection of motherhood'. Brazil's 1988 Constitution explains in Article 6 that protection of motherhood is a social right under the Constitution.

The special contribution that women make to society through maternity and motherhood is recognized in many national constitutions and human rights documents. Under Article 5(*b*) of the Women's Convention, States Parties agree to take all appropriate measures: '[t]o ensure that family education includes a proper understanding of maternity as a social function'. The Universal Declaration of Human Rights in Article 25(2), addressing health and well-being, explains that 'Motherhood and childhood are entitled to special care and assistance.' The American Declaration similarly recognizes that '[a]ll women, during pregnancy and the nursing period . . . have the right to special protection, care and aid'.[106] Through Article 15 of the Protocol on Economic, Social and Cultural Rights to the American Convention, states agree to 'provide special care and assistance to mothers during a reasonable period before and after childbirth'.

Under Article 24(*d*) of the Children's Convention, States Parties commit themselves to ensure appropriate prenatal and postnatal care for mothers. Article 12(2) of the Women's Convention requires provision of free maternity services where necessary: 'States Parties shall ensure to women appropriate

---

[106] Organization of American States (OAS), *American Declaration of the Rights and Duties of Man, 1948 Article VII*; OAS Res. XXX, adopted by the Ninth International Conference of American States, 1998, reprinted in Organization of American States, *Basic Documents Pertaining to Human Rights in the Inter-American System* (Washington, DC: OAS, 1992), OEA/Ser.L.V/ II.82, doc. 6, rev. 1 at 17.

services in connexion with pregnancy, confinement and the post-natal period, granting free services where necessary, as well as adequate nutrition during pregnancy and lactation.' Where services that are appropriate for pregnancy, confinement, and the postnatal period are not provided, States Parties might be encouraged to take steps to provide these services in order that they are in compliance with Article 12(2) of the Women's Convention and Article 24(2) of the Children's Convention (see Pt. I, Ch. 7, Sect. 3.4).

Necessary though these provisions are, their focus tends to link protection of women's health to motherhood and care of infants and children, reinforcing a perception that protection of women's health is an instrumental means of serving children, rather than an inherent right for women to enjoy for themselves. Whatever the motivation is for such provisions, they do obligate states to ensure that motherhood is safe. Legal research is needed to show if and how these provisions have been or could be applied to ensure that women are adequately protected during pregnancy.

4.2.4. *The right to maternity protection during employment*

The Economic Covenant, Article 10(2), states: 'Special protection should be accorded to mothers during a reasonable period before and after childbirth. During such period working mothers should be accorded paid leave or leave with adequate social security benefits.'

The maternal health of women during employment has been an objective of the International Labour Organization (ILO) since its establishment in 1919. The Maternity Protection Convention, No. 3 (1919)[107] was among the first instruments to be adopted. The 1919 Convention stipulates in Article 3(*c*) that the pregnant woman is entitled to free attendance by a doctor or qualified midwife.

In 1952, this Convention was revised[108] to take into consideration developments in national law and practice. The 1952 Convention, Convention No. 103, began to reflect the increasing participation of women in the workforce, as well as rising social expectations regarding the rights of women during their childbearing years, particularly with respect to a growing commitment to eliminate discrimination in employment. The 1952 Convention provides in Article 4(1) for the material support of mother and child through financial benefits and medical care. Article 4(3) explains that medical care includes 'prenatal, confinement and postnatal care by qualified midwives or medical practitioners as well as hospitalisation care where necessary; freedom of choice of doctor

---

[107] ILO, *Convention Concerning the Employment of Women before and after Childbirth* (Geneva: ILO, 1919), ILO Convention C3, 38 UNTS 53, entered into force 13 June 1921, revised in 1952.
[108] ILO, *Convention Concerning Maternity Protection (revised)* (Geneva: ILO, 1952), ILO Convention C103, 214 UNTS 321, entered into force 7 Sept. 1955.

and freedom of choice between a public and private hospital' where applicable. The Maternity Protection Recommendation, No. 95 (1952),[109] provides further guidance on the health protection of employed women with regard to conditions of work, such as the prohibition of work prejudicial to the health of mother and child.

Article 1 of the 1952 Convention suggests that its provisions apply to 'women employed in industrial undertakings and in non-industrial and agriculture occupations, including women wage earners working at home'. However, the provisions of national laws defining the scope of persons to whom the maternity protections apply vary widely from country to country. Even so, a survey of legislation indicates that the scope of women whose maternity protection is covered in most countries approaches or exceeds that prescribed by the Convention, and is moving towards broad coverage for all employed women.[110] Women are generally covered across the industrial and non-industrial sectors, and in both the private and public sectors.[111] However, significant gaps still exist with respect to the agricultural sector, as well as to part-time workers, homeworkers, domestic workers, and casual, contract, and temporary workers.[112] While these gaps are decreasing, much remains to be done to ensure that legal protection available in principle becomes effective in practice.

The 1952 Convention was further revised by the Maternity Protection Convention (Revised), 2000.[113] In addition, the 1952 Recommendation was revised in 2000.[114] These revisions were undertaken, in part, to reflect the growing commitment to eliminate discrimination in the workforce. Through all of these conventions and their accompanying recommendations, member states are obligated to devote attention to the health aspects of maternity protection, since they state that women have the right to medical care as well as to financial benefits.

4.3. *Rights relating to health and the benefits of scientific progress*

4.3.1. *The right to the highest attainable standard of health*

The Economic Covenant, Article 12, states:

---

[109] ILO, *Recommendation Concerning Maternity Protection No. 95* (Geneva: ILO, 1952), ILO Recommendation R95. ILO, *International Labour Conventions and Recommendations*, ii (Geneva: ILO, 1996), at 44.

[110] ILO, *Report V(1): Maternity Protection at Work—Revision of the Maternity Protection Convention (Revised), 1952 (No. 103)* (Geneva: ILO, 1952), Recommendation, 1952 (No. 95).

[111] Ibid. [112] Ibid. at 29.

[113] ILO, *Convention Concerning Maternity Protection (Revised), 2000* (Geneva: ILO, 2000), ILO Convention C183.

[114] ILO, *Maternity Protection Recommendation, 2000* (Geneva: ILO, 2000), ILO Recommendation R191.

1. The States Parties to the present Covenant recognise the right of everyone to the enjoyment of the highest attainable standard of physical and mental health.

2. The steps to be taken by the States Parties to the present Covenant to achieve the full realization of this right shall include those necessary for:

(*a*) The provision for the reduction of the stillbirth-rate and of infant mortality and for the healthy development of the child;

(*b*) The improvement of all aspects of environmental and industrial hygiene;

(*c*) The prevention, treatment and control of epidemic, endemic, occupational and other diseases;

(*d*) The creation of conditions which would assure to all medical service and medical attention in the event of sickness.

The right to health is also protected by regional and other international human rights instruments (see Pt. III, Ch. 4), as well as by various national constitutions. The Constitution of the Federative Republic of Brazil is particularly clear in providing that: 'Health is the right of all and the duty of the State and shall be guaranteed by social and economic policies aimed at reducing the risk of illness and other maladies and by the universal and equal access to all activities and services for its promotion, protection and recovery.'[115]

The CESCR General Comment on Health significantly develops the content of the right (see Pt. III, Ch. 6, Sect. 3). It provides guidance to countries on what they are required to do to comply with this right. The General Comment explains that the right to health contains interrelated features of *availability*, *accessibility*, *acceptability*, and *quality* (see Pt. III, Ch. 6, Sect. 3, para. 12). The Comment provides the following.

Availability of services requires that a state ensures that functioning public health and health care facilities, goods and services, and essential drugs are available in sufficient quantity. While the General Comment recognizes that the precise nature of the services will vary according to country, it requires that the public health services need to consider the underlying determinants of health.

Accessibility of services has four overlapping dimensions:

• Non-discrimination: health services must be accessible to all, especially the most vulnerable or marginalized sections of the population, in law and fact, without discrimination on any of the prohibited grounds.

• Physical accessibility: health facilities and services must be within safe physical reach for all parts of the population, especially for vulnerable or marginalized groups, such as ethnic minorities and indigenous populations, women, children, adolescents, persons with disabilities, and persons with HIV/AIDS.

---

[115] Brazilian Constitution, 5 Oct. 1988, as amended to 4 June 1998, Art. 196.

- Economic accessibility (affordability): health services must be affordable for all. Payments for health care services have to be based on the principle of equity, ensuring that these services, whether privately or publicly provided, are affordable for all, including socially disadvantaged groups.
- Information accessibility: accessibility includes the right to seek, receive, and impart information and ideas concerning health issues.

Acceptability requires that health services are ethically and culturally appropriate, i.e. respectful of the culture of individuals, minorities, peoples, and communities, and sensitive to gender and life-cycle requirements, as well as being designed to respect confidentiality and improve the health status of those concerned.

Quality requires that health facilities' services must be scientifically and medically appropriate and of good quality. This requires, *inter alia*, skilled medical personnel, scientifically approved and unexpired drugs, and hospital equipment.

The World Health Organization (WHO) is developing indicators to determine how fully the substantive elements of the right to health services, namely their availability, accessibility, acceptability, and quality, are satisfied. Laws and policies that unreasonably restrict health services according to these criteria would not comply with this right. For instance, a law or policy requiring unnecessary qualifications for health service providers might limit the availability of a service that contributes to safe motherhood. Examples of such policies are those that require excessive qualifications for health service providers to perform Caesarean deliveries, and that require several specialists to determine satisfaction of criteria for lawful termination of pregnancy. Such policies may be proposed in good faith in order to ensure excellence in women's health care. However, it is poor policy, and may be a human rights violation where health services are jeopardized, to allow the excellent to be the enemy of the good, or the good the enemy of the adequate. The standard of provision should be of adequacy, rising to excellence when possible, rather than of uncompromising but occasional excellence that dysfunctionally denies many women the adequate care their health requires.

Some or all of the standards proposed in the CESCR's General Comment on Health and other general recommendations, such as the CEDAW General Recommendation on Women and Health and those arising out of the Cairo and the Beijing Conferences, are used to determine whether states are in compliance with treaty obligations or in violation. Much work is still required to apply the right to health care effectively so as to ensure the availability, accessibility, acceptability, and quality of reproductive and sexual health services in particular countries. Treaty monitoring bodies, through their Concluding Observations on country reports, have made some significant beginnings. For example, CESCR, in its Concluding Observation on a report by Gambia, explained that: 'Regarding the right to health in Article 12 of the [Economic] Covenant, the Committee expresses its deep concern over the extremely high maternal mortality rate of 1,050 per 100,000 live births. UNICEF identifies the main causes to be haemorrhage and infection related to the lack of access to [appropriate services] and poor services.'[116]

Studies have been undertaken to show how tribunals have addressed the general right to health in different countries, through Concluding Observations and through complaint procedures.[117] These kinds of analyses could similarly be undertaken regarding the right of women to maternity care in general and obstetric services in particular.

4.3.1.1. *Available resources and their fair allocation*

Under the Economic Covenant, states are required to take immediate and progressive steps to achieve specific health standards. States are judged on the extent to which they are moving toward 'the realization' of the right to the highest attainable standard of health. CEDAW's General Recommendation on Women and Health provides that: 'the duty to fulfil rights places an obligation on States parties to take appropriate . . . budgetary, economic and other measures to the maximum extent of their available resources to ensure that women realise their rights to health care' (see Pt. III, Ch. 6, Sect. 2, para. 17).

The Constitutional Court of South Africa has addressed the issue of whether the government is required, under the South African Constitution,[118] to provide long-term dialysis treatment for a claimant's chronic renal failure.[119] The Court found that the government is not so required, because the constitutional obligations regarding access to health care services, which include reproductive health care, 'are dependent upon the resources available for such purposes, and . . . the corresponding rights themselves are limited by reason of the lack of resources'.[120] The Court stated, however, that emergency services cannot be denied in situations where a person 'suffers a sudden catastrophe which calls for immediate medical attention'.[121]

---

[116] UN, Committee on Economic, Social and Cultural Rights, *Concluding Observations on Gambia* (New York: UN, 1994), UN Doc. E/C.12/1994/9 at para. 16.
[117] I. Boerefijn and B. Toebes, 'Health and Human Rights, Health Issues Discussed by the United Nations Treaty Monitoring Bodies', *Netherlands Institute for Human Rights, SIM* special issue, 21 (1998), 25–53.
[118] South African Constitution, section 27(3). Section 27 provides that: '(1) Everyone has the right to have access to—(*a*) health care services, including reproductive health care; . . . (2) The State must take reasonable legislative and other measures, within its available resources, to achieve the progressive realisation of these rights. (3) No one may be refused emergency medical treatment.'
[119] *Soobramoney v. The Minister of Health, KwaZulu Natal*, 1998 (1) SA 765 (Constitutional Court of South Africa).
[120] Ibid. at 771.   [121] Ibid. at 774.

A legal distinction is often drawn between the provision of 'extraordinary care', sometimes described as heroic measures, which may be of unproven effect and dependent upon scarce resources and specialized skills, and of 'ordinary care', which is of proven benefit and is routinely available.[122] Courts find no general duty to provide extraordinary care, but that governments and other health care service providers are required to maintain the availability of ordinary care. The Constitutional Court of South Africa treated the chronic renal failure case as concerning extraordinary care, and so found no duty of provision. In contrast, the Constitutional Court of South Africa has found that anti-retroviral treatment for pregnant women to resist mother-to-child HIV transmission, which was routinely available in some provinces, is ordinary care, which should therefore be available to all pregnant women.[123]

Thus, it would seem that under legal systems such as in South Africa, women seeking essential obstetric care or other forms of life-saving treatment such as treatment for an incomplete abortion, have a right of reasonable access to treatment, in the same way that pregnant women with HIV/AIDS have access to anti-retroviral treatment.[124]

A state's willingness in principle to give effect to women's rights to health and safe motherhood may be deterred by the fear that full implementation will have indeterminate economic consequences for the national health budget. A finding in a World Bank study, however, has 'estimated that providing a standard "package" of maternal and new-born health services would cost approximately $3 per person per year in a developing country; maternal health services alone could cost as little as $2 per person'.[125]

The same World Bank study has also found that family planning and maternal health services are the most cost-effective governmental health interventions, in terms of death and disability prevented.[126] When a mother dies, the economy loses her productive contribution to the workforce, her community loses the domestic and wider caring services of a vital member, and her death puts others around her at risk and impaired capacity to function in social, employment, and other roles. Studies have shown that, when their mother dies, the surviving children are three to ten times more likely to die within two years than children that live with both of their parents.[127]

The study also explains that the savings resulting from investing in maternal health and reduction of maternal morbidity are significant.[128] The population

[122] *Re Quinlan* (1976), 355 Atlantic Reporter 2d 647, 664 (New Jersey Supreme Court).
[123] *Treatment Action Campaign* (see n. 42).
[124] C. Ngwena, 'AIDS in Africa: Access to Health Care as a Human Right', *South African Public Law*, 15/1 (2000), 1–25.
[125] A. Starrs, *Safe Motherhood*, 17, based on a presentation by A. Tinker, 'Safe Motherhood as an Economic and Social Investment', Safe Motherhood Technical Consultation in Sri Lanka, 18–23 Oct. 1997, Colombo, Sri Lanka.
[126] Ibid.   [127] Ibid. at 16.   [128] Ibid. at 15–16.

will have fewer poor women, and the workforce will be healthier and therefore capable of higher productivity. Reducing maternal mortality and morbidity reduces household poverty, and benefits the health system. Moreover, preventative care may save money when its result is that there are fewer sick women. Practical and economically viable solutions to the problem of maternal death and sickness include the purchase of a community ambulance to ensure prompt treatment of pregnancy complications, where resources exist for fuel and maintenance of an ambulance, or financial help is available to a community to cover emergency transport costs.

Women whose governments have failed to address their basic obstetric needs in the allocation of health resources in a fair and transparent way may be able to ground a complaint in the right to procedural fairness in administrative decision-making. Courts are slowly applying the right to procedural fairness to require that health benefits are allocated equitably, or at least are not denied in an unfair or arbitrary way.[129] For example, the European Court of Human Rights has found that a sickness allowance should not be withdrawn, unless the recipient is given a fair hearing.[130] This decision could be applied to require the restoration of reproductive and sexual health services where they have been withdrawn in an unfair and arbitrary way, and governmental explanation and justification of policies that disfavour reproductive and sexual health services against other health expenditures or budgetary allocations. Further, since in the world's prevailing global economy few if any countries exercise full fiscal sovereignty, governments may be amenable to international persuasion and inducement to invest in such services compatibly with their human rights undertakings.

4.3.1.2. *Health sector reform*

The CESCR General Comment on the Right to Health explicitly requires states 'to ensure that privatization of the health sector does not constitute a threat to the availability, accessibility, acceptability and quality of health facilities, goods and services' (para. 35). Moreover, the Comment specifically requires governmental members of international financial institutions to ensure that lending policies and credit agreements ensure respect of the right to health (see Pt. III, Ch. 6, Sect. 3, para. 39).

Some health sector reform initiatives have instituted user fees for health services in order to cover the partial cost of health care. Health sector reform advocates explain that there is a need to raise revenues to be available for health care, but also that user fees might help to prevent selfish or irrational use of publicly funded health services. Moreover, there is a perceived need to

---

[129] V. Leary, 'Justiciability and Beyond: Complaint Procedures and the Right to Health', *International Commission of Jurists Review*, 55 (1995), 105 at 115.

[130] *Feldbrugge v. The Netherlands* (1985), 8 EHRR 149 (European Court of Human Rights).

impress upon users of health services that their use has economic costs. Paying from their own pockets is believed to bring this reality home to them, and to cause them to question whether their request for services is based on a real health need, or is rather a frivolous indulgence at others' expense that they will not allow at their own. There is a market-based perception that people exercise rationality in expenditure of their own resources that they do not exercise in expenditure of others' or of public resources, and that cost-effective utilization of resources can be achieved by imposition of user fees for services.

What effect the imposition of user fees would have on resort to reproductive and sexual health services among poor people in developing countries is uncertain and problematic, particularly regarding whether such fees would deter or prevent poor people's resort to necessary care. A study on safe motherhood funded by the UK Department for International Development and the WHO reported in 1999 that '[t]he paucity of relevant global, let alone local, information on cost poses a challenge to maternal health planners and managers in developing countries, for in the development of health financing schemes, programme costs are critical'.[131] Evidence following removal of user fees by the post-apartheid government elected in South Africa in 1994 'suggests that gains in maternal health care . . . have been relatively modest', and that more deliveries within health facilities and improvements in the quality of services are also required to reduce maternal and perinatal mortality.[132]

Contrasting evidence has come from other countries experimenting with general user fees, including Kenya. A review of maternity services there has observed that:

Cost is known to affect both uptake and delays in seeking care. The GOK [Government of Kenya] introduced cost-sharing in 1989 for specific services, but excluding promotive and preventive services, which includes antenatal care . . . Evidence from other developing countries indicates a direct decline in utilisation of maternity services linked with the introduction of user fees, and this will need to be monitored in Kenya. Fees appear to vary from facility to facility, but generally women are charged in proportion to the service rendered. A caesarean section for example, is more expensive than a normal delivery. This appears logical in terms of the health service inputs but may also be an important deterrent for poor women seeking care.[133]

The inability of impoverished families to pay for the full range of reproductive and sexual health services available only by payment appears evident. When

[131] E. Weissman, O. Sentumbwe-Mugisa, A. K. Mbonye, and C. Lissner, 'Costing Safe Motherhood in Uganda', *Reproductive Health Matters* (1999), 85–91.

[132] H. Schneider and L. Gibson, 'The Impact of Free Maternal Health Care in South Africa', ibid. 93–101 at 100.

[133] W. J. Graham, F. S. Murray, and C. Taylor, 'A Question of Survival: I. A Review of Safe Motherhood in Kenya: II. Two Years after the Review: Accomplishments, Hurdles and Next Steps', ibid. 102–16 at 108.

medical services are themselves free of charge, however, poverty may remain an obstacle to reproductive and sexual health care. It has been observed that:

Even when formal fees are low or nonexistent, there can be other costs that deter women from seeking care. These costs may include transport, accommodation, drugs, and supplies, as well as informal or under the table fees that may be imposed by health staff. When women lack control over resources and are dependent on others to provide funds, fees of any kind can be a serious obstacle to their use of services.[134]

Proposed options to overcome economic barriers to access to health services include making medical services free of charge, having means-related sliding fees, insurance schemes based on community membership, or, for instance, employment and community trust fund or loan schemes, each with advantages and disadvantages concerning coverage and effectiveness.

In responding to the problem of economic barriers to reproductive and sexual health services and to economic conditions that aggravate ill-health and unsafe practices, governments are accountable under the Economic Covenant for denials of the right to the highest attainable standard of health that are due to individuals' poverty. Moreover, Article 12(2) of the Women's Convention, addressing maternity services, requires states to grant 'free services where necessary'. Accordingly, governments will have to explain whether and, if so, to what extent measures of standards of health attainable in their countries include the factors of personal poverty and of national options in the allocation of economic and other resources (see below, Sect. 4.4.1).

4.3.2. *The right to the benefits of scientific progress*

The Economic Covenant, Article 15(1)(b), states: 'The States Parties to the present Covenant recognise the right of everyone . . . [t]o enjoy the benefits of scientific progress and its applications.'

The right to enjoy the benefits of scientific progress and its application has yet to be effectively applied to require governments to give high priority to conducting reproductive health research, including biomedical, social science, and legal research, or to apply the findings of this research. The right could be invoked, for instance, where, for religious or political reasons, women are denied access to drugs that pharmaceutical science has made effective for emergency contraception or for non-surgical abortion (see below, Sect. 4.5.3). The same right may be invoked, although probably with more difficulty, where reproductive and sexual health services are not financially or geographically accessible to individuals who are at high risk of reproductive or sexual ill-health.

The right to the benefits of scientific progress can also support the claim that governments should spend public funds on research designed to benefit

[134] Starrs, *Safe Motherhood*, 42.

reproductive and sexual health. The modern history of ethical regulation of research involving human subjects originated in the trial of physicians who conducted inhumane experiments on vulnerable subjects, including inmates of concentration camps, to serve military and scientific interests in the Second World War. Their trial before the International War Crimes Tribunal in Nuremberg resulted in the 1947 Nuremberg Code on research involving human subjects, which invoked concepts of human rights to prohibit non-consensual medical experimentation. The subsequent decades saw reinforcement of protections against improper medical experimentation in a series of international human rights conventions. Under this inspiration, medical research recovered its moral standing, and its benefits came to be almost universally recognized. In the 1980s it began to be perceived, however, that women were not participating equitably in these benefits.

Human rights protections had been implemented by rigorously excluding women of reproductive age from research initiatives, in order to guard against injuring unborn children. Their exclusion was also economic, since it was costly to have sufficiently large-scale studies to achieve statistically valid data on women of reproductive age at every stage of their menstrual cycle. The effect, however, was that women's health was not seriously studied, except regarding fertility. The health-related factors that predisposed women to reproductive ill-health and morbidity, other than fertility itself and its control, were under-researched.

In the 1980s it came to be realized, however, that women had been denied their collective human right to benefits of progress in medical science. Reversing the Nuremberg-influenced perception that individuals would be protected by their exclusion from medical studies, women's groups showed that women's health protection depended on scientific research, and that exclusion of research on women's health from governmental funding constituted discrimination. Women allied themselves with AIDS activists to require the conduct of medical research, to address and remedy causes of mortality and morbidity of special concern to them. They pointed to states' legal commitments to respect women's rights 'to enjoy the benefits of scientific progress and its applications'.

Health care providers can accordingly rely on this right to argue for governmental funding to achieve equity in the recruitment of members of both sexes into reproductive and sexual health studies. Medical researchers may also invoke this right when seeking public funding for the studies they want to conduct. Similarly, research agencies, health research centres, and, for instance, governmental health departments should remember human rights responsibilities to pursue the goal of reproductive and sexual health through sponsorship and support of appropriate scientific studies. These should include not only biomedical studies, but also epidemiological or public health research, health systems research, and social science and legal research that could expose and remedy underlying causes of reproductive and sexual ill-health.

4.4. *Rights to non-discrimination and due respect for difference*

The Political Covenant, Article 2(1), states: 'Each State Party to the present Covenant undertakes to respect and to ensure to all individuals within its territory and subject to its jurisdiction the rights recognised in the present Covenant, without distinction of any kind, such as race, colour, sex, language, religion, political or other opinion, national or social origin, property, birth or other status.'

This Article is reinforced by Articles 3 and 26 of the Political Covenant. Article 3 requires states to 'undertake to ensure the equal right of men and women to the enjoyment of all civil and political rights set forth' in the Covenant. Article 26 requires that:

All persons are equal before the law and are entitled without any discrimination to the equal protection of the law. In this respect, the law shall prohibit any discrimination and guarantee to all persons equal and effective protection against discrimination on any ground such as race, colour, sex, language, religion, political or other opinion, national or social origin, property, birth or other status.

Article 26 requires states to act against discrimination in all fields of civil and political rights and also of economic, social, and cultural rights, including health. States are also obligated to eliminate laws, policies, and practices that discriminate on specified and unspecified ('other status') grounds. It is therefore necessary to examine the ways in which states ensure that they eliminate discrimination on grounds of race, colour, sex, national, or social origin. These are not the only prohibited grounds of discrimination that are risk factors for reproductive and sexual ill-health. The phrase 'other status' would include such prohibited grounds of discrimination as age, rural residence, and poverty, which can affect individuals' ability to exercise their rights.

While each of these forms of discrimination can be addressed separately, in practice they often overlap. For instance, sex discrimination is frequently aggravated by discrimination on grounds of marital status, race, age, health status, disability, rural residence, and class. Multiple and thus compounding forms of discrimination often leave women of young age, of minority racial groups, and of lower socio-economic status living in rural areas the most vulnerable to the risk of poor reproductive and sexual health. Treaty monitoring bodies are requiring states to address compounding forms of discrimination, whether they be sex and marital status (see Pt. III, Ch. 6, Sect. 4, para. 19), sex, race, colour, language, religion, political or other opinion, national or social origin, property, birth, or other status (see Pt. III, Ch. 6, Sect. 4, para. 30), sex and race (see Pt. III, Ch. 6, Sect. 5, paras. 1–5), and sex and disability.[135]

States are obligated to change laws that discriminate on their face, or in their effect. An example of a law that is discriminatory on its face is a law that requires married women, but not men, to obtain the authorization of their spouses in order to access health services. States are also required to remedy the discriminatory effects of laws that are equal on their face but disproportionately disadvantage one group. Such laws include those that require everyone to pay the same for health care, but that leave services unaffordable by people not in paid employment, such as single mothers who care for dependent children, and single or widowed women who live in cultures where women are not employable outside the home, and cannot earn more than the lowest wage for domestic service. Another example of a policy that is superficially neutral but has a disproportionately harmful impact on women's health interests is a law that denies adolescents reproductive health information and services without parental consent. Such a policy will leave girls, but not boys, at risk of pregnancy. Where laws or policies treat men and women differently with respect to their health needs, whether on the face of such laws or policies or in their effect, states are required to provide reasons, and often compelling justifications, for such differential treatment, since disadvantage due to different treatment or different effects amounts to discrimination.

The general right to non-discrimination requires that we treat the same interests without discrimination, for example, providing all races with equal access to health care. However, the right to non-discrimination also entails treating significantly different interests in ways that adequately respect those differences. The right to sexual non-discrimination requires that societies treat different biological interests, such as in pregnancy and childbirth, in ways that reasonably accommodate those differences. National courts and international tribunals that have been vigilant in applying the right to non-discrimination to require treatment of the same interests without discrimination are beginning to require that states treat differently situated persons according to those legitimate differences. For example, the European Court of Human Rights has recognized that:

The Court has so far considered that the right under Article 14 [of the European Convention on Human Rights] not to be discriminated against in the enjoyment of the rights guaranteed under the Convention is violated when States treat differently persons in analogous situations without providing an objective and reasonable justification . . . However, the Court considers that this is not the only facet of the prohibition of discrimination in Article 14. The right not to be discriminated against

---

[135] UN, Committee on Economic, Social and Cultural Rights, 'General Comment 5: Persons with Disabilities' (1994), *International Human Rights Instruments*, 66–76, para. 19.

. . . is also violated when States without an objective and reasonable justification fail to treat differently persons whose situations are significantly different.[136]

The CEDAW General Recommendation on Women and Health requires that states apply the right to non-discrimination to protect women's distinct interests in reproductive health, such as their distinctive needs to prevent pregnancy, to treat the consequences of unwanted pregnancy, and the needs of safe pregnancy and childbirth.

States are obligated to eliminate not only their own discriminatory practices, but also those of private individuals in all spheres. For example, courts have supported a government's use of its authority to license professionals to require that they provide professional services to under-served populations.[137] Governments can therefore use their authority to make it a condition of licensure of health care professionals that they perform a portion of their licensed services in the interests of social justice, such as by serving for limited times in public hospitals or clinics that provide services to groups that have historically been subject to discrimination.

4.4.1. *Sex and gender*

The Women's Convention, Article 1, states:

the term 'discrimination against women' shall mean any distinction, exclusion or restriction made on the basis of sex which has the effect or purpose of impairing or nullifying the recognition, enjoyment or exercise by women, irrespective of their marital status, on a basis of equality of men and women, of human rights and fundamental freedoms in the political, economic, social, cultural, civil or any other field.

The Women's Convention emphasizes the need to confront the different causes of women's inequality by addressing 'all forms' of discrimination that women suffer. Legal prohibitions cover discrimination on grounds both of sex, which is a biological characteristic, and of gender, which is a social, cultural, and psychological attitude that identifies particular acts or functions only or primarily with one sex, such as religious leaders being male and nurses female. Article 1 of the Women's Convention is reinforced by Article 3 of the Political Covenant. Article 3 requires that: 'The States Parties to the present Covenant undertake to ensure the equal right of men and women to the enjoyment of all civil and political rights set forth in the present Covenant.'

The General Comment on Equality Rights between Men and Women makes clear that Article 26 of the Political Covenant (on the rights to equality before the law and equal protection of the law) requires states to act against discrimination in all spheres of civil, political, economic, social, and cultural

---

[136] *Thlimmenos v. Greece* (2001) 31 EHRR 15, para. 44 (European Court of Human Rights).
[137] *Van der Mussele v. Belgium* (1983) EHRR 163 (European Court of Human Rights).

rights (see Pt. III, Ch. 6, Sect. 4). States are therefore obligated to eliminate all forms of discrimination against women in respect of all rights, for example to life, to family and private life, and to the highest attainable standard of health.

The devastating paradox of many societies' observance of human rights is that they discriminate against women where differences between the sexes should not matter, but ignore the distinction where it is critical. States often discriminate against women's access to educational, political, spiritual, economic, and other opportunities, where sexual difference in capacity for insight, intelligent application of knowledge, compassion, and creative initiative is inconsequential, while ignoring women's vital need for appropriate treatment in maternal health care. If political, professional, religious, and other influential institutions could be inspired to put the effort into respecting women's distinctive needs for reproductive health care that they have historically put into discriminating against women in areas where sexual differences should not matter, considerable advancement would be achieved towards reproductive health.[138]

The prohibition of both sex and gender discrimination obligates states to eliminate sexual stereotyping, which requires initiatives for redressing popular assumptions, such as that responsibility to guard against unwanted pregnancy rests with the couple's female partner. Sexual equality requires that men accept responsibility with women to take measures against unwanted pregnancy and sexually transmitted diseases. In many societies, unmarried motherhood is stigmatizing in ways that unmarried fatherhood is not, and requirements of proof of virginity in eligibility for marriage apply only to females.

Equality requires that we not only treat the same interests without discrimination, for example in access of all young people to education irrespective of race, sex, or class, but that we also treat different interests in ways that adequately respect those differences, such as women's distinct interests in access to prenatal care, care during delivery, and postnatal care. Rights to due respect of sexual difference are violated when health services fail to accommodate the fundamental biological differences in reproduction, as evidenced by the 515,000 women each year who die, often preventably, of pregnancy-related causes.[139]

4.4.1.1. *Sex and gender non-discrimination in the family*

International tribunals have held governments accountable for unequal treatment of women in regard to their right to enjoy family life. The Human Rights Committee has required a state to alter its laws that disadvantaged female citizens by subjecting their foreign husbands' residency and citizenship to

---

[138] R. J. Cook, 'Human Rights Law and Safe Motherhood', *European J. of Health Law*, 5 (1998), 357–75.

[139] WHO and UNICEF, *1995 Estimates of Maternal Mortality* (Geneva: WHO, 2000).

review and refusal while not similarly subjecting that of foreign wives of male citizens. Legal reform has been required in order to ensure equality of women and men with respect to family life.[140] States have also been put on notice to change differential legal ages of marriage, in part because they stereotype women into childbearing and unpaid or low-paid service roles and can disproportionately prejudice their health (see above, Sect. 4.2.2).

In its Concluding Observations on the report of Mexico, the Committee on the Rights of the Child (CRC) expressed its concern that:

the minimum legal ages for marriage of boys (16) and girls (14) in most of the states of the State party are too low and that these ages are different for boys and girls. This situation is contrary to the principles and provisions of the Convention [on the Rights of the Child] and constitutes a form of gender-based discrimination which affects the enjoyment of all rights. The Committee recommends that the State party undertake legislative reform, both at the federal and state levels, to raise and equalize the minimum legal ages for marriage of boys and girls.[141]

CEDAW has addressed how patriarchy, meaning male dominance or leadership, is embedded in many national laws. In its Concluding Observations on the report of Guatemala, CEDAW explained that: 'the legal provision according to which the husband remained the head of the family and a woman needed the husband's permission to take up outside activities was contrary to the provisions of the Convention and extended the patriarchal system'.[142]

Several governments are placing promotion of gender equality in the mainstream of many of their activities and concerns. For example, Nepal has improved the living standards of women at the grass-roots level by facilitating their access to commercial loans from Mothers Groups' bank accounts. Through training, women developed leadership and communication skills that enabled them to make decisions among options in life for themselves. This was the first step in equipping them with the ability to decide freely and in an informed manner how many children to bear, and how closely spaced their pregnancies should be.[143]

4.4.1.2. *Sex and gender non-discrimination in health*

Women's right to equal access to necessary health care, including maternity care, is recognized in Article 12 of the Women's Convention, by which states agree to:

[140] *Aumeeruddy-Cziffra et al. v. Mauritius*, Comm. No. 35/1978, UN Doc. A/36/40 (1981) (United Nations Human Rights Committee).
[141] UN, Committee on the Rights of the Child, *Concluding Observations on Mexico* (New York: UN, 1999), para. 16. UN Doc. CRC/C/15/Add. 112.
[142] UN, Committee on the Elimination of Discrimination against Women, *Concluding Observations on Guatemala* (New York: UN, 1994), para. 71. UN Doc. A/49/38.
[143] UN Population Fund (UNFPA), *Promoting Gender Equality in Population and Development Programmes: Best Practices and Lessons Learned* (New York, UNFPA, 1999) at 5.

1. . . . take all appropriate measures to eliminate discrimination against women in the field of health care in order to ensure . . . access to health care services, including those related to family planning.

2. . . . ensure to women appropriate services in connexion with pregnancy, confinement and the post-natal period, granting free services where necessary, as well as adequate nutrition during pregnancy and lactation.

The content and meaning of this Article has been elaborated in CEDAW's General Recommendation on Women and Health, which includes the observation that:

Studies such as those which emphasize the high maternal mortality and morbidity rates worldwide and the large numbers of couples who would like to limit their family size but lack access to or do not use any form of contraception provide an important indication for States parties of possible breaches of their duties to ensure women's access to health care. (see Pt. III, Ch. 6, Sect. 2, para. 17)

This General Recommendation specifies the information that CEDAW requires reporting states to present on such breaches and on steps taken to achieve remedies. It emphasizes rights of access to confidential family planning services, and notes that: 'In particular, States parties should ensure the rights of female and male adolescents to sexual and reproductive health education by properly trained personnel in specially designed programmes that respect their rights to privacy and confidentiality' (see Pt. III, Ch. 6, Sect. 2, para. 18).

The Recommendation requires that state reports 'must demonstrate that health legislation, plans and policies are based on scientific and ethical research and assessment of the health status and needs of women in that country and take into account any ethnic, regional or community variations or practices based on religion, tradition or culture' (see Pt. III, Ch. 6, Sect. 2, para. 9). It also calls on states to: 'Prioritize the prevention of unwanted pregnancy through family planning and sex education and reduce maternal mortality rates through safe motherhood services and prenatal assistance. When possible, legislation criminalizing abortion could be amended to remove punitive provisions imposed on women who undergo abortion' (see Pt. III, Ch. 6, Sect. 2, para. 31(*c*)).

Ministries of Health concerned about ensuring compliance with the right to non-discrimination in access to health services will need to assess the different ways in which women's rights might be violated in the health care context. Governments have already been put on notice about their failure to reform laws and policies that discriminate against women, such as policies that require women requesting health services to obtain the authorization of their husbands. For example, the CEDAW Concluding Observation on the report of Indonesia explained that laws requiring a married woman to secure her husband's authorization to obtain certain reproductive health services, even in emergency situations, are discriminatory and not in accordance with the Women's Convention.[144]

CEDAW asks states to identify the 'test by which they assess whether women have access to health care *on a basis of equality between men and women* in order to demonstrate compliance with Article 12' (emphasis in the original; see Pt. III, Ch. 6, Sect. 2, para. 19). States are required to report on 'the impact that health policies, procedures, laws and protocols have on women when compared to men'.

Treaty monitoring bodies have also signalled the importance of member states allocating resources fairly in ways that are appropriate to women's particular needs to go safely through pregnancy and childbirth. In its Concluding Observations on the report of Venezuela, for instance, CEDAW noted with concern: 'the reduction of health budgets, the rise in the maternal mortality rate, the lack of and limited access to family-planning programmes (especially for teenagers), and women's limited access to public health services. In addition, legislation that criminalized abortion, even in cases of incest or rape, remains in force.'[145]

CESCR, in its Concluding Observations on a report by Paraguay, expressed its concern about the inequitable distribution of health services between urban and rural areas, which resulted in higher rates of maternal mortality in the rural areas.[146] HRC has required a state to provide women with the same entitlements to social security benefits as men enjoy.[147] The same reasoning could be applied to require states to ensure equal access of men and women to health care appropriate to their needs.

4.4.2. *Marital status*

The Women's Convention requires that women exercise their rights 'irrespective of their marital status'. Articles 2 and 26 of the Political Covenant require the elimination of discrimination on grounds of marital status because they prohibit 'discrimination of any kind, such as . . . sex . . . or other status'. None the less, discrimination on grounds of marital status pervades practices, social attitudes, and laws of many countries, particularly in the area of family law, often called the law of personal status. The stigmatization experienced by women who are pregnant outside marriage, even when they become so through sexual assaults or abuse, may impair their access to care and to good

---

[144] UN, Committee on the Elimination of Discrimination against Women, *Concluding Observations on Indonesia* (New York: UN, 1998), para. 284. UN Doc. A/53/38.

[145] UN, Committee on the Elimination of Discrimination against Women, *Concluding Observations on Venezuela* (New York: UN, 1997), para. 236. UN Doc. A/52/38/Rev. 1.

[146] UN, Committee on Economic, Social, and Cultural Rights, *Concluding Observations on Paraguay* (New York: UN, 1996), para. 16. UN Doc. E/C.12/1/Add. 1.

[147] *Broeks v. The Netherlands*, Communications No. 172/1984, 42 UN GAOR, 1987, UN Doc. A/42/40 at 139 (United Nations Human Rights Committee).

quality in the care they receive, aggravating their vulnerability, for instance, to unsafe motherhood.

Many family and related laws were modelled on families founded according to conservative orthodoxies of legal marriage. Many countries retain legislated provisions, governmental practices, and, for instance, judicial rulings that privilege married couples over unmarried cohabiting, unpartnered, and same-sex partnered individuals. Increasingly, however, human rights entitlements of partners in unmarried unions and single mothers are gaining recognition. CEDAW has expressed its concern, for instance regarding the Dominican Republic, that '[d]iscriminatory provisions regarding unmarried women, as well as single mothers, persist in social security provisions and in land inheritance rights under the agrarian reform law'.[148]

4.4.3. *Age*

The Children's Convention, Article 2, states:

1. States Parties shall respect and ensure the rights set forth in the present Convention to each child within their jurisdiction without discrimination of any kind, irrespective of the child's or his or her parent's or legal guardian's race, colour, sex, language, religion, political or other opinion, national, ethnic or social origin, property, disability, birth or other status.
2. States Parties shall take all appropriate measures to ensure that the child is protected against all forms of discrimination or punishment . . .

Discrimination based on age is a common violation of women's reproductive rights.[149] Young women often suffer in communities that deny or impede the expression of natural adolescent sexuality. This fact takes on a heightened significance in light of the increased risk that premature pregnancy brings. It has been established that women who give birth before age 18 are three times more likely to die in childbirth than women aged over 18 years.[150]

While international law clearly protects children's rights to equal care with adults, young women's reproductive health services are often overlooked, and even opposed. The Children's Convention, which defines a child as a human being below the age of 18 years, provides in Article 24(1) that '[s]tates parties shall strive to ensure that no child is deprived of his or her right of access to . . . health care services'. The interdependence of mother and child is recognized in Article 24(2)(*d*), by which states agree to take measures '[t]o ensure appropriate pre-natal and post-natal care for mothers'. The full realization of these

[148] UN, Committee on the Elimination of Discrimination against Women. *Concluding Observations on Dominican Republic* (New York: UN, 1998), para. 332. UN Doc. A/53/38.
[149] C. A. A. Packer, 'Preventing Adolescent Pregnancy: The Protection Offered by International Human Rights Law', *Int. J. of Children's Rights*, 5 (1997), 47–76.
[150] World Bank, *World Development Report 1993: Investing in Health* (New York: Oxford University Press, 1993), 84–117.

rights is vital for the reduction of maternal mortality and morbidity, as well as for children's survival and health.

Laws that detract from girls' equality with boys often impede adolescent girls' access to protective health services and erode their control over their reproductive lives. Intellectually mature young women's vulnerability to age and sex discrimination is deepened when reproductive health services that females need are made available to them only on the condition of parental authorization, while it is available to adults without need for authorization. Mature adolescents suffer unjust discrimination when they are not free to obtain reproductive health counselling and services with the same confidentiality as adults. The Children's Convention requires that: 'States Parties shall respect the rights and duties of the parents and, when applicable, legal guardians, to provide direction to the child in the exercise of his or her right *in a manner consistent with the evolving capacities of the child*' (Article 14(2); emphasis added).

Modern courts tend to favour interpretation of laws on adolescents' legal powers that takes due account of 'the evolving capacities of the child'. Courts do not generally permit parents to veto their mature adolescent children's access to reproductive health services solely on grounds of minor age. Courts often determine that parental powers over their children are not absolute, but decrease as children's decision-making capacity advances, and parental choices can be overridden by the courts. A common judicial approach is to recognize that parental rights exist not for the benefit of the parents, third parties, or society, but for the benefit of the children. Laws equip parents to discharge their legal responsibilities to protect the best health and related interests of their children, but not to be arbitrary or to pursue their own religious or other convictions by risking their children's health or well-being.

Adolescents' disadvantages in resort to reproductive health counselling and services might be a reason why adolescents often report late for health services, for instance, for pregnancy or STIs. Adolescents may fear that they will not be afforded the same confidentiality as adult women seeking the same services. Many health service providers will recognize minors' rights to health care and confidentiality if the minors demonstrate intellectual and emotional maturity or emancipation. However, clinic policies or laws that set chronological age limits for types of care, and deny reproductive health services to adolescent girls that they are capable of requesting according to their evolving capacities, violate the Children's Convention.[151]

Human rights monitoring bodies are beginning to expose violations of the rights of adolescent girls. For example, the Committee on the Rights of the

---

[151] R. J. Cook and B. M. Dickens, 'Recognizing Adolescents' "Evolving Capacities" to Exercise Choice in Reproductive Health Care', *Int. J. Gynecol. Obstet.* 70 (2000), 13–21.

Child has expressed its concern 'about the relatively high maternal mortality rate, especially as it affects young girls' in Nicaragua. It also noted that clandestine abortions and teenage pregnancies appear to be a serious problem in the country.[152] The Committee recommended that 'the State party consider the possibility of focusing its attention on the organization of a more comprehensive and co-ordinated campaign in order to address the interrelated family and social-related problems of the high number of family separations, the relatively high maternal mortality rate and teenage pregnancies'.[153]

When addressing adolescent maternal deaths, investigators should examine the extent to which governments have implemented laws to protect women's interests, such as laws that prohibit child marriages. The age of marriage will often dictate a woman's ability to exercise choice over the timing of her pregnancies. Failure to enforce minimum marriage-age laws, and legal provisions and practices that condone child marriages, discriminate in effect against girls and women by denying them due protection of the law, so allowing early marriage and the risk of death inherent in premature pregnancy and childbirth.

4.4.4. *Race and ethnicity*

The Race Convention, Article 1, states:

the term 'racial discrimination' shall mean any distinction, exclusion, restriction or preference based on race, colour, descent, or national or ethnic origin which has the purpose or effect of nullifying or impairing the recognition, enjoyment or exercise, on an equal footing, of human rights and fundamental freedoms in the political, economic, social, cultural or any other field of public life.

There is increasing recognition of compounding or interlocking forms of discrimination, such as on grounds of both sex and race, in the area of health generally and reproductive and sexual health specifically. The Committee on the Elimination of Racial Discrimination (CERD) has recommended in its Concluding Observations on the report from Colombia that government programmes need to be more responsive to the needs of indigenous and Afro-Colombian women, explaining that they are subjected to multiple forms of discrimination based on sex, gender, race, or ethnicity, and often their displaced status.[154]

The South African Parliament recognized the contribution of a liberal abortion law to equality of the sexes and races in the country in the Preamble to South Africa's Choice on Termination of Pregnancy Act 1996. The first

---

[152] UN, Committee on the Rights of the Child, *Concluding Observations on Nicaragua* (New York: UN, 1995), para. 19. UN Doc. CRC/C/15/Add. 36.
[153] Ibid., para. 35.
[154] UN, Committee on the Elimination of Racial Discrimination, *Concluding Observations on Colombia* (New York: UN, 1999), para. 15. UN Doc. CERD/C/55/Misc.43/Rev. 3.

paragraph of the Preamble states that its provisions are enacted 'Recognising the values of human dignity, the achievement of equality, security of the person, non-racialism and non-sexism, and the advancement of human rights and freedoms which underlie a democratic South Africa.' The Human Rights Committee's General Comment on Equality Rights between Men and Women requires states to address how discrimination on grounds other than sex, such as race, religion or social origin, affects women (see Pt. III, Ch. 6, Sect. 4, para. 30). The CEDAW General Recommendation on Women and Health encourages states to address discrimination against particular subgroups of women (see Pt. III, Ch. 6, Sect. 2, paras. 6 and 12).

The Committee on the Elimination of Racial Discrimination, in its General Recommendation on the definition of racial non-discrimination, explains that it will consider any act to be discriminatory if it has an 'unjustifiable disparate impact upon a group distinguished by race, colour, descent, or national or ethnic origin'.[155] Its General Recommendation on Gender Related Dimensions of Racial Discrimination amplifies that explanation by requiring states to address:

the relationship between gender and racial discrimination, by giving particular consideration to:
  (*a*) the form and manifestation of racial discrimination;
  (*b*) the circumstances in which racial discrimination occurs;
  (*c*) the consequences of racial discrimination; and
  (*d*) the availability and accessibility of remedies and complaint mechanisms for racial discrimination. (see Pt. III, Ch. 6, Sect. 5, para. 5)

Racial discrimination manifests itself against women of ethnic or racial subgroups in a variety of ways and in different circumstances. These manifestations include a subgroup's poorer access to care and greater vulnerability to abuse and exploitation of their reproductive capacity and sexuality.[156] In many countries, both developing and developed, health status among population groups varies by race and ethnicity, indicating differential access to health care services, information, and education necessary for health protection. Statistics often show disparity in the risk of maternal death between majority and minority populations. In Australia, for instance, the aboriginal population is at up to ten times greater risk of maternal death than the non-aboriginal population.[157] Differences exist even where different racial populations live in the same cities,

---

[155] UN, Committee on the Elimination of Racial Discrimination, 'General Recommendation XIV, Article 1 (definition of racial nondiscrimination)', 1993, *International Human Rights Instruments*, 95–6, para. 2.

[156] T. Banks, 'Women and AIDS: Racism, Sexism and Classism', *New York University Review of Law and Social Change*, 17 (1988–9), 351.

[157] H. K. Atrash, S. Alexander, and C. J. Berg, 'Maternal Mortality in Developed Countries: Not Just a Concern of the Past', *Obstetrics and Gynecology*, 86 (1995), 700–5.

such as in the United States, where the black population has a relative risk of maternal death 4.3 times higher than the non-black population.[158]

Higher rates of reproductive ill-health can result from ethnically marginalized groups having poorer socio-economic status than mainstream communities, and less access to necessary health care. Some groups have genetic traits that can cause more acute problems, such as during pregnancy. For example, certain groups of black women and women from the Mediterranean region who have sickle cell anaemia suffer related difficult and painful problems during pregnancy, labour, and the post-partum period.[159] Sickle cell anaemia comes from a genetic trait that provides beneficial resistance to malaria, but also disposes women to higher risk of maternal morbidity and mortality. The particular health needs of these subgroups of women have to be addressed, and when they are not addressed, the neglect is increasingly seen as a compounded form of discrimination.

The potential to suffer abuse of rights is often greater among ethnic minorities, which suggests that great care and sensitivity need to be applied in the delivery of reproductive health and related services in mixed-race communities. It has been reported, for instance, that some indigenous women in Mexico do not seek delivery care for fear of being sterilized during delivery without their consent or knowledge.[160] The use of permanent or long-acting contraceptive methods without the recipients' free and informed consent has been reported in some countries. These methods may be offered or employed in ways that exploit the powerlessness, vulnerability, and subordinate status of racial minority populations. Control of reproduction in such communities in the United States, for instance, has been attempted through suspect means, such as courts offering minority-group, low-income women offenders early release from imprisonment on probation if they accept long-acting contraceptive implants.[161]

4.4.5. *Health status / disability*

Human rights conventions prohibit discrimination not only on specified grounds such as sex, race, and age, but also on open-ended grounds of 'other status', such as health status and disability. The CESCR through General Comment 14 on the Right to the Highest Attainable Standard of Health has

---

[158] Ibid.

[159] C. AbouZahr, 'Maternal Mortality Overview', in C. J. L. Muray and A. D. Lopez (eds.), *Health Dimensions of Sex and Reproduction* (Cambridge, Mass.: Harvard University Press, 1998), 111–64 at 150.

[160] Cited in A. Yamin and D. Maine, 'Maternal Mortality as a Human Rights Issue: Measuring Compliance with International Treaty Obligations', *Human Rights Quarterly*, 21 (1999), 563–607, 599.

[161] T. Lewin, 'Implanted Birth Control Device Renews Debate over Forced Contraception', *New York Times* (10 Jan. 1991).

interpreted 'other grounds' of prohibited discrimination to include physical and mental disability and health status, including HIV/AIDS (see Pt. III, Ch. 6, Sect. 3, para. 18).

The CESCR's General Comment on Persons with Disabilities adopts the following approach to disability: 'The term "disability" summarizes a great number of different functional limitations occurring in any population . . . People may be disabled by physical, intellectual or sensory impairment, medical conditions or mental illness. Such impairments, conditions or illnesses may be permanent or transitory in nature.'[162] It requires states that are party to the International Covenant on Economic, Social and Cultural Rights to take positive steps to reduce discrimination on grounds of disability.[163] Moreover, States Parties to the Convention on the Rights of the Child are specifically obligated through its Article 23 to address the needs of children with disabilities, including disabilities relating to their health status.

CEDAW has emphasized the need to avoid discrimination against high-risk women when developing national strategies for the prevention and control of HIV/AIDS. In its General Recommendation, CEDAW urges states that are parties to the Women's Convention to implement programmes to combat HIV/AIDS that: 'give special attention to the rights and needs of women . . . and to the factors relating to the reproductive role of women and their subordinate position in some societies which make them especially vulnerable to HIV infection'.[164]

As a result of the CESCR and CEDAW initiatives, the Cairo[165] and Beijing[166] documents and the International Guidelines on HIV/AIDS and Human Rights (see Pt. III, Ch. 7), governments have committed themselves to:

• eliminate discrimination against persons infected with HIV and against their families;
• strengthen services to detect HIV infection, making sure that they protect confidentiality; and
• devise special programmes to provide care and necessary emotional support to men and women affected by HIV/AIDS, as well as counsel their families and near relations.

The texts recognize that HIV infection in women often reflects women's preconditioning disability that, as women, they lack social and legal power to control whether, when, and with what protections they have sexual relations.[167]

---

[162] *International Human Rights Instruments*, para. 3.   [163] Ibid., paras. 8–12.
[164] UN, 'CEDAW General Recommendation 15 (1990): Avoidance of Discrimination against Women in National Strategies on HIV/AIDS', ibid. 109–10.
[165] Cairo Programme, para. 8.34.   [166] Beijing Platform, para. 108.
[167] Cairo Programme, para. 7.34; Beijing Platform, para. 99.

Non-discrimination rights of persons with disabilities, which exist not only for their protection against, for instance, sexual abuse, but also for their achievement of sexual satisfaction and health, present new frontiers for the advancement of human rights.

4.4.6. *Sexual orientation*

Non-discrimination law increasingly includes sexual orientation as a prohibited ground of discrimination. The UN Human Rights Committee explained that sex 'is to be taken as including sexual orientation',[168] and chose not to subsume sexual orientation under the term 'other status'.

With regard to equality in access to health care, the Committee on Economic, Social and Cultural Rights (CESCR) explains that the Economic Covenant prohibits 'any discrimination in access to health care and underlying determinants of health, as well as to means and entitlements for their procurement, on grounds of . . . sexual orientation . . . which has the intention or effect of nullifying or impairing the equal enjoyment or exercise of the right to health' (see Pt. III, Ch. 6, Sect. 3, para. 18). Denying individuals in same-sex relationships services that are necessary to protect their health and that are provided to partners in heterosexual relationships, discriminates against these individuals on grounds of their sexual orientation, offending human rights law. Human rights agencies may develop law and practice in this area, since medical care must be available on a basis of non-discrimination on the ground of sexual orientation. National human rights agencies have, for instance, recognized rights to screened sperm for medically assisted reproduction of unmarried women[169] and women in lesbian relationships.[170]

4.5. *Rights relating to information, education, and decision-making*

4.5.1. *The right to receive and to impart information*

The Political Covenant, Article 19, states:

2. Everyone shall have the right to freedom of expression; this right shall include freedom to seek, receive and impart information and ideas of all kinds, regardless of frontiers, either orally, in writing or in print, in the form of art, or through any other media of his choice.

3. The exercise of the rights provided for in paragraph 2 of this article carries with it special duties and responsibilities. It may therefore be subject to certain restrictions, but these shall only be such as are provided by law and are necessary:

---

[168] *Toonen v. Australia* (see n. 71), para. 8.
[169] *McBain v. Victoria, Commonwealth Human Rights Law Digest*, 3 (2000), 153 (Federal Court of Australia).
[170] *Korn v. Potter* (1996), 134 DLR (4th) 437 (British Columbia Supreme Court, Canada).

(a) For respect of the rights or reputations of others;
(b) For the protection of national security or of public order (*ordre public*), or of public health or morals.

The significance of information to reproductive health is reinforced by Article 10(*h*) of the Women's Convention, which requires that women have access to 'specific educational information to help to ensure the health and well-being of families, including information and advice on family planning'. None the less, in a number of countries it remains a criminal offence, sometimes described as a crime against morality, to spread information about contraceptive methods or to publicize where women can receive pregnancy termination services.[171]

Traditionally, the right to information has been understood to guarantee freedom to seek, receive, and impart information and ideas free from government interference. However, some commentators now argue that the right has evolved to the point where governments have concrete and immediate obligations to provide information that is necessary for the protection and promotion of reproductive health and choice, not just to refrain from interfering with its provision.[172] The claim that governments have positive duties to ensure access to information that is necessary for individuals to protect their health is increasingly supported by decisions of human rights tribunals.

The European Court of Human Rights has examined whether a national court injunction issued to prohibit the provision of information regarding availability of abortion services violated the right to freedom of expression.[173] The Court held that a governmental ban on counselling and on circulation of information on where to find legal abortion services in another country violated the right to impart and receive information. The Court emphasized the connection between limited access to information and health risk, finding that the injunction preventing the provision of information on where to find abortion services

created a risk to health of those women who are now seeking abortions at a later stage in their pregnancy, due to lack of proper counselling, and who are not availing of customary medical supervision after the abortion has taken place. Moreover, the injunction may have had more adverse effects on women who were not sufficiently resourceful or had not the necessary level of education to have access to alternative sources of information.[174]

---

[171] S. Coliver (ed.), *The Right to Know: Human Rights and Access to Reproductive Health Information* (London and Philadelphia: Article 19 and University of Pennsylvania Press, 1995).

[172] S. Coliver, 'The Right to Information Necessary for Reproductive Health and Choice Under International Law', ibid. 38–82.

[173] *Open Door Counselling and Dublin Well Women v. Ireland* (1992), 15 EHRR 244 (European Court of Human Rights).

[174] Ibid., para. 77.

It would seem, therefore, that human rights tribunals will be especially vigilant in reviewing cases alleging infringements on the right to information that is necessary to protect reproductive health, and cases in which such infringements may disproportionately disadvantage women who lack resources or education.[175]

4.5.2. *The right to education*

The Economic Covenant, Article 13, states:

1. The States Parties to the present Covenant recognise the right of everyone to education. They agree that education shall be directed to the full development of the human personality and the sense of its dignity, and shall strengthen the respect for human rights and fundamental freedoms. They further agree that education shall enable all persons to participate effectively in a free society . . .

2. The States Parties to the present Covenant recognize that, with a view to achieving the full realization of this right:

  (*a*) Primary education shall be compulsory and available free to all;
  (*b*) Secondary education in its different forms, including technical and vocational secondary education, shall be made generally available and accessible to all by every appropriate means, and in particular by the progressive introduction of free education;
  (*c*) Higher education shall be made equally accessible to all, on the basis of capacity, by every appropriate means, and in particular by the progressive introduction of free education; . . .

3. The States Parties to the present Covenant undertake to have respect for the liberty of parents and, when applicable, legal guardians, to choose for their children schools, other than those established by the public authorities, which conform to such minimum educational standards as may be laid down or approved by the State and to ensure the religious and moral education of their children in conformity with their own convictions.

There is a strong relation between girls' access to education and literacy, and their capacity to protect and improve their reproductive and sexual health. Key factors in reducing maternal death in a number of countries, including Sri Lanka, Kerala State in India, Cuba, and China have been the combined effects of education and empowerment strategies for girls, and improved access to necessary health services.[176] National courts can contribute to these effects by applying the right to education to require that the state ensure the provision of free primary education to girls.

---

[175] N. Whitty, 'The Mind, Body, and Reproductive Health Information', *Human Rights Quarterly*, 18 (1996), 224–39.
[176] UNICEF, *Programming for Safe Motherhood: Guidelines for Maternal and Neonatal Survival* (New York: UNICEF, 1999), 26–7.

The Supreme Court of India, for example, relying on Article 13 of the Economic Covenant, has explained that the state is obligated to provide every child with free education until he or she reaches the age of 14 years.[177] The Court found that the right to education is implicit in the right to life and personal liberty contained in Article 21 of the Indian Constitution, but is not an absolute right. After children reach the age of 14, their right to education is subject to the limits of economic capacity and development of the state. The Court emphasized that the Indian Constitution requires that 'the State shall promote with special care the educational and economic interests of the weaker sections of the people . . . and shall protect them from social injustice and all forms of exploitation'.[178]

National courts are also requiring that educational authorities ensure equal educational opportunities for girls. For instance, the highest court in England, the House of Lords, has held that a local education authority was treating girls less favourably than boys, contrary to the Sex Discrimination Act 1975, because there were fewer places for girls than boys in secondary schools.[179]

The Cairo and Beijing documents encourage educational systems that eliminate all barriers that impede the schooling of married and/or pregnant girls and young mothers.[180] Such a barrier was removed in 1995, for instance, when the Botswana Court of Appeal ruled unconstitutional a college regulation that discriminated against female students by requiring that they inform the college director of their pregnancy, and would then become liable to suspension or expulsion.[181] Male students who initiated pregnancy were subject to no such regulation.

Where attempts to introduce compulsory sex education into schools are challenged, for instance on moral or religious grounds, courts generally tend to favour such education. For example, the European Court of Human Rights addressed the human rights dimensions of a state requiring a sex education curriculum to be taught in its schools. The Court required sensitivity to parents' views, but upheld a compulsory sex education course in the state's schools because 'the curriculum is conveyed in an objective, critical and pluralistic manner [and does not] pursue an aim of indoctrination that might be considered as not respecting parents' religious and philosophical convictions'.[182]

---

[177]   *Unni Krishnan v. State of Andhra Pradesh*, [1993] AIR 2178 (Supreme Court of India).

[178]   Ibid. 2231.

[179]   *R. v. Birmingham City Council*, [1989] 2 WLR 520 (House of Lords, England), digested in *Commonwealth Law Bulletin*, 15 (1989), 414.

[180]   Cairo Programme, para. 11.8; Beijing Platform, para. 277(a).

[181]   *Student Representative Council, Molepolole College of Education v. Attorney General of Botswana (for and on behalf of the Principal of Molepolole College of Education and Permanent Secretary of Ministry of Education)*, unreported, Civil Appeal No. 13 of 1994, Misca No. 396 of 1993. Judgment delivered on 31 Jan. 1995, reported in E. K. Quansah, 'Is the Right to Get Pregnant a Fundamental Human Right in Botswana?', *Journal of African Law*, 39 (1995), 97–102.

[182]   *Kjeldsen v. Denmark* (1976) 1 EHRR 711, para. 53 (European Court of Human Rights).

The courts tend to favour access to educational opportunities, on a basis of equality of the sexes, because they recognize education as a foundation of individual autonomy and responsibility. Women able to exercise self-determination in their sexual relationships and responsibility in the choice, timing, and spacing of pregnancies increase the likelihood of their improved reproductive and sexual health.

4.5.3. *The right to freedom of thought, conscience, and religion*

The Political Covenant, Article 18, states:

1. Everyone shall have the right to freedom of thought, conscience and religion. This right shall include freedom to have or to adopt a religion or belief of his choice, and freedom, either individually or in community with others and in public or private, to manifest his religion or belief in worship, observance, practice and teaching.
2. No one shall be subject to coercion which would impair his freedom to have or to adopt a religion or belief of his choice.
3. Freedom to manifest one's religion or beliefs may be subject only to such limitations as are prescribed by law and are necessary to protect public safety, order, health, or morals or the fundamental rights and freedoms of others.
4. The States Parties to the present Covenant undertake to have respect for the liberty of parents and, when applicable, legal guardians to ensure the religious and moral education of their children in conformity with their own convictions.

Many of the laws that regulate human reproduction, and information about reproductive options, reflect moral values derived from religious convictions and doctrines. Freedom of religion includes an individual's freedom from compulsion to comply with laws designed only or principally to uphold doctrines of religious faith. Religious freedom is without substance unless individuals are free to act consistently with their own beliefs about religion, and to follow their own conscience regarding doctrines of faiths they do not hold. This view was expressed by the Minister of Health of Chile, Michelle Bachelet, when the courts denied emergency contraception to women in that country. The Minister explained that 'We cannot deny the choice to one part of the population because of the view that another part of the population might have.'[183]

When law is secular, there is accommodation of every individual's own religious conscience. However, when law is based on the belief system of a dominant religion, there is often little accommodation or tolerance of religious dissent or of alternative religious conscience. That is, when laws permit practices offensive to a religion, adherents of that religion are usually allowed a right of conscientious objection, but when laws embody a religious value, conscientious dissent is often denied, and criminalized. This was the case when the Supreme Court of Chile denied women in Chile access to emergency

---

[183] *Lancet* 357 (2001), 1188 (14 Apr. 2001).

contraception based on ideological views of the Court.[184] In contrast, the therapeutic drug regulatory institute of Colombia, INVIMA (Instituto Nacional de Vigilancia de Medicamentos y Alimentos) approved emergency contraception based on the determination of its safety and efficacy for the purposes for which it is promoted.[185]

Freedom to express religious, philosophical, and social convictions regarding reproductive self-determination runs in at least two directions. Individuals enjoy human rights of reproductive choice, and equally health professionals must be free not to participate in practices they find offensive on religious grounds, such as performing abortions and sterilizations and performing procedures relating to *in vitro* fertilization. Where health professionals object on grounds of conscience, they have a professional duty to refer to others who will do the procedures. Moreover, conscience cannot justify a health professional's refusal to participate in life-saving abortion when no other suitable person or method is available, and normally the burden of justifying conscientious objection falls on the health professional who invokes it (see Pt. I, Ch. 5, Sect. 9, on legal aspects). The UK Abortion Act of 1967 makes this explicit, by stating in section 4:

(1) Subject to subsection (2) of this section, no person shall be under any duty, whether by contract or by any statutory or other legal requirement, to participate in any treatment authorised by this Act to which he has a conscientious objection:
Provided that in any legal proceedings the burden of proof of conscientious objection shall rest on the person claiming to rely on it.
(2) Nothing in subsection (1) of this section shall affect any duty to participate in treatment which is necessary to save the life or to prevent grave permanent injury to the physical or mental health of a pregnant woman.[186]

Human rights provisions require maximum respect for and equitable balance between individuals' choices to avail themselves of reproductive services, and health care providers' rights not to participate in delivery of services they consider objectionable on grounds of conscience. Non-participation may require, however, voluntary exclusion from employment opportunities where participation in the provision of such reproductive health services is a central part of employment.[187]

---

[184] *Recurso de Protección, rol C.S. 2186–2001 y otros, 'Phillipi Izquierdo con Laboratorio Chile S.A. y otros'*, 30 Aug. 2001 (Supreme Court of Chile).

[185] INVIMA (Instituto Nacional de Vigilancia de Medicamentos y Alimentos) Resolución No. 2001297067, 15 Nov. 2001, 'Por la cuál se adoptan unos conceptos y recomendaciones de la Sala Especializada de Medicamentos de la Comisión Revisora' (Embracing concepts and recommendations issued by the official review specialized board of medicaments INVIMA; Resolución No. 2002000510, 11 Jan. 2002, 'Por la cuál se resuelve una revisión de oficio de un medicamento' (Stating to carry out the official review of a medicament).

[186] UK Statutes 1967, ch. 87 (as amended).

[187] B. M. Dickens and R. J. Cook, 'The Scope and Limits of Conscientious Objection', *Int. J. Gynecol. Obstet.* 71 (2000), 71–7.

5. *Progress and Challenges*

Because human rights are intended to provide the power of self-defence and self-determination to those who have historically been powerless, and require at least restraint and sometimes allocation of resources by government, they remain resisted by agencies and people who historically have enjoyed privileges and the power of governance. Resistance is often veiled because of the rhetoric that invokes professed adherence to democratic values and individuals' subordination to majority rule. However, political, religious, professional, and other agencies conventionally accustomed to the exercise of power and leadership remain reluctant to yield their power to individuals, and continue paternalistic control of individuals' reproductive choices.

Accordingly, progress towards individual reproductive and sexual health and self-determination faces the continuing challenge of making human rights effective in practice, and of inspiring and requiring governmental compliance. The clustering and detailing of human rights described above is neither definitive nor exhaustive. Human rights are rich, infinitely mouldable raw materials out of which individuals, communities, and societies can shape their reproductive and sexual liberty. Human rights described above, and others including, for instance, the right to freedom of assembly, can be invoked and employed, before governmental and non-governmental agencies, and before tribunals and national and international judicial bodies, to urge that reproductive and sexual health rights be respected, protected, and fulfilled.

Human rights also furnish the critical frame of reference for the work of the international human rights treaty monitoring bodies that present internationally visible commentary on countries' compliance with their human rights obligations, on the basis of governmental submissions and submissions made by non-governmental and other independent organizations. Monitoring bodies provide a valuable resource, accessible to individuals and organizations inspired to speak out against governmental failures to observe their human rights responsibilities, through which human rights abuses and disregard can be exposed. They provide international leadership to require governments to give an account of their conduct, including their advancement of human rights and failures to make human rights effective, and statements of standards against which national compliance with human rights requirements will be measured.

Human rights and statements of standards that determine compliance may also be employed by health care practitioners, and their professional associations and agencies, to guide their own conduct and to inspire and require compliance by the persons and institutions they can influence. Originally aspirational in identifying a high level or ceiling of conduct which conscientious practitioners and associations should strive to reach, they are increasingly appearing as a floor or foundation on which just professional careers and institutions can be built.

7

Implementation of Legal and Human Rights Principles

1. *Overview*

Implementation of the laws discussed in Chapter 5 and the human rights discussed in Chapter 6 requires a collaborative and joint effort by the health and legal professions, women, and social activist groups. A necessary step towards applying human rights to advance women's sexual and reproductive health is to assess the situation and the need in the particular community and culture. Assessment will include clinical care, health systems, and underlying social, economic, and legal conditions. Compliance with standards, measurement of indicators over time, and progress towards stated goals will help in this assessment.

Laws are enforceable at the level of national courts and institutions. Many human rights principles are given the force of law through national legislation and judicial and other institutions, and developed by agencies that monitor international human rights conventions. Where efforts to obtain justice fail at the national level, appropriate remedies can be pursued through international and regional human rights tribunals. Before international judicial tribunals can become involved in enforcement of rights, complainants are usually required to exhaust such national judicial and other remedies as exist for them.

Where health professionals enjoy the privilege and public trust of maintaining self-discipline, the ethical principle of justice requires professions themselves to act as moral agents and to require their members to observe the law.

Preparatory strategies for presentation of claims and complaints at national and international levels have much in common. This chapter will first address factors that assist the effective development of claims. They include identifying and documenting the alleged wrongs and their causes, determining which laws and human rights principles are implicated by what standards, and, finally, assessing what kinds of remedies might be appropriate for the effective remedy of the violations. Then, the chapter will consider how legal (including human rights) claims may be advanced through national mechanisms such as ombudsmen, national human rights commissions, regulatory and professional approaches, and finally courts of law. Human rights claims will then be more briefly addressed, regarding how they might be prepared for presentation before regional and international agencies and human rights convention monitoring bodies. The International Court of Justice and comparable international judicial tribunals are too remote to warrant attention here, since, although some may receive petitions by individuals against their own countries, their essential role concerns litigation among nation-states and international institutions.

2. *Human Rights Needs Assessment*

A necessary step towards applying human rights to advance reproductive and sexual health is to make an assessment of the scope, causes, and consequences of reproductive and sexual ill-health in a particular community and culture, based on the collection of relevant new data or on available data sources (see Pt. III, Ch. 1). Local assessment should identify laws, including the language of enacted laws and any subordinate regulations made under the authority of such laws, interpretive and other relevant decisions of courts, and policies of governments, health care facilities, and other influential agencies that facilitate or obstruct availability of and access to reproductive and sexual health services.[1] A determination should be made of the extent to which laws that would facilitate access are actually implemented, and, if they are not adequately implemented, of how they might be. Laws and policies that obstruct individuals' autonomy and choice regarding their reproductive and sexual health, and the availability of and access to services, should also be identified, along with laws that facilitate individuals' empowerment.

An assessment should be made of what must be done in a district or country to foster compliance with human rights at different levels, including regarding:

- clinical care,
- operation of health systems, and
- underlying conditions, including social, economic, and legal conditions of observance of human rights.

These levels are not necessarily distinct. Often there is overlap between them, in that failure to respect human rights at one level can exacerbate problems at another level. Examples follow of application of human rights to clinical care, health systems, and underlying health conditions, but these are far from exhaustive.

---

[1] See generally Human Rights Impact Assessment in L. O. Gostin and Z. Lazzarini, *Human Rights and Public Health in the AIDS Pandemic* (New York: Oxford University Press, 1997).

2.1. *Clinical care*

An assessment of the degree to which patients' human rights are respected in clinical care contexts might show lack of respect for their dignity and their own judgement of their circumstances. Rights of privacy in the delivery of reproductive and sexual health services are liable to be ignored. Health care providers need to be trained in the importance of maintaining confidentiality of patients seeking and receiving services. Breaches of confidentiality are violations not only of service providers' professional ethical duties, but also of the laws on patient confidentiality (see Pt. I, Ch. 5, Sect. 7.2).

There is need to assess how well clinical care incorporates due attention to diseases or conditions specific to, or more prevalent among, certain subgroups of pregnant women, such as malaria, sickle cell trait, hepatitis, and HIV/AIDS. Steps need to be taken to ensure that requested lawful abortion services are provided, and also to ensure that these underlying conditions are treated, or that affected women are referred for accessible appropriate treatment. A challenge is to address such reproductive health problems in non-discriminatory, constructive ways. There is also a need to examine conditions that present clinical manifestations specific to certain subgroups of women, such as domestic violence resulting, for instance, in unwanted pregnancy. Emphasis should be given to finding ways to reduce the stigma of victimization in the clinical care context by ensuring respectful treatment of all patients seeking services, irrespective of their reasons, circumstances, or, for instance, socio-economic status.

2.2. *Health systems*

An assessment of the degree to which patients' rights are respected throughout the health system might be approached through an examination of systemic barriers to the availability of care, and to laws, policies, and practices that might deter those in need of care from seeking it. First, there is need to examine the *barriers to availability* of reproductive and sexual health services, such as

- lack of implementation of laws and policies that are beneficial to reproductive health, such as failure to give effect to legal permission of abortion when pregnancy is due to rape;
- lack of skilled health personnel due to legal prohibition or restriction of procedures or, for example, abuse of conscientious objection to participation in lawful services by health personnel;
- lack of good quality reproductive and sexual health services, due, for example, to low priority given to these services in health facilities, or in allocation of necessary governmental or other budgetary resources;

- gendered barriers, such as lack of availability of institutional services at times when it is possible for women to attend, and lack of facilities to care for their young or otherwise dependent children while they receive counselling and treatment; and
- health laws and policies that require excessive qualifications for health care providers to provide reproductive and sexual health services.

Secondly, there is need to examine the *deterrents to access* to available reproductive and sexual health services, particularly for women or certain subgroups of women, such as

- lack of protection of confidentiality, or perceived lack of protection;
- poor quality of care, including providers' disrespectful or punitive attitudes;
- third-party authorization requirements, such as spousal authorization requirements;[2]
- failure to treat adolescent girls according to their 'evolving capacity' to exercise mature choice in reproductive sexual health care;[3] and
- payment or co-payment requirements, particularly for adolescent girls.

2.3. *Underlying conditions, including social, economic, and legal conditions*

Barriers to improving reproductive and sexual health are often rooted in social, economic, cultural, legal, and related conditions that offend human rights. A human rights needs assessment might show social obstacles to reproductive health that include lack of literacy and of educational or employment opportunities that deny individuals such as young women alternatives to early or repeated pregnancy, and deny them economic and other means of access to reproductive and sexual health services. Women's vulnerability to sexual and other abuses, in and out of marriage, increases their risks of unsafe pregnancy and mental illness.[4] Social, religious, and economic customs become embedded in laws, and historically have been invoked to provide a justification for discrimination against women. A gender-sensitive approach to social science and legal research can help to identify how underlying socio-legal conditions can have positive or negative effects in advancing women's independence and access, for instance, to lawful and safe abortion services.

---

[2] R. J. Cook and D. Maine, 'Spousal Veto over Family Planning Services', *American Journal of Public Health*, 77 (1987), 339–44.

[3] R. J. Cook and B. M. Dickens, 'Recognizing Adolescents' "Evolving Capacities" to Exercise Choice in Reproductive Health Care', *Int. J. Gynecol. Obstet. (World Report on Women's Health)*, 70 (2000), 13–21.

[4] L. Gulcur, 'Evaluating the Role of Gender Inequalities and Rights Violations in Women's Mental Health', *Health and Human Rights*, 5 (2000), 47–66.

A human rights needs assessment will be able to examine the underlying conditions that increase risk factors for reproductive and sexual ill-health that are common particularly to women or certain subgroups of women, such as:

- violence against women;
- sexual abuse;
- poverty;
- different forms of discrimination against women; and
- different social and economic conditioning of women's powerlessness.

There are several comparative studies that provide information on laws in various countries[5] and regions.[6] Legal research can help to identify how laws advance or compromise women's interests in their personal, family, and public lives, with indirect effects on women's health. Family law frequently expresses communities' basic cultural values, such as rights to inheritance of land. Cultures that deny they are resistant to women's equality with men have often unselfconsciously perpetuated women's subordination and powerlessness. They consider women's lesser status a 'natural' condition of family life and social order so profoundly as to render women's disadvantage invisible. Where women's subordination and powerlessness are perceived, they are considered not just a feature but a necessary requirement of the maintenance of social order and stability.

Laws that entrench women's inferior status to men, and interfere with women's access to health services, seriously jeopardize efforts to improve women's health. These laws take a variety of forms, such as those that obstruct economic independence by impairing women's education, inheritance, employment, or acquisition of commercial loans or credit, but they all infringe

---

[5] For instance, W. Nowicka (ed.), *The Anti-Abortion Law in Poland: The Functioning, Social Effects, Attitudes and Behaviors* (Warsaw: Federation for Women and Family Planning, 2000).

[6] See e.g. V. Bermudez, *La Regulacion Judica del Abortio en America Latina y el Caribe* (Lima: Comité de América Latina y el Caribe para la Defensa de los Derechos de la Mujer (CLADEM), 1997); Center for Reproductive Law and Policy (CRLP), and Demus, *Estudio para la Defensa de los Derechos de la Mujer. Women of the World: Laws and Policies Affecting their Reproductive Lives—Latin America and the Caribbean* (New York: CRLP, 1997); Centro Legal para Derechos Reproductivos y Politicas Publicas y Demus, *Estudio para la Defensa de los Derechos de la Mujer, Mujeres del Mundo: Leyes y Politicas que Afectan sus Vidas Reproductivas-America Latina y el Caribe, Suplemento 2000* (New York, CRLP, 2001); CRLP and International Federation of Women Lawyers—Kenya Chapter; *Women of the World: Laws and Policies Affecting their Reproductive Lives: Anglophone Africa* (New York: CRLP, 1997); CRLP, *Women of the World: Laws and Policies Affecting their Reproductive Lives: Anglophone Africa—2001 Progress Report* (New York: CRLP, 2001); CRLP and Groupe de recherche femmes et lois au Sénégal, *Women of the World: Laws and Policies Affecting their Reproductive Lives: Francophone Africa* (New York: CRLP, 1999; also available in French); CRLP, *Women of the World: Laws and Policies Affecting their Reproductive Lives—East Central Europe* (New York: CRLP, 2000). See also references at Women's Human Rights Resources website at: www.law-lib.utoronto.ca/diana, last accessed 7 May 2002.

on women's ability to make their own choices about their lives and health.[7] Account should be taken of criminal laws that condone or neglect violence against women, and, for instance, of inequitable family, education, and employment laws that deny adolescent and adult women alternatives in life to marriage, or that limit women's self-realization on marriage and motherhood.

Investigation should determine, for instance, whether laws adequately protect girls and women from sexual coercion, including sexual abuse. Studies show that forced first intercourse is prevalent in many communities, affecting as high as 32 per cent of girls and women.[8] Laws that inadequately protect girls and women from coercion in sexual relations undermine women's independence and ability to protect themselves from unwanted pregnancies. Laws must be identified and enforced that allow women effective defence or self-defence, and to control the timing and number of their births.

3. *Development of Legal Claims*

Preparation of legal claims, for violations of general laws or laws protecting basic human rights, is assisted when the following factors are addressed and, as far as possible in individual circumstances, resolved.

3.1. *Identify the wrong, its causes, and the wrongdoer*

Leaders of institutions accustomed to the exercise of authority in their communities, including office holders in governmental, religious, educational, health care, and other institutions, may not recognize that their familiar practices constitute injuries or wrongs to reproductive and sexual health. They may believe that protection of these familiar practices preserves necessary social values including family integrity, private and public morality, and social order. For instance, denying unmarried adolescent girls access to contraceptive means may be seen as necessary to maintain girls' respect for family and social disapproval of sexual misconduct evidenced by pregnancy. Accordingly, advocates of remedies for legal and human rights violations may bear an initial burden of persuasion to show how legitimate interests in reproductive and sexual health have been violated.

The human rights discussed above in Chapter 6 may be applied to the identification of wrongs to reproductive and sexual health. The principles embodied in human rights may indicate that prevailing local laws are disrespectful of

---

[7] CRLP, *Reproductive Rights 2000: Moving Forward* (New York: CRLP, 2000).

[8] L. Heise, M. Ellsberg, and M. Gottemoeller, 'Ending Violence Against Women', *Population Reports*, series L., 11 (1999), 9–18, 10–11.

these rights, and require review, and perhaps repeal or amendment. Accordingly, the wrong may require challenge not simply to particular practices that violate human rights, but to the laws that condition those practices. Causes of wrongs often extend beyond laws, however, and are to be found in social customs and attitudes, particularly those that equate expressions of sexuality outside marriage as sinful. Causes may be identified by reference to different time frames, ranging from the immediate precipitating cause of an injury to reproductive health, such as lack of essential obstetric care, to long-standing socio-cultural practices, such as women's subordination to the authority of husbands and parents. Similarly, wrongdoing can be identified at different levels of immediacy, from schoolteachers who are required to punish students for possessing condoms, to government officers who decline to allocate resources favourably to reproductive health interests. An ultimate wrongdoer may be a government or sovereign state itself, for instance when it fails to punish and deter acts of domestic violence and spousal rape.

The development of legal claims presents a variety of decisions that activist individuals and agencies have to make. They have choices in identifying the wrongs of which to complain, the level at which they identify the causes of those wrongs, and the persons or institutions they claim have violated reproductive and sexual rights. As initiators of legal action, they bear the burden of proving the facts and establishing the legal basis of their claim. Their advantage is that they can choose their target, and set the agenda of the legal claim to their own advantage. They can identify the most obvious outrage and injustice of which to complain, the most demonstrable cause, and the most culpable party responsible for the violation. If, however, there are obstacles (such as unavailable evidence), or legal doctrines (such as immunity protecting governmental officers or institutions), they can cater their claim to the facts they can establish and to defendants who are amenable to the jurisdiction of the tribunal before which the claim is to be presented. They can set the agenda of the claim, time and locate the proceedings to maximum advantage, for instance through news media coverage, and require defendants to react where they consider the defendants most vulnerable.

3.2. *Document the alleged wrongs*

Documentation of alleged violations of legal and human rights is a necessary step in holding governments and other institutions and officers accountable. Data, whether events-based or standards-based,[9] can play an instrumental role in advancing claims.

---

[9] T. B. Jabine and R. P. Claude (eds.), *Human Rights and Statistics: Getting the Record Straight* (Philadelphia: University of Pennsylvania Press, 1992).

Meticulously documented events-based data, such as the repeated sexual abuse of schoolchildren by public school employees and rapes of women in military, police, or prison custody, can demonstrate that human rights abuses represent trends rather than individual aberrations. Cases can highlight the absence of efforts required of responsible agents to eliminate and remedy abuses, and can be employed to analyse trends over time. Cases before national and international tribunals, and events that are publicized by non-governmental human rights organizations, can direct attention beyond their facts to the underlying conditions of abuse. Individual testimony can be more effective than explanations of the history and dimensions of violations of rights relating to reproductive and sexual self-determination. A case puts a human face, identity and history to a representative human rights violation, and can be multiplied in common understanding to its statistical dimension.

Standards-based data, such as the country data presented in Part III, Chapter 1, are used particularly in international human rights monitoring, where states' discharge of their programmatic obligations are the focus of analysis. Standards-based data are most useful when they include accompanying references to the defined standards that are in issue, and that states and other agents are accused of violating.[10] Breaking down data by reference to sex is usually essential to prove a violation of recognized standards that measure discrimination against women. Advocates for reproductive self-determination can employ existing data for the construction or support of arguments, for instance where maternal mortality ratios are high (see Pt. III, Ch. 1). In addition, however, activists may have to generate new standards, based on available credible data, through objective investigation of suspicions of discrimination. This may have to be done in order to determine whether suspicions have demonstrable substance, and to show violations of rights relating to reproductive self-determination by reference to favourable standards of practice that prevail in comparable national and international experience. For instance, country authorities can be called to account if rates of maternal mortality and morbidity significantly exceed rates in neighbouring countries, or countries of similar economic development and resources.

The nature of a violation intended to be investigated may define the data to be employed. For instance, sexual abuse of women detained in state prisons can be demonstrated by medical reports of examinations of victims. Data can also show neglect to protect certain reproductive rights. Evidence of high rates of abortion,[11] for example, can be used to require governments and other institutional or private agencies to explain why they are not effectively providing

---

[10] Ibid. at 9–10.
[11] WHO, *Unsafe Abortion: Global and Regional Estimates of Incidence of and Mortality due to Unsafe Abortion with a Listing of Available Country Data* (Geneva: WHO, 3rd edn., 1998).

contraceptive services, including emergency contraception. Reports, including those developed by the United Nations and its specialized agencies,[12] and by non-governmental organizations,[13] can demonstrate how action and neglect by accountable agencies and officers implicate rights relating to reproductive self-determination. Events-based and standards-based data can be used in evaluating how effectively a right in question has been protected, and whether an alternative approach to protection would be more effective in preventing instances of violation or in reducing the incidence of their occurrence.

3.3. *Determine which laws are implicated*

National, regional, and international judicial tribunals are increasingly willing to treat human rights as interdependent, and to recognize that infringement of one right frequently implicates another. Nevertheless, advocates must specify which legal and/or human right or rights they claim have been violated in a particular injury and complaint. Specification is necessary in all claims of legal violations, such as of negligence in delivery of care or delay in diagnosing a condition in need of treatment, or assault when an intervention a patient refused was imposed. Specification of a right alleged to have been violated is of particular significance before human rights tribunals, because national, regional, and international human rights instruments may be applied in different ways. Depending on the way a right is invoked, agencies might be able to escape liability on the technical claim that the instrument alleged to have been violated is not binding on the agency, or was not binding at the time of incidents alleged to have caused injuries.

Rights are rarely expressed in language that is directly applicable to reproductive and sexual health. The advocate must show the relevance of a particular right to an alleged failure of reproductive or sexual health. This can be done by drawing on documents of national and of international authority, such as the Cairo and Beijing documents and their five-year reviews, General Recommendations and Concluding Observations on national reports and performance made by treaty monitoring bodies, such as CEDAW, and legal literature, including judicial decisions. Because general principles of law and human rights have been applied only infrequently to reproductive health problems, the challenge is to achieve collaboration among colleagues who can bring their individual knowledge of medicine, law, health system organization, governmental structure, and local culture and practice to the task.

---

[12] UN, *The World's Women: 2000 Trends and Statistics* (New York: UN, 2000).

[13] See e.g. Latin American and Caribbean Committee for the Defence of Women's Rights (CLADEM) and CRLP, *Silence and Complicity: Violence against Women in Peruvian Public Health Facilities* (New York: CLADEM CRLP, 1999; also available in Spanish); The Women's Rights Project of Human Rights Watch, *Criminal Injustice: Violence against Women in Brazil* (New York: Human Rights Watch, 1991; also available in Portuguese).

3.4. *Identify standards by which to determine whether and how laws are violated*

Performance standards are needed to determine whether governments and other accountable agencies and officers are meeting their legal obligations to respect, protect, and fulfil human rights. Different standards, indicators, and stated or agreed goals exist that can be relied upon to show whether obligations are being met with regard to laws that implement rights related to reproductive and sexual health. They include, but are not limited to:

- standards in national legislation and developed by national courts, for example, that require access to certain kinds of care such as emergency treatment[14] or respect for confidentiality;
- goals in international documents, such as those developed by the Cairo and Beijing processes, for example ensuring that at least 50 per cent of all births should be assisted by skilled attendants by the year 2010;[15] and
- standards that have evolved through the human rights treaty monitoring bodies, such as those requiring availability, accessibility, and acceptability of health services (see Pt. III, Ch. 6, Sect. 3, para. 12).

Indicators are needed to measure whether standards set by different bodies are being met. For example, the World Health Organization and other United Nations agencies have developed the Reproductive Health Indicators for Global Monitoring (Global Indicators).[16] As discussed above in Chapter 2, they include:

- total fertility rate
- contraceptive prevalence
- maternal mortality ratio
- antenatal care coverage
- births attended by skilled health personnel
- availability of basic essential obstetric care
- availability of comprehensive essential obstetric care
- perinatal mortality rate
- low birth weight prevalence (<2500 g)
- positive syphilis serology prevalence in pregnant women

[14] *Paschim Banga Khet Mazdoor Samity v. State of West Bengal* (1996), 4 SCC 37; (1996), 3 SCJ 25, digested in *Commonwealth Human Rights Law Digest*, 2 (1998), 109 (Supreme Court of India).
[15] United Nations, General Assembly, *Report of the Ad Hoc Committee of the Whole of the Twenty-First Special Session of the General Assembly: Overall Review and Appraisal of the Implementation of the Programme of Action of the International Conference on Population and Development*, A/S-21/5/Add.1 (New York: United Nations, 1999) (hereinafter Cairo+5), para. 64.
[16] WHO (Division of Reproductive Health), *Reproductive Health Indicators for Global Monitoring: Report of the Second Interagency Meeting* (Geneva: WHO, 2001) (hereinafter *Global Indicators*).

- prevalence of anaemia in women
- percentage of obstetric and gynaecology admissions owing to abortion
- reported prevalence of women with female genital cutting
- prevalence of infertility in women
- reported incidence of urethritis in men
- HIV prevalence in pregnant women
- knowledge of HIV-related prevention practices.[17]

Table III.1.1 provides country data on these bulleted indicators and adolescent fertility rates. The advantage of the Global Indicators is that WHO and other UN agencies maintain country databases on them. Efforts are under way to coordinate the different databases and to develop new more sensitive indicators and databases, such as for adolescent fertility rates.

In general, these indicators have been developed to measure the effectiveness of health interventions. Some measure the effectiveness of health interventions by reference to health status, such as maternal mortality and morbidity. Others measure the effectiveness of health interventions by references to health services, such as the percentage of births attended by skilled birth attendants.

To illustrate how indicators would work in a human rights context, WHO estimates that only 55 per cent of women in the developing world are attended at delivery by a health worker who has received at least the minimum of necessary training.[18] A skilled birth attendant can ensure hygiene during labour and delivery, provide safe and non-traumatic care, recognize and manage complications, and, if needed, refer the mother to a higher level of care. The Cairo plus Five document offers a standard by which to measure the degree of compliance with the right to the highest attainable standard of health:

In order to monitor progress towards the achievement of the Conference's goals for maternal mortality, countries should use the proportion of births assisted by skilled attendants as a benchmark indicator. By 2005, where the maternal mortality rate is very high, at least 40 per cent of all births should be assisted by skilled attendants; by 2010 this figure should be at least 50 per cent and by 2015, at least 60 per cent. All countries should continue their efforts so that globally, by 2005, 80 per cent of all births should be assisted by skilled attendants, by 2010, 85 per cent, and by 2015, 90 per cent.[19]

Other goals agreed upon in the Cairo plus Five document are presented in Chapter 3.

Use might be made of these Global Indicators in both national and international tribunals to determine whether the standards on availability, accessibility,

---

[17] UN *Global Indicators*, ibid. at 17–18.
[18] WHO, *Coverage of Maternity Care: A Listing of Available Information* (Geneva: WHO, 1997). WHO/RHT/MSM/96.28.
[19] Cairo+5, at para. 47.

acceptability and quality of reproductive health services, established by CESCR's General Comment on the Right to Health (see Pt. III, Ch. 6, Sect. 3, para. 12), are being met (see Pt. I, Ch. 6, Sect. 4.3.1). However, great care has to be used in transposing them to a legal and human rights context, because these indicators were developed with the objective of measuring health interventions. Where health status indicators show, for instance, that women in a country are in poor reproductive health, this may suggest that the government and/or other accountable agencies and officers need to do more to comply with their obligations to ensure the right to equality in access to health services. However, the health status indicator might not necessarily be used as proof of a violation of the right to non-discrimination in access to health care.

Indicators can also be used to show trends over time. Where trends show improvement, this suggests that responsible bodies are progressing towards the realization of the right to the highest attainable standard of reproductive health. Where the trends do not show improvement, or where they indicate continuing poor reproductive health, the data could then shift the burden to those accountable for reproductive and sexual health status to explain the situation. If the indicators show default in satisfying performance standards, an agency could be said to be not adequately complying with the duty to ensure that individual patients or community members achieve the highest attainable standard of reproductive health. As a result, the agency will need to give greater priority to protection of this right.

No single indicator can reflect the complete reproductive health situation of a community, whether it reflects the health status of that community or the level of services and the degree to which they are used. Even though indicators are subject to some uncertainty and limitations, however, they can tell something about the extent to which laws are actually implemented. For example, high perinatal mortality rates in a country indicate that women are not receiving adequate maternity care and nutrition during pregnancy (see Table III.1.1 for country data on perinatal mortality rates).

In addition to the relatively well-developed health service and health status indicators, there are health policy indicators that measure the extent to which a policy or law is implemented. For example, the percentage of adolescent girls who marry below the legal age of marriage, or data on age at first birth within marriage, can indicate the extent to which a government is vigilant in enforcement of minimum age-of-marriage laws, which could positively affect the outcomes of pregnancy and childbirth. Where data show that a high percentage of girls marry under the legal age of marriage, or have their first birth below the legal age of marriage, the data shift the burden to government to explain its actions and proposals to implement the law effectively.

These indicators could be supplemented by other kinds of indicators or guidelines, such as the Guidelines for Monitoring the Availability and Use of Obstetric Services by women with life-threatening complications.[20] Alternatively, where data exist at a community level, such as data on hospital admissions due to unsafe abortions (see Table III.1.3.2 for country data on hospitalizations due to abortion complications), the data indicate inadequate availability of and accessibility to contraceptive services (see Table III.1.1 for country data on contraceptive prevalence).

3.5. *Assess how to pursue effective remedies*

Since not every available initiative may be effective to secure every result, the outcome desired from a complaint must be clearly identified. For instance, the aim to achieve future supply of governmental services may require consultation with government. The aim to achieve compensatory or even punitive remedies may require proceedings in law courts. The aim to hold governments to their international commitments may require action before international treaty monitoring agencies that can determine governmental failures and call for improved performance.

Desired outcomes must be conditioned by the identified causes of injuries to reproductive or sexual health. The effectiveness of remedies, even when successfully pursued, depends on the proper identification of causes of injuries. Nevertheless, best remedies may not be possible to pursue, and root causes of reproductive ill-health may be too complex or culturally ingrained to be changed by outcomes less than fundamental social change. Therefore, within the limits of resources, personnel, time, and other practical constraints, outcomes may have to be targeted and remedies pursued that are less than perfect, but that will achieve significant advances in reproductive health.

For example, a study in the US state of Washington showed that two-thirds of a sample of 535 young women who became pregnant were so as a result of sexual abuse committed by older men.[21] These findings show that governments in general and law enforcement and child welfare agencies in particular need to address the problem of sexual abuse of adolescent girls. An approach that provides contraceptive services to adolescents in order to reduce the incidence of pregnancy, or that improves their access to educational opportunities, does not remedy such abuse. Criminal law enforcement and parental and other protection of vulnerable adolescents, reinforced by judicial and welfare agency initiatives, are required for an effective remedy.

[20] D. Maine, T. M. Wardlaw, V. M. Ward, J. McCarthy, A. Birnbaum, M. Z. Akalin, and J. E. Brown, *Guidelines for Monitoring the Availability and Use of Obstetric Services* (New York: UNICEF, 2nd edn., 1997 (hereinafter UN *Guidelines*).

[21] D. K. Boyer *et al.*, 'Sexual Abuse as a Factor in Adolescent Pregnancy and Child Maltreatment', *Family Planning Perspectives*, 24 (1992), 4–11.

3.6. Determine which agencies or individuals are bound to provide remedies

Governmental agencies are usually bound to provide some sort of remedy for neglect or violation of their obligations to implement rights. Subordinate agencies and officers may be liable to mandatory orders of compliance issued by courts of law or appropriately empowered tribunals or commissions, and liable to institutional sanctions and even, in a case of wilful defiance, punishment or legal charges of contempt of court. Remedies can be monetary, such as a damage payment as compensation for harm resulting from a violation of a right, or they can be non-monetary, such as the undertaking or requirement to change a law in a certain way to bring it into compliance with a constitutional or treaty obligation. Obligations may originate by force of law, through reforming legislation or orders of judicial tribunals under existing law, and can be established at national, regional, or international levels. Obligations may also originate through political pressure that may be brought to bear by legal action, through political persuasive power wielded by political, religious, and other institutions including news media, and at times through the force of public opinion, particularly where governments respect democratic principles. The highly restrictive laws against contraception and abortion in Ireland, for instance, became liberalized due to public opposition to religiously supported restrictions.

The advantage of bringing proceedings under national laws is that they may be conducted before courts or administrative bodies with the power to compel partics to attend proceedings and defend accusations of misconduct made against them, and the power to enforce judgments designed to compensate or remedy proven wrongs. Some regional human rights agencies are developing comparable authority, such as the Inter-American Commission and Court of Human Rights. Generally, the higher the level at which remedies are pursued through national, regional, and international agencies, the weaker the compulsory powers to enforce compliance become. The bodies that monitor regional and international human rights conventions often depend upon the power of moral persuasion or condemnation, political embarrassment, and national pride to induce reform, since they lack the legal authority that court officers, police, and constitutional agencies enjoy in countries' national laws.

Governmental officers who want to be shown to act within the rule of law may be persuaded by advocacy and findings of judicial and other inquiries that the administrations in which they participate are failing in the protection of legal and human rights in general, and reproductive rights in particular. Governments widely recognize that the greatest assets of their countries are the people themselves, especially their children. By demonstrating that the interests of the people, families, and children are compromised through neglect or political policies that harm reproductive health, advocates may inspire or oblige reform. In order to be successful, advocates should not necessarily focus on compensation or punishment, but remember that the task remains to guide or direct reform towards specified goals that more directly advance reproductive health.

4. *Advancement of Legal Claims*

Procedures available at the national, regional, and international levels to compel the observance of duties to remedy, prevent, and/or punish violations of reproductive rights may be undertaken by a spectrum of means, ranging from more consensual, non-confrontational discussions and inquiries, to sharply adversarial political and legal action. Deciding which means are used will be a matter of political and social judgement, and of how comfortable committed agencies and individuals feel in initiating procedures to compel compliance with legal and human rights standards before particular tribunals.

4.1. *National procedures*

The least invasive, most collegial approaches are to inquire of agencies that control reproductive and sexual health services or service funding levels if they are satisfied that the results of their practices meet legally required and human rights standards. They may be presented with data from other agencies or countries on levels of performance that meet such standards, and asked if they are performing at this level or have programmes in place to do so. If public data exist indicating that they are not meeting such standards, they can be asked how they propose to raise their performance to these standards of achievement. This approach supposes that questioners and agencies share common purposes, and questioners may offer assistance or advice on developments towards the satisfaction of standards.

Responsible agencies may claim that their performance is satisfactory, or that they have no obligation or means to satisfy higher standards than they profess to be achieving. A response may be to call for an inquiry into the prevailing standards of agency performance, the methods of determining the level and adequacy of the standards that agencies meet and intend to meet, and the source and extent of the obligations that agencies are required to discharge. The conduct of such inquiries may be inquisitorial, in which an appointed investigator asks questions and seeks evidence, or adversarial, in which opposing interests present their evidence, and question the evidence presented by others, before independent fact-finders.

4.1.1. *Implementation of legal and human rights principles*

Legal systems frequently provide a variety of means to encourage and if necessary enforce observance of legal principles. Indeed, historic theories of law claim that the law is distinguishable from other systems of normative ordering by its means of enforcement. That is, a rule unenforceable through a legal duty or sanction is not a true rule of law but may be, for instance, a moral rule. In practice, however, means of law enforcement available in theory are frequently inoperative in practice. Such means are inaccessible to individuals who feel that they have been injured or victimized by health care providers' misconduct, because they lack knowledge of relevant law and how to gain advice of their legal entitlements, and of procedures to compel observance of the law. Similarly, professional, governmental, and other agencies may not monitor health service providers' conduct. Not all legal systems require health care providers to inform patients of errors or legally substandard care, or other breaches of patients' lawful entitlements that providers realize have occurred. As against this, health care providers in some countries feel oppressed by patients' capacity to misuse law to pursue unjustified grievances, and courts' liability to be unduly sympathetic to patients' claims that lack merit.

Where professionals such as physicians, nurses, and comparable health care providers enjoy the privilege and public trust of maintaining professional self-discipline, the ethical principle of justice, to which the law claims primarily to devote itself, requires professions themselves to act as moral agents and to require their members to observe the law. Professional bodies are usually concerned about members' possible violations of the law, and behave very conservatively to deter not just legal violations, but any risks of violations. Where the public trust appears to have been inadequately respected or to have been betrayed, however, societies may consider it necessary to promote legislation that reinforces the requirement that professionals maintain legal and human rights standards. Such legislation might replace or supplement professional self-discipline that has failed the public by laxity or professional protectionism. This response is not particular to health professionals, but applies to all self-regulating professions, including that, for instance, of lawyers.

More serious outrages, whether deliberate or negligent, may attract criminal proceedings, usually initiated by public law enforcement officers, and punishment (see below, Sect. 4.1.3). In societies where patients have relatively convenient access to courts, they will more probably prefer to initiate civil, meaning non-criminal, proceedings, in order to obtain financial compensation for injuries suffered to their physical integrity and well-being and for financial costs or losses, and perhaps also for the infliction of indignity. Civil complaints may also be managed without court proceedings, through means of alternative dispute resolution (ADR). These means may resolve patients' dissatisfaction by negotiated settlements reached with their health service providers, usually without the publicity that attends proceedings in courts of law (see below, Sect. 4.1.5).

As members of a senior profession with a historical record of conscientious dedication to those they serve, physicians in many countries have been particularly active in organizing their observance of the law and of human rights within their profession. Most countries' confidence in the capacity of physicians to maintain professional self-regulation has been justified. Professional licensing authorities, primarily directed by physicians, discharge the legal function delegated to them by governments of applying professional self-discipline, ensuring that licensed members conduct themselves in accordance with legal and ethical standards. Further, through participation in the work of licensing authorities, voluntary national and regional medical professional associations and specialized medical professional associations, for instance of obstetricians and gynaecologists, physicians have actively advocated for laws that better serve the goals of reproductive and sexual health. Although often conservative in requiring members' compliance with prevailing law, many have been courageous in advocacy of legal reform to advance the frontiers of health care in general and to remove obstacles to protection and promotion of reproductive and sexual health in particular.

International medical associations tend to be cautious about undue involvement in the legal affairs of individual countries. They have been active, however, in development of international standards, including respect for universal human rights, that member national associations are expected to adopt and enforce among individual practitioners. The World Medical Association's periodically amended Declaration of Helsinki, for instance (see Pt. I, Ch. 4, Sect. 8, and Pt. III, Ch. 2), is widely respected as a basis for the ethical review and conduct of biomedical research involving human subjects, and has influenced countries' legal requirements for research. Similarly, the Council for International Organizations of Medical Sciences (CIOMS), jointly constituted by the WHO and UNESCO, has published guidelines for both biomedical research[22] and epidemiological studies.[23]

In the reproductive health specialty, the International Federation of Gynecology and Obstetrics (known through its French and Spanish acronym FIGO) has been active, particularly through its Committee on Ethical Aspects of Human Reproduction and Women's Health and its Committee for Women's Sexual and Reproductive Rights. These Committees are strongly engaged in promoting understanding of how to apply ethics and human rights among its

---

[22] Council for International Organizations of Medical Sciences (CIOMS), *International Ethical Guidelines for Biomedical Research Involving Human Subjects* (Geneva: CIOMS, 2002).

[23] CIOMS, *International Guidelines for Ethical Review of Epidemiological Studies* (Geneva: CIOMS, 1991).

membership, reproductive health practitioners, and beyond. The FIGO Committee on ethics has developed guidance on a range of issues related to the ethical delivery of sexual and reproductive health services and research in human reproduction.[24] The FIGO Women's Sexual and Reproductive Rights Committee is developing a Reproductive Rights Code. Among international non-governmental organizations, the International Planned Parenthood Federation (IPPF) has published a Charter on Sexual and Reproductive Rights[25] that offers directions for fostering compliance with such rights.

National agencies, including courts of law, may consider CIOMS and FIGO guidelines and, for example, the IPPF Charter to indicate the levels of performance and expected procedures that are part of national providers' legally applicable standards of care and of conduct. Such agencies may translate internationally derived standards and processes into national laws.

Accordingly, providers of reproductive and sexual health services have guidance from colleagues within and sympathetically related to their own professions on observance of prevailing laws, and on reform of law to advance reproductive and sexual health. They also have opportunities for contribution to, and leadership in, promotion and protection of reproductive health through law. Law is a weapon that empowers those capable of employing it, and it can be employed both against and on behalf of providers of reproductive health services. Law can discipline inadequate practice, and also provide grounds to challenge and remove rules and practices that impair good medical care directed to patients' reproductive and sexual health. The sword of legal justice is double-edged.

It has been seen that human rights are recognized through legal systems at both national and international levels. Legal ways to implement internationally recognized human rights principles are not necessarily different from implementation of national laws. Many human rights are expressed in national laws, including the constitutional laws of many countries, and international human rights instruments have derived much of their substance from national laws. Nevertheless, the modern international human rights movement, commencing after 1945, is a reaction to national laws and courts denying human rights under the influence of totalitarian governments, and tolerating oppression of countries' nationals on racial, religious, political, economic, and military grounds.

Human rights claims may be advanced by individuals in the same way as they would pursue other legal claims, but enforcement of human rights claims has several distinctive features. Because human rights are expressed in leading

---

[24] FIGO, Committee for the Ethical Aspects of Human Reproduction and Women's Health, *Recommendations on Ethical Issues in Obstetrics and Gynecology* (London: FIGO, 2000). Also available at website http://www.figo.org, last accessed 7 May 2002.

[25] IPPF, *Charter on Sexual and Reproductive Rights* (London: IPPF, 1996).

international conventions by which countries have agreed to be bound, claims tend to be brought against states themselves on the ground that state agencies or officers have violated human rights. A promising development is recognition that states themselves can be considered at fault when a human rights outrage is perpetrated by a private person or agency, but the state facilitated or accommodated the violation by its own lack of due diligence to prevent or deter the violation. For instance, when a member of her family commits an 'honour killing' of a woman believed to have had sex outside marriage, the state can be implicated in that murder for not acting adequately to prevent or deter such killings.

States are represented by their governments, which may enjoy immunities under their own national laws and invoke their national sovereignty to resist international and national criticism of conduct undertaken within their territorial jurisdiction. Claimants may have the support of non-governmental organizations and other activists in developing their claims. They take on the powerful legal, research, and other defences that governments can amass by grass-roots activism and the committed energy of dedicated individuals with different types and levels of skills. Qualified lawyers are usually required to draft necessary documents and conduct the procedural stages of resort to courts and other tribunals, but they are guided by the evidence and arguments gathered by and on behalf of the claimants they represent. How those supporting and fashioning human rights claims might prepare materials for their lawyers is outlined above (Sect. 3).

4.1.2. *Courts of law*

Best used as a measure of last resort, when consensual approaches have failed or been prevented, national courts of law may be mobilized to conduct hearings according to civil law, administrative law, or criminal law processes. National courts of law can compel participation of agencies that will not agree to informal resolution of disputes, such as by alternative dispute resolution (ADR). In some countries, separate constitutional courts exist, which can determine claims regarding rights contained in constitutional documents.

Courts of law conduct proceedings according to publicly available rules of practice, and are usually open to the public and reportable in news media. According to their traditions, they may conduct their hearings by adversarial or inquisitorial procedures, but will usually accommodate the arguments and evidence of parties to which they award standing to be heard. It is usually expected that judges give reasons for their decisions, that their decisions be issued publicly, and that decisions be enforceable by the authority of the tribunals themselves.

The status of international human rights law and ratified conventions will be different in the courts of law of each country. Some require their legislatures specifically to enact legislation implementing a treaty into national law before it is applicable domestically. In the United Kingdom, for instance, the Human Rights Act was enacted in 1998 to give the force of national law to the European Convention on Human Rights, by which the United Kingdom had previously been bound internationally but not by its domestic law. In others, such as Colombia,[26] the constitution gives priority over national law to an international treaty that the country has ratified.

The transcending problem with courts of law is that the justice they offer is frequently practically inaccessible to many people and interests. Access often depends on the purchase of expensive legal skills, knowledge of detailed procedures, drafting and interpretation of complex documents, and willingness to be patient for many months or years for the completion of sequential procedural steps leading to a judgment. Trial judgments are often open to appeal, which further prolongs the process to resolution, and increases complexities and costs. Important initiatives are under way to educate national court judges in the domestic application of international human rights conventions, such as the Convention on the Rights of the Child.[27] Similar work could usefully be initiated to train judges about the application in their own legal systems of national, regional, and international human rights concerning reproductive and sexual health.

National courts are beginning to apply international human rights standards, particularly where there is a gap in national law.[28] For example, the Indian Supreme Court has applied CEDAW General Recommendation 19 in an important decision on sexual harassment.[29] A group of social activists and non-governmental organizations went to court with the aim of preventing sexual harassment of all women in all workplaces, by filling a vacuum in existing legislation. The immediate cause for bringing the case was the acquittal of the accused in a criminal case brought on behalf of a social worker employed by the Ministry of Health of the Government of Rajastan, who had been subjected to a brutal gang rape in a Rajastani village. In line with other gender-sensitive decisions,[30] the Supreme Court of India recognized that sexual harassment is a clear violation of the national Constitution (Articles 14 (sexual

---

[26] Constitution of Colombia, Art. 93: 'International treaties and agreements ratified by the Congress that recognize human rights and that prohibit their limitation in states of emergency have priority domestically.'

[27] V. Yolles, *The United Nations Convention on the Rights of the Child: A Practical Guide to its Use in Canadian Courts* (Toronto: UNICEF Canada, 1998).

[28] A. Byrnes, J. Connors, and L. Bik, *Advancing the Human Rights of Women: Using International Human Rights Standards in Domestic Litigation* (London: Commonwealth Secretariat, 1997).

[29] *Vishaka v. State of Rajasthan* (1997), 6 SCC 241 (Supreme Court of India).

[30] S. P. Sathe, 'Gender, Constitution and Courts', in A. Dhanda and A. Parashar, *Engendering Law: Essays in Honour of Lotika Sarkar* (Lucknow: Eastern Book Co., 1999), 117–35.

non-discrimination), 19(1)(*g*) (pursuance of an occupation), 21 (life and liberty), and 42 (just and humane working conditions)), and merits an effective remedy. Recognizing that existing Indian laws had not adequately protected women from workplace-related sexual harassment, the Court issued guidelines on the prevention of sexual harassment, and explained that they would be judicially enforceable until suitable national legislation is enacted. The guidelines define sexual harassment, and outline the duty of employers to prevent, punish, and remedy sexual harassment.

In fashioning this remedy, the Court relied on the CEDAW General Recommendation 19 on Violence against Women (see Pt. III, Ch. 6, Sect. 1). The Court explained that:

The international conventions and norms are to be read into [the fundamental rights guaranteed in the Constitution of India] in the absence of enacted domestic law occupying the field when there is no inconsistency between them. It is now an accepted rule of judicial construction that regard must be had to international conventions and norms for construing domestic law when there is no inconsistency between them and there is a void in the domestic law.[31]

The Court gave content and meaning to Indian constitutional principles by relying on the CEDAW General Recommendation. Perhaps even more significantly, the Court also affirmed the international significance of the work of agencies like CEDAW, thus forging a path for other courts to follow in the use of international standards as interpretative guides in giving substance to principles of national human rights law. Other courts will recognize the potential to apply this General Recommendation and other similarly developed international law standards in addressing the underlying causes of violations of women's rights. The Court's initiative and vision give reason to think that other international clarifications of required standards of protection could be similarly adopted into national laws in addressing other affronts to human dignity, such as the neglect of preventable causes of reproductive and sexual ill-health.

4.1.3. *Criminal law approaches*

Criminal laws directed to society at large are obviously also applicable to health care providers. Accordingly, if their practices violate such general laws they will be liable to criminal proceedings. Applications of criminal law to compel health care providers' observance of laws specifically related to health care have been unusual. However, there are cases, some of historic significance, in the field of reproductive health law, concerning contraception and abortion. More common are exemptions from legal liability that allow

---

[31] *Vishaka* (see n. 29), at 251, para. 14.

physicians to do what non-physicians cannot, such as conduct physical examinations of unconscious people. Legislation is increasingly proposed to control new reproductive technologies, and to prohibit anticipated developments such as human reproductive (as opposed to therapeutic) cloning. These laws may be reinforced, in extreme circumstances such as deliberate defiance, by criminal sanctions. Where any form of professional practice is permitted only under licence, unlicensed practice is usually criminally punishable.

Criminal law tends to be a rather crude instrument that society may direct against the more severe violations of standards of social conduct and safety. It governs deliberate wrongs such as assaults, gross negligence causing bodily harm, and recklessness in care of others when they are in peril. For instance, an anaesthetist has been convicted of manslaughter when death was caused by his grossly negligent inattention during surgery.[32] Licensed physicians are privileged to conduct physical examinations and invasive procedures, such as surgery, but unqualified practitioners may face criminal penalties for conducting invasive procedures, even with consent of recipients of care who know that they are not medically qualified. Mentally competent individuals, both adults and mature adolescents who have not reached the age of legal majority, are usually considered competent to give legally effective consent for medical interventions on themselves. Parents can usually consent for examinations and treatments that are medically indicated for their children, and often have legal duties to ensure that their children receive necessary medical care. This may include termination of pregnancy, for instance when young girls have been victims of sexual assaults (see Pt. I, Ch. 5, Sect. 6.3.2, and Ch. 6, Sect. 4.4.3).

In many jurisdictions, parents and other guardians of children are not free to authorize medical treatments unless they are intended to serve a therapeutic or orthodox preventive health care purpose. This may present difficulties when investigators propose non-therapeutic research procedures on children, or on mentally compromised adults. Circumcision of infant and young males, for instance on religious grounds, has been judicially considered to be within parental power to approve,[33] but female circumcision is considerably more contentious. In several countries, health professional rules of conduct prohibit the practice, and increasingly criminal law prohibitions are being enacted (see Pt. I, Ch. 5, Sect. 11).

Similarly, professional and legal prohibitions are increasing against contraceptive sterilization procedures on young, non-consenting females and those who suffer mental impairment and are under parental or other guardianship. Where guardians are not legally empowered to authorize such procedures, such as by courts of law or specifically created legislation, providers who undertake

[32] *R. v. Adomako*, [1994] 3 All ER 78 (House of Lords, England).
[33] *R. v. Brown*, [1993] 2 All ER 75 (House of Lords, England).

them lack lawful consent, and are liable to criminal and professional disciplinary proceedings. If providers are convinced that procedures are of positive benefit to the females for whom they are proposed, such as to control menstruation that they cannot learn to cope with and causes them alarm or serious distress each month, they may afford evidence of their assessment to guardians, who may then have authority to give approval of the procedures on the ground that they are therapeutic. If guardians' approval is granted, providers may undertake these procedures with legal security. Hysterectomy will leave the females sterile, but the procedure is not intended for the purpose of reproductive control as such. It remains professionally hazardous, however, to conduct such a procedure without prior judicial or other specific legal approval.

In criminal law, liability for assault arises from touching another person without legal authority, from that person if he or she is competent, or another legally empowered to consent, such as a guardian or a judge. A special concern for gynaecologists, and urologists, is that some legal systems provide that sexual assault is more severely punishable than ordinary or common assault, and that the distinction between common and sexual assault is the objective or impersonal nature of the unauthorized touching. It is no defence to a charge of sexual assault that it was not motivated by any sexual purpose. Accordingly, if a gynaecologist touches a person's genitalia in the course of a medically regular but legally unauthorized examination, a criminal charge may be considered for sexual assault, which is more socially stigmatizing than the lesser charge for common assault and may attract greater attention and sanction by medical associations and licensing authority disciplinary tribunals. However, public prosecutors have to exercise professional responsibility in laying charges, having regard to their duty to act in the public interest. That interest is not served by making reproductive (or any other) health care providers reluctant to conduct necessary care, and so restraint is usually used regarding laying criminal charges, except in the most egregious cases. Agents under whose authority public prosecutors act, such as Ministers of Justice or Attorneys-General, are politically accountable for their prosecutorial practice, and may make declarations of what practices will and will not be prosecuted as criminal. For instance, the Attorney-General of England has stated that undertaking emergency contraception within seventy-two hours of unprotected intercourse will not be governed by provisions of the abortion law.[34]

4.1.4. *Civil (non-criminal) law approaches*

Where members of communities enjoy convenient and affordable access to lawyers and courts, health care providers may be concerned that allegations of

---

[34] Sir Michael Havers, Written Answer, *Parliamentary Debates (Hansard)* 6th series, vol. 42, cols. 235–6, 10 May 1983.

their failure to observe legal principles or standards governing patient care will result in civil litigation, and that they will be sued particularly for financial compensation called 'damages'. Courts finding them liable will, at a minimum, require return of fees charged for services that were improperly delivered, and beyond this may award nominal damages. They will award substantial damages where patients suffered distress, physical and/or psychological harm, and other injuries such as loss of employment or professional opportunities. In addition, courts may award further compensation, called exemplary or punitive damages, where improper care was delivered with indifference or callousness towards patients' interests, or caused them humiliation, indignity, or loss of self-esteem.

The most common basis of civil liability arises from professional negligence (see Pt. I, Ch. 5, Sect. 8). However, treating patients without legal authorization is also a legal wrong, frequently called battery or assault, which is usually a lesser form of criminal assault. This is not necessarily serious enough to punish under criminal law, but justifies an award of compensation to the patient, even if the injury that resulted was minor. Battery may arise when treatment is different from what a patient consented to, or when it exceeds the procedure approved, such as performing a sterilization when the patient requested only abortion. The fact that sterilization was medically indicated and in the patient's interests to have performed at the same time as surgical abortion is no defence, except when life-saving procedures are necessary. The touching itself is a wrong even if the procedure was competently undertaken. It is no defence to a civil charge of battery that it was skilfully performed.

Chapter 5 explains that, if a procedure is performed negligently, even with full legal authorization to undertake it, a practitioner will be liable if injury is caused. Patients give informed consent to the inherent risks of the procedure, but do not consent to the risk of it being performed negligently.[35] When a practitioner bears a legal duty of care, liability to pay compensation will arise if the duty is not performed according to the legally set standard of care, causing harm to a person to whom a duty of care is owed. In law, negligence is addressed only as a transient incident, although identification of what constitutes negligence can guide practitioners on the difference between acceptable and unacceptable practice. However, health care providers sometimes overreact to an allegation of negligence, treating it as if it claims an enduring defective personality trait in the practitioner.[36]

When a patient is injured from a procedure that bears an irreducible level of inherent risk, the occurrence of the injury risked is not evidence that the

---

[35] See n. 32.
[36] American College of Obstetricians and Gynecologists (ACOG) Committee Opinion (Committee on Professional Liability), 'Coping with the Stress of Malpractice Litigation', *Int. J. Gynecol. Obstet.* 74 (2001), 65–6.

provider who performed the procedure was negligent. However, the provider's explanation that the patient knowingly assumed that level of risk, and accordingly cannot prevail in a claim that negligence was involved, depends on the patient having been adequately informed of the risk, and having been competent and free from the provider's improper pressure to accept it. A patient who consents to performance of a procedure cannot succeed in a claim for battery if it results in injury, but may succeed in a claim for negligence by showing that the patient was not provided with adequate information about the irreducible level of risk inherent in the procedure. Injury may not have been due to any lack of skill or care by the practitioner in performance of the procedure. It may be shown to have been caused, however, by defective disclosure of information because, had relevant information been given, the patient would have chosen not to have the procedure, and therefore would not have been exposed to its irreducible risk. The practitioner must avoid negligence not only in performance of the procedure, but also in ensuring that appropriate information is provided to assist the decision by or on behalf of the patient concerning what, if any, treatment to receive.

As a general rule, providers are not taken to guarantee the effectiveness or the complete safety of procedures they propose to undertake. However, in some cases, providers or their clinics enter into undertakings or contracts with patients, and terms are included (which courts may find implicit when they are not in written language) that guarantee certain outcomes, or that particular events will not occur. A provider may have given an assurance, for example, that a procedure will terminate a pregnancy, or that a sterilization procedure will exclude the risk of pregnancy, or that the drug Viagra will ensure a man's sexual capacity and be safe to take. Such terms are binding, and their breach justifies compensation, even if there was no negligence on the part of the practitioner in performing the procedure in question, and the outcome was impossible to achieve or guarantee, or the harm was unavoidable. Parties to contracts who give guarantees that are impossible to perform are nevertheless liable for breach of the guarantee. Practitioners should therefore risk no misunderstanding about the limits within which the procedures they propose to undertake can be safe and effective. They should remain vigilant for instance in abortion cases, and also alert patients, to watch for signs of continuation of pregnancy, and inform sterilization patients about risks of future pregnancy. Women should be warned of the continuing risk of, for instance, tubal pregnancy, and vasectomy patients should be warned about unprotected intercourse too soon after the procedure.

4.1.5. *Alternative dispute resolution*

The capacity of legal systems to accommodate non-judicial resolution of disputes is receiving emphasis in modern practice in the quest to reach convenient, private, prompt, and less expensive settlements of disputes about observance of legal duties. Many legal systems retain historical, customary, and communal methods of dispute resolution that avoid the costs, delay, and adversarial winner-take-all processes of dispute resolution that characterize judicial outcomes in many modern legal systems. Judicial proceedings reflect individualism and adversarial relationships between strangers. Techniques of alternative dispute resolution (ADR) reflect how disagreements may be overcome when they arise between parties who expect to be in continuing relationship with each other, such as members of families and residents in the same communities, and who do not want a dispute to become a distracting preoccupation in their enduring collaborative relationship.

The aim of ADR is that parties to a dispute achieve resolution by negotiation that leaves them all satisfied in the outcome. A focus of negotiators may be on how injuries or service failures are best overcome, rather than on identification of who is to blame, and on how hurt emotional feelings can be overcome and all parties regain their self-esteem and pay due respect to the feelings of other parties. Prolonged judicial proceedings can be countertherapeutic in that they provide incentives for plaintiffs to preserve signs of injury, disability, and distress until judgment, whereas in ADR injuries can be quickly acknowledged in pursuit of steps towards recovery. ADR avoids the worst excesses of adversarial conflict, including exaggerated claims to injury and insult by plaintiffs and to virtue by defendants, which may be distasteful to those who make them as well as to those against whom they are made.

Unlike in courts of law, important aspects of ADR may concern sincere apology, such as for oversights and lack of due respect to another party's dignity. In addition, ADR may facilitate factual inquiries when legal principles are not in contest, and bring in scientifically qualified mutually approved assessors rather than opposing parties' witnesses to determine facts in dispute through 'battle of the experts'. In many legal systems, courts of law are the only resort for patients resentful that their emotional comfort and dignity were degraded by health care providers who seem to act as managers of sophisticated technologies and conduits of drugs that have unpronounceable names and uncertain effects, rather than as patients' concerned care-givers. Litigation is used as a means to gain such aloof providers' attention and respect, and to bring them down to patients' levels. Alternative dispute resolution may achieve parties' mutual respect in a manner that is less public, adversarial, and expensive, and that addresses the relationships among different parties in personal terms. All parties may prefer ADR to judicial processes that are impersonal and require employment of the special language, descriptions, and documents, frequently alien to the experience of both patients and providers, which characterize formal judicial proceedings.

ADR cannot be employed when an agency that is complained against refuses to recognize the capacity of the complainant to question its performance or to call it to account. ADR is consensual, depending upon mutual recognition, respect, and collaboration among parties willing to approach each other as equals.

4.1.6. *Regulatory and disciplinary approaches*

Professional discipline may be imposed by associations of health care providers to which members belong voluntarily. Voluntary professional associations such as national medical associations are often influential in their countries in representing the interests both of the medical profession and of the patients their members serve. They afford their members the prestige of membership on the understanding, agreed in the contractual exchange of membership privileges for payment of membership fees, that members will submit to scrutiny of their practice and to the judgement of their professional peers. Associations' ethics or discipline committees tend to include senior and particularly respected members of the profession, as well as peers in status of regular members. Committees may act on complaints made by members, and by others such as patients, and initiate their own inquiries into members' conduct.

Members voluntarily accept their liability to censure and even expulsion for proven misconduct. Such discipline may be imposed for misconduct that is not itself a breach of the law, such as failure to respond promptly to professional association requests for information. Misconduct may also be demonstrated, however, by conduct that violates the law, such as treating patients in non-emergency cases without appropriate consent, and failure to maintain professional confidentiality. Members may also be required, for instance, to give an account of their invocation of rights of conscientious objection to decline to provide particular services in public hospitals which they perform in private clinics.

Whether or not providers are members of voluntary professional associations, their professional status often depends on licensure. Licensing authorities are usually constituted and their members appointed by governments under legislation that allows the authorities to license appropriately qualified persons to practise as licensed professionals, and allows the authorities to regulate and discipline practitioners who are subject to their jurisdiction. Such authorities are usually constituted with heavy reliance on members of the licensed profession itself, but with some governmentally appointed lay members. Their legal mandate is usually to protect the public interest against unqualified practice, and against incompetent or unethical conduct by licensed providers. Professional licensure includes legal liability of providers to submit to the scrutiny of the licensing authority on the regulatory ground of fitness to practise, and the disciplinary ground of personal integrity. Failure to maintain professional standards of competence and, for instance, confidentiality may accordingly lead to regulatory or disciplinary proceedings.

Regulatory proceedings focus on a person's knowledge, capacity, and fitness to fulfil the functions of the profession, so as to be permitted or renewed to practise it. Disciplinary proceedings concern whether a licensed provider has observed the professional code of conduct, which will include the duty to observe the law and ethical standards. Regulatory and disciplinary proceedings are to be conducted in accordance with principles of administrative law, which focus on procedural fairness. These principles address the composition of the tribunal conducting a hearing on fitness or integrity, for instance to exclude the risk of bias or prejudice, the fair presentation of evidence and argument, and rights of recourse to courts of law on matters of law and procedure. They may include subsequent access to regular courts of law to appeal against tribunal decisions, or to seek review of the propriety of the tribunal's conduct of the proceedings or, for instance, the disciplinary sanctions imposed.

4.1.7. *The international exception*

Many judicial decisions relevant to reproductive health care come from civil courts in the United States. Health care providers in other countries often fear that acceptance of legal principles declared by US courts will lead to the same flood of medical malpractice litigation that has appeared there. The same concerns arise about affordability of medical malpractice insurance premiums and their inflation of physicians' fees that make services unaffordable to many people, and the same compromises of patient care and affordability of services associated with so-called defensive medicine. Judges in even the highest courts of other countries have echoed some of these concerns.[37] However, the principles that US courts have applied are little different from those in other countries with similarly qualified and organized medical practitioners,[38] but there has been no similar flood of medical malpractice litigation in those countries. The volume of US medical malpractice litigation is not due to any distinctive legal principles its courts apply, but to procedural rules governing access to US courts that are found in very few, if any, other countries. The US experience is an unrepresentative exception.

Perhaps the key reasons that explain the exceptionally high volume of US medical malpractice litigation are that, in its legal system, it usually costs nothing to lose a case, and US physicians have sufficient insurance to pay sizeable compensation awards if a patient wins a case. In order to facilitate people's access to the courts in a country where governments do not supply or subsidize

---

[37] See, for instance, Lord Scarman in *Sidaway v. Bethlem Royal Hospital Governors*, [1985] 1 All ER 643 at 650 (House of Lords, England).
[38] D. Giesen, *International Medical Malpractice: A Comparative Law Study of Civil Liability Arising from Medical Care* (Dordrecht: Martinus Nijhoff, 1988).

legal services for private persons in civil claims, governments and the legal profession permit lawyers to offer services on the basis that, if the claims they conduct are unsuccessful, their clients do not have to pay their fees or expenses. This is the contingency fee, or 'no win, no pay' system. If a claim is successful, the lawyer's fees are paid as a proportion of the compensation awarded. Lawyers therefore become partners or stakeholders in their clients' claims. Professional associations have sliding scales of permissible recovery, often ranging from, for instance, 40 per cent of small amounts recovered to 10 per cent or less for very large, multi-million dollar awards. Both professional associations and the courts monitor lawyers' rates of recovery from compensation awards. Lawyers' entitlements from successful cases tend to be relatively high, because their fees cover their expenses in conducting unsuccessful claims.

Further, unsuccessful litigants are not ordered to pay successful litigants' legal costs. In other countries, the common rule is that litigants must pay the costs they cause. That is, wrongdoers who deny their liability, and so cause injured persons to sue them, are ordered to pay compensation for the wrongs they did, and also to pay the legal costs incurred by the victims because the victims were compelled to sue them. Those who sue others without just cause, shown by failure of their claims, are ordered to pay the legal costs they caused those they wrongfully sued to incur in self-defence. However, perhaps uniquely, US courts do not usually order losers to pay winners' legal costs. Accordingly, losers may pay neither their own legal costs nor those of the parties they sue. This encourages people to sue, because financially they cannot lose, although they may not win.

Physicians in the USA are usually worth suing. That is, lawyers working on contingency fees find them attractive targets of claims. Whether or not physicians have personal means, they almost invariably have insurance, purchased as commercial services. Physicians who maintain their own practices or clinics usually have insurance. Those who work in or through hospitals, for instance with admission and treatment privileges, are usually required by the hospitals to carry insurance, in order to be able to indemnify them for any costs the hospitals incur in litigation due to the doctors. In addition, the US Constitution entitles litigants to trial by jury, and juries composed of lay people tend to be sympathetic to sometimes genuinely damaged patients, and more so when physicians are presumed to be wealthy and are presented by claimants' lawyers as mercenary, aloof, uncaring or callous, and exploitive. Juries are also empowered to award compensation or 'damages' not only for financial losses shown to have been caused and for patients' pain and suffering, but also punitive damages, to express their communal sense of outrage at the enormity of the wrongs and indignities they have found proven.

Jury trials can be very costly to defend, legal costs of successful defences are not recoverable from those who unjustifiably initiated the proceedings, and jury awards in successful claims can be large because, even though the patients' injuries may be minor, juries can award sizeable punitive damages. Damage awards are open to reduction only through equally expensive appeals to higher courts, which may dismiss such appeals or, if granting them, order the original claim to be retried. Physicians' commercial insurance companies may therefore prefer to settle claims quickly out of court, even when confident that the claims would fail if tried in court. Lawyers for patient-claimants know that, even if their claims are unlikely to succeed, the claims may still have a 'settlement value', meaning that defendant physicians' insurance companies would rather offer payments to settle them without trials than fight them in courts. Lawyers for patient-plaintiffs therefore find that they can profit from taking patients' cases, even if they would fail at the end of court proceedings.

Insurance companies in the US may settle claims for a very modest percentage of the sums for which patients sue, and pass on the expense to physicians through premiums they charge for insurance cover. Physicians pass on these insurance costs to patients in fees for their services. Thus, other patients who, by themselves or their employers, can afford medical care will collectively furnish the means to satisfy individual patients' claims. In other countries, people who have financial means collectively pay for others' misfortunes by governmental taxation of their incomes, transferred to less fortunate people through social insurance payments, for instance for disabled and unemployed people. In the US this occurs indirectly, left to private enterprise through medical malpractice litigation and commercial insurance. Insurance premiums charged to physicians are passed on to patients or to their employers' health insurers in costs for care. A consequence is that care is unavailable for tens of millions of US citizens, who have no means to cover its costs. It was estimated in 2000 that 38.7 million Americans lacked health care insurance.[39] Further, a national study found that half of all personal bankruptcies filed in 1999 involved a medical problem.[40] Beyond publicly funded health care for the elderly and the very poor, there is no publicly funded health care in the US, almost alone among developed countries. The US experience of medical malpractice litigation is unique, and its effects on individuals' access to health care services make it a system not liable to be deliberately copied elsewhere.

4.1.8. *Legislative approaches*

Where confidence does not exist that health service providers will observe their legal and human rights obligations, legislation may be proposed and enacted that prescribes how health service providers are to behave, and how

---

[39] R. Pear, 'Number of Uninsured Drops for 2nd Year', *New York Times* (28 Sept. 2001), A20.
[40] M. B. Jacoby, 'Rethinking the Debates over Health Care Financing: Evidence from the Bankruptcy Courts', *New York University Law Review*, 76 (2001), 375–416 at 377.

their practice will be scrutinized through professionally qualified or other inspectors. Legislation may also define under what circumstances, and by which categories of practitioners, restricted drugs may be prescribed for use.

Where enforcement of law usually entrusted to professional self-regulatory authorities is believed liable to be inadequate in some regards, practices that have aroused public concern may become subject to control by specific legislation. For instance, where undisclosed conflict of interest appears through providers' ownership of clinical laboratories to which they refer patients for costly tests, legislation may be enacted to prohibit such ownership or to require provider-owners to inform patients of their ownership interests and provide alternative options. Where clinical procedures have been undertaken on mentally impaired patients without their guardians' approval, or upon guardians' insistence but not clearly in patients' best interests, such as contraceptive sterilization, legislation may be enacted to regularize consent procedures. Legislation may, for instance, require reference of each proposed procedure to an appropriate public officer or tribunal, or a court of law.

In countries where medically assisted reproduction is available, particularly by employment of recently developed biotechnologies, legislation may be enacted that specifies the conditions and limitations under which such assistance may be requested, supplied, and advertised. Some countries fearful of attempts at human reproductive cloning, for instance, have proposed laws to ban and punish such attempts. Legislation may be enforceable through such means as criminal proceedings or professional disciplinary proceedings, or through a licensing system. Licenses may be granted on approval of governmentally appointed authorities that specify conditions, undertake inspections, and monitor the practice of individual licence holders and the evolving state of the art concerning the safety and efficacy of techniques and practices.

In the United Kingdom, for instance, legislation of 1990[41] establishes the Human Fertilisation and Embryology Authority, which has strong medical and scientific representation, sets standards for and monitors professional practice of assisted reproduction and facilitates the public's informed access to services.[42] Individual health care providers, professional associations and others may urge legislation, and even propose its language, to preserve and advance interests considered to serve the public. This may be, for instance, by compelling or prohibiting particular conduct, or creating capacity for the exercise of professional judgement. An example of how medical professional understanding and practice can be expressed in legislation is found in the UK, where subsection 2(3) of the Human Fertilisation and Embryology Act 1990

---

[41] Human Fertilisation and Embryology Act 1990, UK Statutes, ch. 37.
[42] See the Human Fertilisation and Embryology Authority (HFEA), Code of Practice (London: HFEA, 4th edn., 1998).

provides that 'For the purposes of this Act, a woman is not to be treated as carrying a child until the embryo has become implanted.' Consistently, attempts to prevent implantation, such as by post-coital emergency contraception, do not fall under the Abortion Act, 1967.

4.1.9. *Human rights commissions*

National human rights commissions, such as those in India, the Philippines, and Sri Lanka, and regional human rights commissions, or national commissions more narrowly concerned with patients' or women's rights, provide other opportunities for investigations to promote legal and human rights to reproductive and sexual health. Some of these commissions are beginning to focus on the protection of economic, social, and cultural rights,[43] and may provide platforms to explore how these rights can be more effectively applied to advance reproductive and sexual health. They may conduct public investigations into issues they find of public concern, and *in camera* enquiries into complaints of legal and human rights violations it would be stigmatizing for those not in breach or at fault to have unduly publicized. That is, they are usually vigilant to safeguard the human rights and reputations of those whose actions are under investigation.

4.1.10. *Ombudsmen*

In some countries, officers exist who are appointed by government agencies or more privately, such as by hospitals or health service agencies, and equipped to conduct inquiries into complaints of injustice, and perhaps to receive representations on behalf of agencies and interests in dispute about facts and standards. The model of the Swedish Ombudsman has been widely adopted. Ombudsmen are persons of either sex, who usually act by predetermined procedures to hear complaints of injustice due to maladministration, to determine facts through their own inquiries and the receipt of evidence from interested parties, and to present their conclusions. They may make recommendations for reform, and for correction of any improprieties disclosed by an investigation.

The Human Rights Ombudsman in Colombia, for example, has held hearings to develop strategies to enable the provision of health services, including reproductive and sexual health services, to adolescents based on their evolving capacities, and not on an arbitrary age limitation.[44] The Women's Ombud in Costa Rica, for example, has reported significant lapses in gynaecological and

---

[43] Canadian Human Rights Foundation and Philippine Commission on Human Rights, *The Role of National Human Rights Commissions in the Promotion and Protection of Economic, Social and Cultural Rights* (Montreal: Canadian Human Rights Foundation, 1999).

[44] Correspondence with the executive director of PROFAMILIA, Bogotá, Colombia, 8 May 2002.

obstetric care, including lack of attention to privacy and failure to follow through on tests for detection of cervical cancer.[45] The model of the ombudsman is a systematic example of alternative dispute resolution, through an officer established in advance of any particular dispute arising.

4.2. *Regional and international approaches*

There are several procedures in regional[46] and international[47] human rights conventions through which national observance of human rights to reproductive and sexual health may be scrutinized and assessed. Some of these procedures, such as reporting, can be pursued by regional and international tribunals or committees simultaneously with national efforts; others, such as the complaint procedure available to individuals, usually require the exhaustion of domestic remedies before regional and international tribunals will agree to become involved. These procedures provide important means by which to develop norms and standards on sexual and reproductive health at the regional[48] and international level.[49]

---

[45] International Women's Rights Action Watch, *The Women's Watch*, 12/2–3 (1998), 7.

[46] D. Shelton, 'The Promise of Regional Human Rights Systems', in B. H. Weston and S. P. Marks (eds.), *The Future of International Human Rights* (New York: Transnational Publishers,1999); C. Medina, 'Toward a More Effective Guarantee of the Enjoyment of Human Rights by Women in the Inter-American System', in R. J. Cook (ed.), *Human Rights of Women: National and International Perspectives* (Philadelphia: University of Pennsylvania Press, 1994), 257–84, tr. into Spanish, available from PROFAMILIA, Bogotá, Colombia; C. Beyani, 'Towards a More Effective Guarantee of the Enjoyment of Human Rights by Women in the African System', in Cook (ed.), *Human Rights of Women*, 285–306; R. J. Cook, 'Fostering Compliance with Women's Rights in the Inter-American System', *Revue Québécoise de Droit International*, 111 (1998), 129–42; F. Viljoen, 'Application of the African Charter on Human and Peoples' Rights by Domestic Courts in Africa', *Journal of African Law*, 43 (1999), 1–17.

[47] A. Byrnes, 'Towards a More Effective Enforcement of Women's Human Rights through the Use of International Human Rights Law and Procedures', in Cook (ed.), *Human Rights of Women*.

[48] M. C. Calderón, M. I. Plata, J. Lemaitre, *et al.*, *El Sistema Interamericano de Derechos Humanos: Derechos Sexuales y Reproductivos en Acción* (Bogotá: Profamilia Legal Services for Women, 4 vols., 2001); A. Carbert, J. Stanchieri, and R. J. Cook, *Advocating for Reproductive and Sexual Health Rights in the African Regional Human Rights System* (Chapel Hill, NC: Ipas, 2001); J. Stanchieri, I. Merali, N. Rasmussen, *et al.*, *The Application of Human Rights to Reproductive and Sexual Health: A Compilation of the Work of the European Human Rights System* (Warsaw: Federation for Women and Family Planning and ASTRA—Central and Eastern European Women's Network for Sexual and Reproductive Rights, 2 vols., 2002).

[49] I. Boerefijn and B. Toebes, 'Health and Human Rights: Health Issues Discussed by United Nations Treaty Monitoring Bodies', Netherlands Institute for Human Rights, *SIM, special issue*, 21 (1998), 25–53; J. Stanchieri, I. Merali, and R. J. Cook, *The Application of Human Rights to Reproductive and Sexual Health: A Compilation of the Work of International Treaty Bodies* (Ottawa: Action Canada for Population and Development, 2001). Available at www.acpd.ca, last accessed 7 May 2002; J. Zajkowski, K. H. Martinez, and R. J. Cook, *Bringing Rights to Bear on Reproductive and Sexual Rights: An Analysis of the Work of UN Treaty Monitoring Bodies* (New York: CRLP 2003).

4.2.1. *Reporting procedures*

Countries that are members of different international and regional human rights conventions are obligated to report national performance in discharge of their duties to each appropriate treaty monitoring body, on a periodic basis. For example, as of April 2002, 168 states had committed themselves through the Women's Convention (see Pt. III, Ch. 5) to report regularly to CEDAW on what they have done to: 'take all appropriate measures to eliminate discrimination against women in the field of health care in order to ensure . . . access to health care services, including those related to family planning . . . pregnancy, confinement and the post-natal period, granting free services where necessary, as well as adequate nutrition during pregnancy and lactation' (Article 12). Countries are assisted in fulfilling their reporting obligations by a series of General Recommendations developed by the treaty monitoring bodies.[50] In explaining the content and meaning of treaty provisions, the Recommendations also outline the kind of information that treaty monitoring bodies find useful to receive when reviewing reporting countries' compliance records. For example, the CEDAW General Recommendation on Women and Health provides that:

in order to enable the Committee to evaluate whether measures to eliminate discrimination against women in the field of health care are appropriate, States Parties must report on their health legislation, plans and policies for women with reliable data disaggregated by sex on the incidence and severity of diseases and conditions hazardous to women's health and nutrition and on the availability and cost-effectiveness of preventive and curative measures. (see Pt. III, Ch. 6, Sect. 2, para. 9)

This Recommendation also stresses that: 'reports to the Committee must demonstrate that health legislation, plans and policies are based on scientific and ethical research and assessment of the health status and needs of women in that country and take into account any ethnic, regional or community variations or practices based on religion, tradition, or culture' (see Pt. III, Ch. 6, Sect. 2, para 9). In addition to requiring observance of its General Recommendations, CEDAW also agreed to apply the Cairo Programme in developing performance standards[51] to determine whether states are in compliance with their obligations under the Women's Convention.

Monitoring committees are mandated to be vigilant in their scrutiny of states' reports to investigate evidence of failures to meet responsibilities. For this purpose, most treaty monitoring committees, including CEDAW, are

---

[50] UN, *International Human Rights Instruments, Compilation of Central Comments and General Recommendations Adopted by Human Rights Treaty Bodies* (New York: UN, 1996), HRI/Gen1/Rev.2.

[51] UN, *Report of the Committee on the Elimination of Discrimination against Women (14th Session)* (New York: UN, 1995), A/50/38.

willing to receive alternative reports or comments on state performance submitted by non-governmental organizations.[52] These reports may incorporate significant findings of states' failures to protect and promote reproductive and sexual health. Such findings may result from medical, public health, or social science research, including events-based and standards-based data. Accordingly, a committee may investigate an individually documented case or incident, to see whether it discloses a representative failure of a state to protect a human right.

In its Concluding Observations on a report that a member state's government has submitted, a treaty monitoring committee notes the achievements the state has made in taking steps to bring its laws, policies, and practices into compliance with its treaty obligations, as well as the concerns the committee has with lack of compliance.[53] For example, CEDAW's Concluding Observations on the 1996 report of the government of Hungary included the following points with regard to reproductive health and related matters: 'the state of health of the female population was unsatisfactory when judged by international standards. In particular, the high cost of contraceptives prevented women from freely planning when to have children. The very high increase in the rate of abortions was of concern to the Committee.'[54] As a result, CEDAW requested that the government offer sex education programmes to all young people, and subsidize contraceptives in order to promote family planning and reduce the number of abortions.[55] CEDAW also requested that the government take urgent legislative and concrete measures to provide female victims of violence with protection and appropriate services.[56] CEDAW further noted with concern the scale of the problem of prostitution, which affected girls and women of ethnic minorities in particular,[57] and urgently requested the government to take all necessary measures to rehabilitate and reintegrate prostitutes into society.[58]

4.2.2. *Complaint procedures*

Procedures under some conventions, such as the American Convention on Human Rights, the European Convention on Human Rights, the

---

[52] See for instance CEDAW Alternative Report by Indian Non-Governmental Organizations (NGOs): Article 12 Health Care, CHETNA, Ahmedabad, India, in *Women's International News Network*, 23/3 (1997), 23–4; CLADEM, CRLP, and Estudio para la Defensa de los Derechos de la Mujer, *Women's Sexual and Reproductive Rights in Peru: A Shadow Report* (New York: CRLP, 1998); CRLP and Women's Legal Aid Centre, *Women's Reproductive Rights in Tanzania: A Shadow Report* (New York: CRLP, 1998).

[53] See n. 49.

[54] UN, *Concluding Observations of the Committee on the Elimination of Discrimination against Women, Hungary* (New York: UN, 1996), para. 254, A/51/38.

[55] Ibid. at para. 260.   [56] Ibid. at para. 259.
[57] Ibid. at para. 255.   [58] Ibid. at para. 261.

International Covenant on Civil and Political Rights, and the Women's Convention, enable individuals or in some cases groups of individuals to bring international complaints against their own states for alleged violations. However, these procedures can be employed only by individuals or national groups whose own states voluntarily consent to their right to employ them.

A normal condition of regional and international tribunals receiving individuals' petitions is that such individuals have exhausted all reasonable possibilities of achieving remedies before national tribunals of the states against which their petitions are presented. This condition respects the legal duties and opportunities of states first to afford remedies for wrongs through their own procedures. Once complainants have exhausted domestic procedures available to them without a remedy they find adequate, they can then proceed to either regional or international human rights tribunals to claim remedies for alleged violations. While complaints are brought by individuals or groups of individuals on their own behalf, their successful complaints can have the effect of requiring governments to change laws to the benefit of their entire societies, since other complainants equally aggrieved would be likely to enjoy the same success.

4.2.3. *Inquiry and communications procedures*

The Optional Protocol to the Women's Convention allows for a procedure of inquiry, which may be by experts appointed by CEDAW making a visit to a state that is a party, if reliable information is received indicating grave or systematic violations there of rights under the Convention. This procedure would allow, for example, for visits to appropriate sites to investigate allegations of governmental neglect of high rates of preventable maternal mortality, or failure to provide treatment to HIV-infected pregnant women.

Outside the treaty regimes, the UN Special Rapporteur on Violence against Women has facilitated clarifications of both international and national standards of protection against such violence. The UN Commission on Human Rights appointed the Special Rapporteur on Violence against Women in 1994 with a broad mandate to eliminate such violence and its causes, and to remedy its consequences, by recommending ways and means to eliminate gender violence at national, regional, and international levels.[59] The Special Rapporteur receives communications about alleged incidents of gender-specific violence against women that have not been effectively addressed through national legal systems. In ways that are similar to those of an ombudsman working at the national level, the rapporteur uses information showing violence to initiate and conduct dialogue with governments about finding resolutions.[60] Reports

---

[59] UN Doc. E/CN.4/1995/42, 22 Nov. 1994.
[60] UN Doc. E/CN.4/1997/47/Add. 4, 30 Jan. 1997.

of the Special Rapporteur[61] show that such violence may be an offence by a state itself against a broad range of accepted rights expressed in international human rights treaties and already binding on the state in question.[62]

In 2002, the UN Commission on Human Rights established a Special Rapporteur on the Right of Everyone to the Highest Attainable Standard of Physical and Mental Health. The role of the Special Rapporteur is to report to the Commission on the realization of the capacity of everyone to exercise this right.[63]

---

[61] See particularly country mission reports of the United Nations Special Rapporteur on Violence against Women: *Report on the Mission to the Democratic People's Republic of Korea, the Republic of Korea and Japan on the Issue of Military Sexual Slavery in Wartime* (New York: UN, 1996), E/CN.4/1997/47/Add. 1; *Report on the Mission to Poland on the Issue of Trafficking and Forced Prostitution of Women* (New York: UN, 1996), E/CN.4/1997/47/Add. 1; *Report on the Mission to Brazil on the Issue of Domestic Violence* (New York: UN, 1997), E/CN.4/1997/47/Add. 2; *Report on the Mission to South Africa on the Issue of Rape in the Community* (New York: UN, 1997), E/CN.4/1997/47/Add. 3.

[62] See e.g. *Velasquez v. Honduras* (1988), OAS/Ser.L/V/III.19, doc. 13 (Inter-American Court of Human Rights); *X and Y v. The Netherlands* (1985), 8 EHRR 235 (European Court of Human Rights).

[63] UN, Commission on Human Rights Res. 2002/31, The Right of Everyone to the Enjoyment of the Highest Attainable Standard of Physical and Mental Health.

PART II

From Principle to Practice

1

Overview

Through a series of case studies, Part II applies principles of medicine, ethics, law, and human rights to a series of representative fact situations in reproductive and sexual health. The purpose is to explore approaches to integrating medicine, ethics, and law in responding to these scenarios. The previous chapters are drawn upon and selectively expanded to show how reproductive and sexual health care might be enhanced by the application of ethical, legal, and human rights principles. The approaches involve duties in clinical care, obligations for the health care systems, and societal obligations of collaborating to address the underlying conditions of reproductive and sexual ill-health. It is hoped that integrating these related perspectives in responding to the cases will enhance the professional development of human rights-based codes of ethical care.

The objective of the exercise is not simply to address the proficient practice of medicine and related health care disciplines, but to indicate how dialogue can be initiated between practitioners of the same and other disciplines to advance the agenda of women's reproductive rights and health. The 1999 statement on The Role of the Ob/Gyn [Obstetrician/Gynecologist] as Advocates for Women's Health issued by the International Federation of Gynecology and Obstetrics (FIGO) Committee for Ethical Aspects of Human Reproduction and Women's Health opens with the observation that 'Obstetrician-Gynecologists have an ethical duty to be advocates for women's health care.'[1] Paragraph 6 of the statement urges practitioners to promote debate to improve health practices and laws, and provides that '[t]he debate should include a broad spectrum of society, such as other medical associations, women's organisations, legislators, educators, lawyers, social scientists and theologians'.[2]

Accordingly, one of the aims of Part II is to help to equip health care providers to interact with others in their communities to promote reproductive rights and health. The goal is to advance good human rights-based clinical

---

[1] The FIGO Committee for the Ethical Aspects of Human Reproduction and Women's Health, 'General Issues in Women's Health and Advocacy', in FIGO, *Recommendations on Ethical Issues in Obstetrics and Gynecology* (London: FIGO, 2000), 6, para. 1.

[2] Ibid. 7, para. 6.

practice, to stimulate discussion among health care providers through common perceptions, and to equip providers to undertake social advocacy, meaning advocacy within the wider community they serve, to identify and overcome barriers to women's reproductive and sexual rights and health. In the language of ethics, the aim is both microethical, concerned with interactions between providers and recipients of services, and macroethical, concerned with the discharge of responsibilities that professional groups as such owe to patient populations, related professional colleagues, and official and non-official actors who influence health care policies. The 1999 FIGO statement ends with the observation that 'obstetrician-gynecologists are obligated to organise themselves and other professional groups to ensure that essential health services are available for disadvantaged and underprivileged women'.[3]

The case studies are not specific to individual countries, but drawn from experiences that reflect a number of critical issues that are often faced. They bring together medical, ethical, and legal issues, sometimes in harmony and sometimes in apparent conflict. In preparing to respond professionally to circumstances such as are described in these case studies, practitioners should consult, when feasible, with local health authorities and lawyers, perhaps in collaboration with local societies of obstetricians and gynaecologists and more general medical associations.

1. *Methodology*

Approaches to the following case studies are developed through initially placing each case study in a social context affecting health, followed by a closer review of the medical aspects relevant to care of the central person, usually a female patient, in the case study. The case is then set in an ethical framework, including an identification of the ethical principles the case raises and, for instance, a review of the ethical implications of the options for its management. Legal aspects are then addressed, including basic components such as consent to care and confidentiality, and some of the wider legal dimensions of options of medical and ethical management. Before approaches to the particular case study are considered, the critical human rights dimensions of the circumstances are addressed, including availability of and access to services, and the regard paid to the status and dignity of women in general and the potential recipient of care in particular. Approaches to management of cases identify:

---

[3] The FIGO Committee for the Ethical Aspects of Human Reproduction and Women's Health, 'General Issues in Women's Health and Advocacy', in FIGO, *Recommendations on Ethical Issues in Obstetrics and Gynecology* (London: FIGO, 2000), 7, para. 6.

- the clinical duties of health care providers (that is, obligations of a doctor–patient relationship),
- the treatment and prevention obligations of health care systems, and
- social action available to health care providers and others to redress and prevent repetition of the underlying conditions that created the hazards to health to which case studies are directed.

Medical and health data often need to be analysed in order to produce knowledge, and knowledge must be placed in the setting of abstract principles to determine possible and preferable approaches. Knowledge may show how the prioritization of one ethical orientation, principle, or level of analysis over another can lead to different practical responses. Similarly, knowledge may show how an outcome results from application of a law, and how a different application of that law, or prioritization of a different law, perhaps inspired by human rights values, may achieve a preferable approach.

Health care providers may be considered to discharge their responsibilities within the strict confines of their roles by attending to ethical and legal concerns in their clinical practice. That is, their responsibility to their patients, at the microethical level, requires that they observe basic responsibilities. These are to ensure, for instance, that they have the adequately informed choice of their patients who are cognitively and judgementally capable, that they observe due confidentiality, treat their patients with respect for their dignity, and practise medicine with due regard for required standards of practice in accordance with the law on negligence. If in addition to clinical responsibilities they have administrative responsibilities for resource allocation, they must also resolve ethical and legal dilemmas concerning conflict of interest, such as when care for their patients may compromise just allocation of scarce resources among patients in general.

Within the conditions of their own countries, health care providers may have sources of reference to address issues of clinical ethics and law. For instance, clinical practitioners may find assistance by analysing cases according to the medical indications for treatment options, patients' preferences, quality of life considerations, and some contextual features such as patients' family circumstances, patients' financial means, and institutional resource implications of treatment options.[4] The purpose of these case studies is to include but go beyond clinical analysis, to encourage and enable readers to consider wider dimensions. The case studies identify medical, ethical, and legal sensitivities that must be brought to bear upon clinical problems, but also focus more widely on human rights dimensions, which may be reflected in law but which in particular countries may also be compromised by law. Resolution

---

[4] A. R. Jonsen, M. Siegler, and W. J. Winslade, *Clinical Ethics* (New York: McGraw-Hill, 4th edn., 1998); presented in the context of US law and practice.

must be sought of each case-study problem that is immediately presented, but the problem must also be addressed in terms of the capacity of the prevailing health system to cope with the clinical resolution, and in terms of social action for underlying conditions.

Those responsible for clinical care are encouraged to want to be more than satisfactory clinicians. As practitioners with a capacity for professional and social leadership in their communities, they are encouraged to employ individual cases to measure how their health care systems could be improved better to resolve individual health care problems and prevent their recurrence, and to develop their social conscience. Although presented as clinical problems, the case studies are situated within wider frameworks of personal, cultural, economic, gender, and other dimensions of justice and injustice. Health care providers approach patients as potential recipients of medical services, but medical care is only part of health care. There is universal subscription to the World Health Organization's description of health as a state of physical, mental, and social well-being, and health care providers must accordingly take account not only of patients' physical well-being, but also of their mental and social well-being. This can be advanced through reform of patients' personal and social circumstances, including their entitlement to cultural, economic, and other equity. The background concern is not simply that individuals satisfy criteria of physical health, but that they have maximum, equitable opportunities to enjoy their lives. That individuals can enjoy their lives is a principal goal of human rights.

The wider human rights dimensions of how ethical and legal provisions are applied may lead to recognition of how outcomes conform to, or violate, transcending human rights principles.[5] In short, the methodology of considering case studies is to show how, by exposing reproductive health care data to ethical and legal review, knowledge can lead to acknowledgement of human rights values that need to be protected, respected, or fulfilled, and how reproductive health care providers can prevent and remedy their breach. It is obvious that if health care practitioners want to be credible and effective advocates of women's reproductive and sexual health rights, they must respect them in their own practice. Furthermore, practitioners will be judged at two levels. Individual practitioners must observe human rights in their dealings with patients, professional colleagues, and community members and organizations, but must also contribute to the protection and promotion of human rights through their professional associations. It is insufficient that individual practitioners should behave conscientiously in dealings with their patients, communities, and others, when local health services exclude women in need of care from

---

[5] British Medical Association, *The Medical Profession and Human Rights: Handbook for a Changing Agenda* (London: Zed Books, 2001).

necessary services. It is similarly a failure of professionalism when deficiencies in services that practitioners could remedy through collective action, including advocacy to governmental, institutional, social, or other agencies, remain unaddressed.

In approaching each case study, it must be remembered that the local law, even when conforming to human rights requirements, is only a minimal ethic. Keeping the law is necessary, but ethics usually require more than mere compliance with law. It is not a satisfactory answer to the question of whether behaviour is ethical to reply that it is lawful. The law often provides legitimate discretions of how to act, and of whether to act or not. The exercise of lawful discretions must be assessed by reference to individual and professional ethical judgements. Accordingly, approaches to each case study must be sensitive to ethical values and human rights principles that can be implemented through local laws.

2. *Choice and Sequence of Case Studies*

Case studies worthy of consideration may be derived from many sources of experiences and be scrutinized at many levels of analysis. They may be viewed from every perspective from the microscopic to the telescopic, focus upon particular cultures or historically linked countries,[6] and be almost limitless in number.[7] For the sake of economy, the fifteen case studies selected here are based on rudimentary fact patterns, derived from experience in largely, although not exclusively, resource-poor settings, and aimed at health care providers, health activists, ethicists, lawyers, and others dedicated to protecting and promoting reproductive and sexual health. Their interests are addressed across a spectrum of concerns, from distressed patients in need of clinical care to inequitable societies in which neglect of human rights and social justice contributes significantly to the distress patients experience in lack of access to appropriate care.

The case studies build on the different perceptions introduced in the different chapters in Part I of the book. The resources in Part I cannot be fully mined in the following case studies, and are employed selectively, non-exhaustively, and to the critical reader perhaps contentiously. The purpose is not to 'solve' the cases, but to show how they can be opened up to medical, ethical, legal, and

[6] Commonwealth Medical Association Trust, *Training Manual on Ethical and Human Rights Standards for Health Care Professionals* (London: Commonwealth Medical Association Trust, 1999).
[7] European Network of Scientific Co-operation on Medicine and Human Rights, *The Human Rights, Ethical and Moral Dimensions of Health Care: 120 Practical Case Studies* (Strasbourg: Council of Europe Publishing, 1998).

human rights analysis, and how perceptions within those areas can be brought to bear upon the achievement of satisfactory remedial and preventive resolution. Readers are invited to take up the challenge of achieving superior analysis and resolution to that proposed here.

The case studies are presented to reflect the sequence of the human life-cycle, beginning with the reproductive disabilities imposed on girl children by female genital cutting, moving to culturally and legally conditioned barriers to adolescent reproductive and sexual health care and the vulnerability of women to sexual assault and the need for relief from its consequences. Sometimes related to sexual assault, but going beyond to social gender inequities, is the concern of hymen reconstruction. The request for medically assisted reproduction often concerns advanced reproductive technologies, but concerns with infertility are universal, and perhaps more urgent in resource-poor countries. Women's vulnerability is addressed through two concerns. The first addresses women's vulnerability to involuntary sterilization, which is often associated with powerlessness and dependency. The second concerns HIV, including HIV-positive patients' claims to clinical care, and also to counselling regarding entry to studies of experimental, unproven products, raising the issue of the need for promotion of, but also protection against, HIV drug research. The issue of abortion remains inescapable among the challenges of reproductive health care. It is addressed in itself, and through the related concerns of pre-natal genetic diagnosis, requests for sex selection services, and treatment of incomplete abortion, both induced and spontaneous. So pervasive have abortion concerns become that they furnish bases for consideration of matters that in principle are unrelated, in these case studies the issue of confidentiality. Unfortunately, common experience requires a case study that addresses domestic violence against women. The final case study concerns the medical and wider instruction that can be derived from the tragedy of maternal death.

The following sequence of case studies aims to be logically defensible, but it is arbitrary in that a sequence of case studies could be presented according to other criteria. Case studies on reproductive health might range, for instance, from the more to the less grave in their consequences, in which case they would begin with maternal death, and proceed according to individual authors' visions of priority. Readers are not required developmentally to address the following case studies in the sequence in which they are presented, but might select to read first the studies that appear most familiar to their experience. It is hoped, however, that on completion of reading all of the case studies, readers will acquire a sense of representative experiences in the treatment and pursuit of reproductive and sexual health, and a sense of how they may empower themselves to react to denials of health at different levels of social reform and effectiveness.

It is emphasized that the analysis and proposed approaches presented in the case studies are not claimed to be definitive. There are different ethical approaches, and several human rights may be applied to the same case. Readers are invited to consider how they would order preferences and priorities in the circumstances of their own health care and legal systems, and the social conditions of their communities, seen in light of the respect they afford to human rights values.

2

Female Genital Cutting (Circumcision/Mutilation)

Case Study

A mother brings her 9-year-old daughter to Dr D requesting that she be 'circumcised'. The mother explains that she wants the procedure done for fear that the daughter will not be eligible for marriage in her community if it is not done. The mother further explains that she wants the procedure to be medically performed because procedures conducted on her older daughters by a traditional birth attendant (TBA) resulted in their severe bleeding and infection of the wounds. The mother says that, unless Dr D consents to perform the procedure, her mother-in-law will insist on taking the girl to the TBA. What should Dr D do, taking into consideration medical, ethical, legal, and human rights aspects of the case?

1. *Background*

The terminology used to describe this procedure varies. The term 'female circumcision' has been used historically. However, as the harm that such procedures caused to girls and women became increasingly recognized, and because this procedure in whatever form it is practised is not at all analogous to male circumcision, the term 'female circumcision' gave way to the term 'female genital mutilation'. The term 'female genital mutilation' has been adopted by many women's health organizations, such as the Inter-African Committee on Traditional Practices Affecting the Health of Women and Children, and intergovernmental organizations, such as the World Health Organization. However, the use of the term may offend women who have undergone the procedure and do not consider themselves mutilated or their families as mutilators.[1]

---

[1] A. Rahman and N. Toubia, *Female Genital Mutilation: A Guide to Laws and Policies Worldwide* (New York: Zed Press, 2000), 4.

The term 'female genital surgery' is used by some.[2] Health care professionals consider this usage is incorrect because they use the term 'female genital surgery' to describe surgical procedures performed for therapeutic purposes, such as for removal of tumours from the internal or external genital organs. This case study uses the term 'female genital cutting' (FGC) in an attempt to find language that is value neutral, but which adequately describes the nature of the procedure.

WHO estimates that in the world today about 2 million girls undergo some form of the procedure every year[3] (see Table III.1.2). About 6,000 girls are 'circumcised' every day. The procedure is commonly performed on girls between the ages of 4 and 12 years of age, but it is also known to be performed in some communities on infants a few days after birth, and in others just prior to marriage or after the first pregnancy.[4] Most of these girls and women live in East and West Africa, and parts of the Arabian Peninsula, although some live in Asia, and some are found in immigrant population groups living in Europe, the USA, Canada, Australia, and New Zealand.[5] The prevalence among and within these countries varies. The variation in prevalence between countries ranges from 5 to 99 per cent.[6]

The clitoris has been a victim of assault, as a result of society's view of female sexuality. Clitoridectomy has a different history and background in the West and in the East.[7] In England, Europe, and the USA, many clitoridectomies were performed by gynaecological surgeons in the second half of the nineteenth century on allegedly medical grounds. Clitoridectomy was considered necessary not only to cure such sexual deviations as 'nymphomania' but also to prevent masturbation and to cure a number of disorders, some of which were thought to have been caused by masturbation, such as hysteria, epilepsy, melancholia, and insanity. Also, it was unthinkable that any decent woman should derive pleasure from sex.

The origin of female circumcision is lost in antiquity. The prevailing reasons for FGC are complex, multifaceted, and interwoven with socially constructed concepts of gender and sexuality. Reasons include custom and practice,

---

[2] C. M. Obermeyer, 'Female Genital Surgeries: The Known, the Unkown and the Unknowable', *Medical Anthropology Quarterly*, 13 (1999), 79–106.

[3] WHO, *Management of Pregnancy, Childbirth and the Postpartum Period in the Presence of Female Genital Mutilation: Report of a 1997 WHO Technical Consultation* (Geneva: WHO, 2001), 2.

[4] N. Toubia, *Female Genital Mutilation: A Call for Global Action* (New York: Rainbo, 2 edn., 1995), 9.

[5] British Medical Association, *Female Genital Mutilation: Caring for Patients and Child Protection: Guidance from the BMA* (approved by Council Jan. 1996, revised Apr. 2001, www.bma.org.uk/pulbic/ethics.nsf/, accessed 31 Nov. 2001.

[6] Ibid. 3; http://www.who.int/frh-whd/FGM, accessed 14 July 2001.

[7] M. F. Fathalla, *From Obstetrics and Gynecology to Women's Health: The Road Ahead* (New York and London: Parthenon, 1997).

control of women's sexuality, and social pressure.[8] FGC is performed as a rite of passage from childhood to adulthood, connecting women to cultural traditions and family values of present and past generations. The reason for the procedure to control women's sexuality is to reduce sexual desire, thus allegedly 'saving' the girl from temptation, and preserving her chastity before marriage and fidelity after marriage. In many situations, social pressure created through social ostracism of uncircumcised girls and men's refusal to marry them perpetuates the practice.

2. *Medical Aspects*

The immediate and long-term damage inflicted on young girls and women ranges, according to the degree of removal of the female genitalia, from an insignificant cut, to removal of the clitoris, up to a major procedure in which the clitoris and labia minora are removed and the opening of the vagina is stitched together (infibulated). Since none of these procedures has a therapeutic purpose, there are no medical definitions. They are usually performed by non-professionals who do not even know the anatomy of the female genitalia. Based on observation of women who have undergone a version of these procedures, the different forms of female genital cutting are classified into four types. The categories are not distinct, as in practice they commonly overlap:[9]

Type I, usually known as clitoridectomy, involves the partial or entire removal of the clitoris;
Type II, known as excision, refers to the removal of the clitoris and the labia minora;
Type III, known as infibulation, removes the clitoris, the labia minora and sometimes the labia majora and stitches or seals together (infibulates) the vagina, leaving a small opening for the flow of urine and menstrual blood;
Type IV refers to unclassified procedures, such as pricking, piercing, cutting or stretching the clitoris and/or the labia; cauterization by burning of the clitoris and surrounding tissues; scraping (angurya cuts) of the vaginal orifice or cutting (gishiri cuts) of the vagina; introduction of herbs or corrosive materials to cause bleeding or to narrow or tighten the vagina.

It should be clear that FGC bears no relationship to male circumcision.[10] In male circumcision, the part removed is the prepuce (a fold of skin that covers the tip of the penis). Its removal has a possible health benefit (such as protection against HIV infection[11]) and carries little (though some) risk of harm.

---

[8] Rahman and Toubia, *Female Genital Mutilation*, 5–6.
[9] WHO, *A Systematic Review of the Health Complications of Female Genital Mutilation Including Sequelae in Childbirth* (Geneva: WHO, 2000), 11.
[10] Fathalla, *From Obstetrics*, 210.
[11] UNAIDS, *Report on the Global HIV/AIDS Epidemic* (Geneva: UNAIDS, 2000), 70.

The practice of male circumcision is authorized by the Jewish and Islamic religions.

The degree of cutting in female circumcision is anatomically much more extensive than male circumcision. The male equivalent of clitoridectomy, in which all or part of the clitoris is removed, would be the cutting off of most of the penis. The male equivalent of infibulation—which involves not only clitoridectomy, but the removal or closing off of the sensitive tissue around the vagina—would be the removal of all the penis, its roots of soft tissue, and part of the scrotal skin.[12]

In addition to the physiological differences, there are also differences in how the respective procedures construct men and women in terms of their gender roles. Male circumcision affirms manhood with its superior social status and associations to virility. A purpose of FGC is to reinforce the passive gender role of girls and women by confining women socially and restraining their sexual desires.[13]

The part removed in so-called female circumcision varies widely, but the procedure commonly aims to remove the clitoris, which plays an important role in sexual arousal and female orgasm. The procedure carries no health benefit, and can be associated with physical and psychological harm and sexual and reproductive dysfunctions. Unlike male circumcision, FGC is neither supported by any religion nor bears any relationship to the geographical distribution of any religion.

All types of FGC have immediate and long-term health complications. The medical complications include bleeding, which may necessitate emergency medical interference. There are health hazards generally related to the fact that the procedure is often performed outside health care facilities by non-professionals. Serious sepsis may occur, particularly where unsterile cutting instruments are used. If the genital area becomes contaminated with urine or faeces, infection can also develop within a few days of the procedure. Infection can lead to septicemia if the bacteria reach the bloodstream, and may be fatal. Acute urine retention can result from the swelling and inflammation around the wound.[14]

Long-term complications can arise from all types of FGC, but the severest complications arise with the Type II and III procedures. Common complications of Type III (infibulation) include repeated urinary tract infection and chronic pelvic infections, which may cause irreparable damage to the reproductive organs and result in infertility. Excessive growth of scar tissue may be

[12] N. Toubia and S. Izett, *Female Genital Mutilation: An Overview* (Geneva: WHO, 1998), 9.
[13] N. Toubia, 'Evolutionary Cultural Ethics and Circumcision of Children', in G. Denniston, F. M. Hodges, and M. F. Milos (eds.), *Male and Female Circumcision: Medical, Legal and Ethical Considerations in Pediatric Practice* (New York: Kluwer Academic and Plenum, 1999).
[14] Toubia and Izett, *Female Genital Mutilation*, 26.

disfiguring. A cyst (implantation dermoid) at the site of the cutting can also result from inadvertent imbedding of a piece of skin in the wound. Such cysts may distress the girl and her parents, who suspect a condition of intersex.

Complications of FGC in childbirth include complications during pregnancy, and before, during, and after delivery.[15] Pain usually results during and after deinfibulation, where an anterior incision of the vulva is generally needed to enable delivery to take place. Antenatal complications and complications in early labour, prolonged or obstructed labour, obstetric fistulae (holes or tunnels between the bladder and the vagina and between the rectum and the vagina) are complications that arise particularly with Type III FGC. Foetal distress and foetal death (stillbirth or early neonatal death) may also result. Foetal deaths appear to be related to the obstruction to delivery posed by the vulva scarring that occurs in Type III procedures or the extra scarring that can happen with complicated Types I or II procedures.[16] Post-partum haemorrhage is significantly more common in women with FGC, usually arising from the extra incisions made and the perineal tears experienced as a result of the scarring resulting from all types of FGC.[17] FGC has been reported as a contributing or causal factor in maternal death, usually resulting from unattended or inappropriately treated obstructed labour caused by the vulval scarring.[18]

3. *Ethical Aspects*

The International Federation of Gynecology and Obstetrics (FIGO) has taken an uncompromising position in opposition to female circumcision, describing it as 'mutilation'. A resolution unanimously adopted by the FIGO General Assembly in 1994 recognized that 'female genital mutilation is a violation of human rights, as a harmful procedure performed on a child who cannot give informed consent'.

Many countries have already passed laws or regulations forbidding the performance of the procedure, leaving little ethical choice. Nevertheless, ethical explanations and guidance can reinforce prohibitory legislation. In the United Kingdom, for instance, the Prohibition of Female Circumcision Act 1985 (Statutes, chapter 38) creates an offence but permits registered medical practitioners to undertake otherwise prohibited acts either during childbirth or for the physical or mental health of the patient. The British Medical Association has provided guidance on enforcement of the law, and also on what constitutes serious professional misconduct found by the General Medical Council.[19] Where there are no prohibitory local laws or regulations, or ethical statements

---

[15] WHO, *Systematic Review*.   [16] Ibid. 51.   [17] Ibid. 46.
[18] Ibid. 48.   [19] BMA, *Female Genital Mutilation*.

by national medical associations with disciplinary sanctions, and physicians have an ethical choice, they may find several principles to be in conflict. Parents' power to impose their preference on young daughters denies the girls their right to autonomy in their future adult lives, and denies them immediate defence as children against parental insistence on the performance of a non-therapeutic, irreversible and risk-laden procedure.

There is concern about overplaying the medical complications because they are largely the result of the FGC, of whatever type, being performed by unqualified people in unsafe settings. One approach to address these complications is to ensure that FGC is done by qualified people in safe settings. However, medicalization of any type of FGC cannot be justified because it has no therapeutic purpose. The 1994 FIGO General Assembly resolution recommended that obstetricians and gynaecologists 'oppose any attempt to medicalize the procedure or to allow its performance, under any circumstances, in health establishments or by health professionals'.[20]

The ethical principle of non-maleficence, which prohibits doing harm, requires that physicians not undertake the procedure. However, the same principle requires that any risk of harm should be minimized, and for a physician to perform a limited form of symbolic genital cutting is less harmful than for a much more invasive procedure to be performed by an untrained person, such as a traditional birth attendant. However, while this approach might reduce the medical harm to a particular individual, it still causes a profound social injury to women more generally. Performing any type of FGC is in fact an approval of the practice of societal control of women's sexuality and an affront to women's bodily integrity and dignity of the person.

The ethical approach taken by the medical profession, as indicated in the FIGO General Assembly and the World Health Assembly of WHO,[21] is that more efforts should be undertaken to address the practice at the macroethical or societal level. The profession characterizes the procedure as individually and socially harmful to women's and girls' health and dignity, and of no compensating medical advantage. The profession remains unpersuaded by the fact that in some cultures the procedure is considered beneficial and described as 'purification', perhaps because of the inference of this description that women and girls not subjected to it are in some way impure. Accordingly, the ethical opinion of organized medicine is that physicians and health facilities should not participate in this procedure, since it implicates health care providers in a procedure of unrelieved harm.

[20] M. F. Fathalla, 'The Girl Child', *Int. J. Gynecol. Obstet.* 70 (2000), 7–12, at 7.
[21] World Health Assembly Resolution: Maternal and Child Health and Family Planning; Traditional Practices Harmful to the Health of Women and Children (WHA 47.10, 1994), partially cited in Toubia and Izett, *Female Genital Mutilation*, 62.

The harm is twofold, in that vulnerable young girls are subjected to risk-laden cutting procedures that afford them no health, hygienic, or other benefit. The procedure also perpetuates a form of sexual control of women that demeans them as members of their communities with the same rights to protection as men. The claim that physicians should participate in order to limit injury, since if physicians refuse to perform such procedures they may be performed more harmfully by unqualified persons, is rejected, in much the same way that medical professional organizations prohibit medical participation in torture and execution of judicial sentences of flogging, amputation, and death.

4. *Legal Aspects*

There are general criminal law prohibitions against unjustified assault that can be applied to punish FGC. For instance, the Penal Code of Kenya provides that '[a]ny person who unlawfully assaults another is guilty of a misdemeanour' (section 250) and that 'any person who commits an assault occasioning actual bodily harm is guilty . . . and is liable to imprisonment for five years' (section 251). The Code defines 'grievous harm' as 'harm which amounts to a maim or dangerous harm, or seriously or permanently injures health', and provides for punishment of up to life imprisonment (section 234).

Kenya reinforced this general provision in the Children Act 2001 (No. 8 of 2001). Section 14 provides that: 'No person shall subject a child to female circumcision, early marriage or cultural rites, customs or traditional practices that are likely to negatively affect the child's life, health, social welfare, dignity or physical or psychological development.' In December 2000, the Kenya District Court for Keiyo condemned the practice on wider grounds, finding it repugnant to morality and a violation of human rights as stipulated in the national constitution, and granted a permanent injunction restraining the defendant and those associated with him from undertaking the practice.[22]

Some countries, such as Burkina Faso,[23] Ghana,[24] Senegal,[25] and the United Kingdom[26] have also progressed beyond the application of general criminal laws by enacting laws that specifically outlaw FGC. The degree of punishment and enforcement of these targeted laws varies. Burkina Faso imprisons for a minimum of six months and up to three years, and fines at least 150,000 and up

---

[22] Decision of 13 Dec. 2001, Keiyo District Court, Kenya, Magistrate Ochenja.

[23] Law No. 43/96/ADP of 13 Nov. 1996 on the Penal Code, Arts. 380–2, *Journal Officiel du Burkina Faso*, 27 Jan. 1997, reprinted in Rahman and Toubia, *Female Genital Mutilation*, 115.

[24] Criminal Code (Amendment) Act, 1994 (Ghana), reprinted in *International Digest of Health Legislation*, 47 (1996), 30–1.

[25] Law No. 99-05 of 29 Jan. 1999 amending various provisions of the Penal Code, Art. 299b, *Journal Officiel* (27 Feb. 1999), No. 5847, 832.

[26] Prohibition of Female Circumcision Act 1985 (UK) Statutes 1985, ch. 38.

to 900,000 francs (about $240–1,440) '[a]ny person who violates or attempts to violate the physical integrity of the female genital organ, either by total ablation, excision, infibulation, desensitization or by any other means'. If the procedure results in death, the minimum punishment is imprisonment for five years, the maximum ten years (Article 380 of the Penal Code). If the offender is a member of the medical or paramedical field, maximum punishments shall be imposed, and a licence to practise medicine may also be suspended for up to five years, perhaps from completion of the custodial sentence (Article 381). Further, any person having knowledge of the offence who fails to advise proper authorities will be fined 50,000–100,000 francs (about $80–160) (Article 382).

While the law has been enforced through numerous prosecutions of perpetrators and accomplices, the sentences of imprisonment have been minimal, and in some cases suspended.[27] A chief law enforcement officer in the capital of Burkina Faso, Ouagadougou, working on the elimination of FGC, has observed that effective law enforcement is needed, since his experience shows that education alone is often ineffective to curb FGC. He explains that excisors 'will not stop unless they are afraid of repercussions' from law enforcement, the potential for which affords health care professionals and law enforcement officers the legitimacy to intervene when parents, excisors, and others propose FGC.[28]

National courts are playing an increasing role in applying laws or Ministry of Health policies to prohibit FGC. For example, in 1997, the State Council, Egypt's highest administrative court, upheld a 1996 Ministry of Health order prohibiting the performance of female genital circumcision in public and private hospitals and clinics, except in cases of medical necessity. The State Council upheld the Ministry of Health order even when performance of the operation has the consent of the woman and her parents, ruling that circumcision is not an individual right that emanates from the shariah (Islamic law). It stated that there is nothing in the Quran (the Holy Book of Islam) that authorizes female genital circumcision.[29]

Because FGC serves no medical or health-related purpose, physicians who perform it are not covered by the medical justification or explanation of surgical necessity that protects acts that, when performed by unqualified people, are criminal offences. Parental consent does not relieve physicians' liability, since parents can consent to medical interventions on their dependent children only to discharge their parental duties to provide medical and health-related

---

[27] Rahman and Toubia, *Female Genital Mutilation*, 115.
[28] WHO, *Female Genital Mutilations—Programmes to Date: What Works and What Doesn't: A Review* (Geneva: WHO, 1999), 16, statement of Mr Issa Kabré, June 1998.
[29] Decision of 28 Dec. 1997, published in *Annual Review of Population Law*, 23–4 (1996–7), 128.

care, and this procedure is outside the scope of such care. It exposes children to immediate and future risks to their health and welfare, unlike such lawful minor cosmetic procedures as ear-piercing that allows young children to wear decorations.

If a mature woman requests this procedure as her freely made choice, a physician with no conscientious objection to performing it might still face legal obstacles. Various forms of body piercing are legally tolerated, but not all forms of voluntary bodily invasion are lawful. The historic law against maim (or 'mayhem') expresses itself in legal tolerance of male circumcision, whether on religious or hygienic grounds, but prohibition of sado-masochistic mutilation.[30] Courts might be equally restrictive of all but the most minor voluntary genital cutting, on grounds of public policy or morals, or *ordre public*. An adult applicant for this procedure might be hard-pressed to obtain judicial approval.

Complying with a woman's request to be re-sutured following childbirth, in order to be restored to the way she was accustomed to be, may at first appear relatively non-contentious. Moreover, denying her the procedure may be difficult psychologically for the woman, because her identity and status might be embedded in her infibulated appearance. However, re-suturing is professionally opposed, on grounds of objectionable medicalization of the procedure, and may constitute an offence by a physician or other health care provider legally bound to provide services only according to health professional codes of ethical conduct.[31]

In addition to liability under the general law, physicians are legally answerable to medical licensing and disciplinary authorities for allegations of professional misconduct. Many such authorities have declared FGC to constitute professional misconduct, and others that have not so declared it may be persuaded to do so by resolutions such as FIGO adopted in 1994. Licensing bodies and medical professional associations may lawfully impose sanctions for professional misconduct that is not itself a breach of the law, which empowers their disciplinary authorities to enforce codes of ethical conduct. Accordingly, physicians can face legal sanctions for undertaking female genital cutting even where it does not clearly constitute an independent breach of the law.

5. *Human Rights Aspects*

FGC of any type, irrespective of the medical complications, cannot be justified. Many human rights are violated by imposition of FGC on infants,

---

[30] *R. v. Brown*, [1993] 2 All ER 75 (House of Lords, England).
[31] WHO, *Female Genital Mutilation—The Prevention and Management of Health Complications: Policy Guidelines for Nurses and Midwives* (Geneva: WHO, 2001), 11–12.

adolescents, and others incapable of providing autonomously given informed consent. The more obvious include the rights to health and security of the person, in light of the many health problems associated with the procedure, particularly when performed by medically untrained people. The gravest is death due to excessive bleeding or infection, but others focus on obstructed urination and menstruation in Type III and possibly less invasive procedures, impaired enjoyment of sexual intercourse and of prenatal care and delivery, and enduring psychological reactions to the trauma of the procedure. Risk of death due to infection or other related factors violates women's right to life. In some contexts, it might be appropriate to argue that the procedure violates the right of girls and women to be free from inhuman and degrading treatment. At a wider level, the procedure violates the right of girls and women to be free from all forms of discrimination, since a justification of FGC is its reinforcement of women's chastity and fidelity by rendering sexual intercourse non-pleasurable for them, when men are liable to no such constraints. The Committee on the Elimination of Discrimination against Women is vigorous in its condemnation of FGC, taking countries to task for neglect of the problem and weak law enforcement.[32]

Although FGC may be undertaken on adult and adolescent women, its major prevalence involves exploitation of vulnerable girl children, who are dependent on parental care and incapable of the intellectual or social exercise of choice. Beyond violations of the general human rights conventions, this violates several provisions of the Children's Convention, which reinforce prohibitions under the general conventions but also demonstrate the aggravated character of violations of rights of defenceless children. A violation is particularly outrageous when perpetrated by those on whom children depend for protection and the exercise of prudent judgement to defend their interests and physical integrity. The fact that parents believe FGC to be in their young daughters' immediate and longer term interests illustrates parental subservience to harmful and even life-endangering customs, which lack religious foundation but embody generations of acceptance of sex discrimination as normal or even desirable. The Committee on the Rights of the Child is persistent in its denouncements of countries where FGC continues unabated and urges them to combat and eradicate the practice.[33]

[32] See Concluding Observation on the Report of Ethiopia to the Committee on the Elimination of Discrimination against Women, 9 May 1996, A/51/38, para. 148, published in Action Canada for Population and Development, *The Application of Human Rights to Reproductive and Sexual Health: A Compilation of the Work of International Treaty Bodies* (Ottawa: Action Canada for Population and Development, 2000), 97, available at website: http://www.acpd.ca, last accessed 6 May 2002.

[33] See Concluding Observation on the Report of Benin to the Committee on the Rights of the Child, 12 Aug. 1999, CRC/C/15/Add. 106, para. 26, published in Action Canada, *Application of Human Rights*, 187, available at website: http://www.acpd.ca, last accessed 6 May 2002.

The FIGO resolution that 'Female Genital Mutilation is a violation of human rights'[34] supports provisions of the Children's Convention and the Women's Convention. Both contain prohibitions of non-discrimination on grounds of sex, and the latter requires parties '[t]o modify the social and cultural patterns of conduct . . . with a view to achieving the elimination of . . . customary . . . practices which are based . . . on stereotyped roles for men and women'. Where FGC is a cultural condition of women's marriage, when men are subject to no comparably invasive and harmful procedure, it violates this provision. Similarly, if the purpose of FGC is to reduce women's sexual appetite or ensure pre-marital chastity, it serves a stereotyped image of female sexual virtue or passivity that is not expected of or enforced on men.

A countervailing human rights claim that may be raised in support of parents' requirement that the procedure be undertaken is based on their religious freedom. This claim may support ritual circumcision of newborn males, for instance in the Islamic and Jewish traditions, but health risks of male and female procedures are not comparable. Under human rights conventions, states must balance competing concerns, so that any states whose legal systems allow FGC may do so, but may face opposition on behalf of girl children on the ground that such states condone violence against children and perpetuate discrimination against women. Disallowing parental requests based on their wish to enhance their daughters' prospects of marriage is not inconsistent with allowing the girls themselves to make their own decisions when intellectually capable and free from family, communal, and cultural constraints.

6. *Approaches*

6.1. *Clinical duty*

Dr D cannot comply with the mother's request, nor succumb to the fear that refusal will result in a more harmful procedure being undertaken by an unqualified provider. Dr D satisfies ethical, legal, and human rights responsibilities at the clinical level by simply refusing to perform the procedure, and strongly advising the mother to protect her daughter against exposure to the injuries her older daughters have suffered. Dr D should inform the mother and the father, if possible, of the harmful consequences of the procedure, and explain the potential legal consequences, despite parental consent. Dr D may also suggest that, if the daughter wishes to have the procedure performed when she is of an age and condition to give her free and informed consent to it, the matter may be raised at that time. Nevertheless, Dr D should observe any

---

[34] Female Genital Mutilation Resolution, FIGO General Assembly, Montreal Canada, 1994: www.figo.org/default.asp?id=/00000086.htm, last accessed 6 May 2002.

applicable prohibitory laws and respect the condemnation expressed by international medical and intergovernmental agencies against individual concessions to pressures to undertake FGC that contribute to legitimising FGC as a medical procedure.

6.2. *Health care systems obligations*

Dr D may alert the health-care community to the immediate and long-term consequences of the procedure by, for example, helping to develop and use curricula on the prevention and management of FGC for health care providers, including nurses and midwives.[35] Dr D may encourage medical licensing authorities whose mandate is to protect the public against unqualified and unethical practice to urge more systematic and transparent approaches to enforcement of criminal law and other prohibitions, including the suspension of licences to practice medicine of those qualified practitioners who perform FGC.

6.3. *Social action for underlying conditions*

The many different programming strategies undertaken to reduce the incidence of FGC include the following.[36]

6.3.1. *The health approach*

It stresses the health advantages of not doing the procedure. Using the health approach alone has led to a number of problems, including overplaying the complications and side effects associated with the procedure. This has led to disbelief about the harmful consequences of FGC among some excised women who have not experienced any complications. This approach, if not supplemented by other approaches, has tended to medicalize the practice since many people believe they can avoid side effects by taking their daughters to health clinics or hospitals which they pressure to perform the procedure.[37]

6.3.2. *The cultural approach*

It examines how alternative local traditions and cultures that are not detrimental to women could be reinforced. This includes supporting and celebrating the social meaning of rites of passage that are positive for women, while condemning and eliminating FGC as a harmful act. This approach also tries to

[35] WHO, *Female Genital Mutilation: Integrating the Prevention and the Management of the Health Curricula of Nursing and Midwifery: A Teacher's Guide* (Geneva: WHO, 2001); WHO, *Female Genital Mutilation: Integrating the Prevention and the Management of the Health Curricula of Nursing and Midwifery: A Student's Manual* (Geneva: WHO, 2001).
[36] WHO, *Female Genital Mutilations—Programmes to Date.*   [37] Ibid. 74.

support other forms of expression that celebrate women's sexuality in positive terms, not in ways like FGC that attempt to control their sexuality. For
example, in some countries, traditional wedding songs are a rich source of
positive cultural expressions of women's sexual life.[38]

6.3.3.   *The women's empowerment approach or the development/ gender approach*

It seeks to find positive roles for adolescent girls through education, training, and, for example, sports. It can also include finding alternative sources
of income and status for those traditional excisors, who generally tend to be
women. This is a wider approach and needs to involve community leaders,
schoolteachers, and even religious leaders.

6.3.4.   *The ethical/legal/human rights approach*

It provides normative languages by which to say the procedure is wrong. The
authoritative nature of the ethical, legal, and human rights languages legit-
imizes efforts to advocate the eradication of FGC. A challenge of using this
approach is, occasionally, that local activists are not familiar with these languages. In particular, local activists can be alienated by arguments based on
international human rights conventions. The challenge is to train people in the
use of human rights that are protected by national constitutions, local laws,
and ethical norms.

Given the strengths and weaknesses of these approaches, a particular
approach might be more useful in one context than in another. Moreover, the
approaches are overlapping and not mutually exclusive. Each approach has
different means of implementation, for instance through community education and engagement, including roles for religious and political leaders, training of youth, and the use of the media.

Where parents are deferential to religious leaders, physicians may urge such
leaders to declare the practice to lack religious authority, and be harmful.
Where reactionary religious leaders subscribe to the culture of male dominance and enforced female chastity, however, physicians may urge that girls
be encouraged and inspired to sexual modesty and abstinence in other ways,
and that males restrain themselves similarly. Families may be persuaded
that their daughters' virginity can be adequately protected in ways that are
not so damaging to their health, to their prospects of safe motherhood, and to
survival of their children. The Convention on the Elimination of All Forms
of Discrimination against Women (the Women's Convention) requires the
reform of cultural practices that demean or endanger women, and Dr D and
the professional society of which Dr D is a member may invoke this provision

[38] WHO, *Female Genital Mutilations*, 74, 112, 120.

to resist parental favour of this practice. Dr D may also collaborate with governmental and non-governmental agencies that oppose violence against women and child abuse to restrain this practice, and to educate families in its harms and service of no legitimate interest.

The FIGO General Assembly resolution of 1994 on female genital mutilation invited member societies to 'urge their governments to take legal and/or other measures to render this practice socially unacceptable by all sectors and groups in society' and to 'collaborate with national authorities, non-governmental and inter-governmental organizations to advocate, promote and support measures aiming at the elimination of female genital mutilation'.[39] In the same resolution, FIGO recommended that obstetricians and gynaecologists: 'explain the immediate dangers and long-term consequences of female genital mutilation to religious leaders, legislators and decision makers, educate health professionals, community workers and teachers about this harmful traditional practice . . . [and] [a]ssist in research for the documentation of the prevalence of the practice and its harmful consequences'.[40]

[39] Female Genital Mutilation Resolution, FIGO General Assembly, 1994.
[40] See R. J. Cook, B. M. Dickens, and M. F. Fathalla, 'Female Genital Cutting (Mutilation/Circumcision): Ethical and Legal Dimensions', *Int. J. Gynecol. Obstet.* 79 (2002), 281–7.

3

An Adolescent Girl Seeking Sexual and Reproductive Health Care

Case Study

Miss B, an unmarried 15-year-old young woman, has come to Dr CD's office and asked for contraceptive care. She explains that for several months she has been sexually active with a young man a few years older than she is whom she intends to marry, but the social circumstances of both of them preclude marriage before two years' time. A pregnancy would be socially disastrous in her situation. Her family knows about her relationship with the young man, but not its sexual nature. When asked, she replies that she believes that her boyfriend had sexual experience with other girls before they met, but that she is confident that she is now his only sexual partner. What are Dr CD's responsibilities, given medical, ethical, legal, and human rights considerations?

1. Background

Adolescence has been defined by the WHO as being between the ages of 10 and 19 years, and youth as between 15 and 24 years.[1] The Convention on the Rights of the Child defines a 'child' as a human being who is below the age of 18 years. Adolescence is the period of transition from childhood to adulthood. National definitions of a child, an adolescent, and a youth vary markedly, as do laws and policies governing adolescents' access to reproductive and sexual health services.[2]

Biologically, adolescence is a period of health. The principal risks to adolescent health are not due to biomedical conditions, but to social health hazards. The social health morbidities of adolescence include substance abuse, injury

---

[1] WHO, *The Health of Young People* (Geneva: WHO, 1993), 1.
[2] Center for Reproductive Law and Policy, *Reproductive Rights 2000: Moving Forward* (New York: CRLP, 2000), 57–67.

from accidents and violence, sexual exploitation and abuse, sexually transmitted diseases (STDs), and adolescent pregnancies.

Young people are a sizeable group of the world population. In the year 2000, people aged 10–24 accounted for 27 per cent of world population, 20 per cent in more developed regions, and 29 per cent in less developed regions.[3] The proportion is projected to decrease in the next century, but the numbers overall will increase. By 2025, the number is expected to increase from about 1,663 million in 2000 to about 1,796 million. In more developed regions, the number is projected to decrease from about 241 to 198 million. In less developed regions, the number is expected to increase from about 1,423 to 1,597 million.

During the period of adolescence, three developments take place.[4] Biological development progresses from the initial appearance of the secondary sex characteristics to that of sexual maturity; psychological processes and cognitive and emotional patterns develop from those of a child to those of an adult; and a transition is made from the state of total socio-economic dependence to one of relative independence. Two trends are taking place in almost every society, though at different paces: a trend towards an earlier onset of biological maturation, and a trend towards delay in socio-economic maturation, with a resultant wider bio-social gap in human development. Today, girls everywhere are becoming sexually mature at an earlier age than in previous generations. Genetic, health, and socio-economic factors influence the wide variations in age of menarche among different countries. Since boys and girls have now to spend more years in school, learning, and training, before they can enter the complex labour market, the period of socio-economic dependence is often prolonged.

Adolescents are left with difficult choices in socio-sexual behaviour: premarital sex, early marriage, or abstinence. The different patterns predominate in different countries, and patterns of transition exist. Premarital sex is now the predominant pattern in developed countries and some parts of the developing world including parts of Latin America and the Caribbean. There is also evidence of a similar trend in other regions. This choice often carries with it an increased prevalence of sexually transmitted infections, unwanted pregnancy, and abortion, with adverse health and social consequences. There is often a double standard between boys and girls. Early marriage is a predominant pattern in many parts of the developing world, notably Asia and Africa. It carries with it a curtailing of the socio-economic development of girls, often limiting their role and opportunities in life to a career of childbearing and childrearing,

[3] Population Reference Bureau, *The World's Youth 2000 Data Sheet* (Washington, DC: Population Reference Bureau, 2000), 10, 18.

[4] M. F. Fathalla, *From Obstetrics and Gynecology to Women's Health: The Road Ahead* (New York and London: Parthenon, 1997), ch. 17, 'Adolescent Sexual and Reproductive Health', 215–21.

and the assumption of parental responsibility before social maturity. Abstinence and delayed marriage seems to be a declining pattern, with the possible exception, at least until recently, of China.

In addition to the widening bio-social gap in human societies today, the family no longer serves in the dominant role of transmitting intergenerational knowledge. Communication between parents and adolescents has greatly decreased. The problem of communication is not in adolescence itself, but in the need to come to grips with the new realities of adolescence, with which parents may be unfamiliar. Misconceptions are contributing to turning what should be a normal, positive phase in growth and development into a problem.

While female adolescents are clearly more likely to face adverse reproductive health consequences than adult women are, it is misleading to lump all adolescents together. It is important to indicate that adolescents are not a homogeneous group, and that younger female adolescents are particularly disadvantaged in terms of adverse health consequences.

2. *Medical Aspects*

2.1. *General points*

Adolescents have reproductive health needs related to sexuality, protection from sexually transmitted infections, fertility regulation, and pregnancy. The response should not be fragmentary. Irrespective of the reason for contact with the reproductive and sexual health system, adolescents' needs should be addressed in their totality. Respect, confidentiality, and privacy should be observed. An adolescent girl seeking a method for fertility regulation would not be well served if her needs for protection from sexually transmitted infections are not addressed. It should also be kept in mind that the adolescent seeking non-specific medical advice may have a 'hidden agenda' and may be waiting for the health professional to bring up the subject of sexuality. Accordingly, health professionals should be prepared to offer and provide comprehensive reproductive and sexual health advice and care.

2.2. *Sexuality*

The female adolescent's approach to a sexual relationship is often different from that of the adolescent boy. It is usually directed to the search for love, tenderness, and closeness, rather than for sexual release. In time, she will learn to enjoy and seek sex as much as the male, and the male may also begin to develop a more caring and loving approach towards the female. Until recently, the subject of adolescent sexual activity was too sensitive to discuss. Information is now available from a number of surveys, however, to indicate that the trend in most countries is for earlier sexual initiations among both boys and girls.

Statistics on rape from several countries suggest that between one-third and two-thirds of rape victims worldwide are 15 years old or younger.[5] Male adolescents need to be educated about responsible sexual behaviour. Studies have also shown high rates of adolescent pregnancies to result from older males' sexual abuse of younger girls.[6] The males may be related to them, or be in positions of authority or influence over them. When adolescent females seek contraceptive or other reproductive health care, the question of whether their sexual relationships are voluntary or involuntary is relevant.

2.3. *Sexually transmitted infections and contraception in adolescents*

Young people aged 15 to 24 have the highest rates of sexually transmitted infections, including HIV.[7] Adolescents should be informed that any sexual relationship, other than a stable mutually monogamous one, carries a risk of sexually transmitted infections; a partner may be infective without having any lesion or even being aware that he or she is infected. A condom should be used in any sexual intercourse carrying a risk of transmission of infection.

For the non-married adolescent, in terms of protection, saying NO is the best oral contraceptive when refusal of sexual advances is a realistic option. The condom is the best method of contraception if there is a risk of STD transmission and an adolescent can require her partner to use it. When she cannot and does not have access to the female condom, provision of contraception for her may leave her exposed to STDs. Emergency contraception is a useful backup method after unprotected intercourse that, unfortunately, is greatly under-utilized. It can prevent many unwanted pregnancies, and should be more widely taught and learned.

2.4. *Adolescent pregnancy*

Thirty-three per cent of women in developing countries give birth before the age of 20, ranging from a low of 8 per cent in East Asia to 55 per cent in West Africa.[8] In more developed countries, about 10 per cent of women give birth by age 20; however, in the United States, the level of teen childbearing is significantly higher, at 19 per cent. Only a few of the teenage pregnancies are really wanted by the young mothers. Many have been coerced by social pressure into early marriage and early pregnancy, or pregnancy has resulted from

---

[5] Fathalla, *From Obstetrics and Gynecology to Women's Health*, 215–21.

[6] L. Heise, M. Ellsberg, and M. Gottemoeller, 'Ending Violence Against Women', *Population Report Series L.*, 11 (1999), 9.

[7] Population Reference Bureau, *2000 Data Sheet*.   [8] Ibid. 1.

unmarried adolescents being denied free access to contraception. Adolescents account for at least 10 per cent of all induced abortions.

Marriage occurs earlier in developing than in developed regions, with regional variations ranging from 4 to 37 per cent.[9] The percentage of women aged 15–19 who are currently married is estimated at 19 per cent worldwide, 6 per cent in developed countries, 21 per cent in developing countries, and 26 per cent in developing countries excluding China. The young bride will be under societal pressure to prove her fertility, which in some societies is the basis of her worth.

Births to unmarried adolescents are increasing. This is due both to an increased exposure to the risk of pregnancy and to limited access to information and means for protection. Opportunities for sexual activity without and outside of marriage have increased, social mores are changing, and in some areas, young women exchange sexual favours to meet their material needs. Access to contraception, including information and education, is still limited for the unmarried adolescent in many societies.

Complications of pregnancy, childbirth, and unsafe abortion are major causes of death for women aged 15–19 in less developed regions. Adolescent pregnancy can have short-term and long-term adverse health consequences. In the short term, the outcome of pregnancy is more likely to be unfavourable. One reason is biomedical. The pregnant adolescent girl is more likely to suffer from toxemia of pregnancy and cephalo-pelvic disproportion (when the bony pelvis did not have enough time to complete its growth), and is more likely to have a low birth weight baby. Another reason for an unfavourable outcome is the poor utilization of health services and poor compliance with medical advice among adolescents. A third reason for an unfavourable outcome is social, since adolescent pregnancy is more common among lower socio-economic levels of communities. There is evidence that the nutritional needs of the adolescent mother increase, to satisfy the cumulative needs of the still growing young girl and the nutritional requirements of the growing foetus, and poor nutrition will affect both.

The impact of unwanted pregnancy on the mental health of the adolescent should not be under-estimated. If the girl decides to terminate an unwanted pregnancy, and safe abortion services are not available or accessible, the girl may risk her health and her life. In the long term, adolescent pregnancy may have adverse social consequences, particularly for the unmarried adolescent. The girl is likely to drop out from school, and in some cases becomes liable to expulsion. In addition, as a single parent, the girl may have economical problems in rearing her child and making a living. She may be forced into an undesirable marriage. An unmarried mother can be a social outcast in some

---

[9] Population Reference Bureau, *2000 Data Sheet.* 10, 18.

countries, and she may even be at risk of being killed by a member of her family 'to bury their shame' and assert their honour. In several countries, so-called 'honour killings' are exempt from punishment or where they are punishable they are rarely investigated or prosecuted, or are only lightly punished.[10]

Teenage girls facing unwanted pregnancies often seek abortions. Teenagers are more likely than older women to be forced to have an unsafe abortion. They also tend to delay obtaining the procedure until later in pregnancy, when the procedure becomes more difficult and may carry more risk. Adolescents, therefore, account for a disproportionate number of abortion complications.

3. *Ethical Aspects*

The ethical principle of justice, that like cases be treated alike and different cases differently, raises the question of whether adolescents are to be treated like mature adults, or children. The answer may be that they are like both, to different degrees. Sexually active adolescents who request contraceptive protection appear to exercise adult prudence, and may be treated as adults regarding both information of their options for prevention of pregnancy and STD infection, and protection of their confidentiality. However, some parent-like protection, or paternalism, is often an appropriate element in their care. Their inexperience in adult relationships makes it ethical to warn them of their vulnerability to exploitation and abuse, even in relationships with partners they trust, and for instance that their protection against unplanned pregnancy may not be protection against STDs, including HIV infection.

Protection in their family and community settings may also be appropriate. In cultures where unmarried adolescent sexual activity is recognized, even if not condoned, as an aspect of courtship preceding marriage, the consequences of adolescent sexuality, for educational, family, and comparable security will usually be less severe than in cultures where sex before marriage is unacceptable and heavily punished. In the latter case, however, both advice against violating social expectations and protection against pregnancy are likely to be more urgent, recognizing that the sanctions against pregnancy outside marriage are more threatening to the female who experiences it than to the male responsible for causing it.

Where adolescent health care involves payments that the adolescents cannot make, their parents' involvement may be necessary for payment, directly or through private or public insurance plans. Parents may therefore learn of gynaecological treatment, but ethically the adolescent patients' confidentiality

---

[10] See the laws of Jordan, Pakistan, and Syria, discussed in CRLP, *Reproductive Rights*, ch. 6 on 'Rape and Other Sexual Violence', 45–50.

must nevertheless be protected. Disclosure of the particular forms of care requested and given should not be made without patients' clearly given consent. If patients inform their medical service providers that they require protection against sexual involvements to which they are being compelled involuntarily to submit, however, notification of others such as parents or police authorities that are obliged to provide protection will be ethically appropriate.

4. *Legal Aspects*

Laws differ among countries about the legal definition of an individual who can give informed, legally effective consent. The governing legal rule is that mentally competent individuals such as adults may act according to their wishes, even when what they wish to do appears contrary to their best interests. When legal minors wish to act in ways that appear against their interests, there is a tendency to presume that this shows that they are not competent to make decisions for themselves. However, some legal systems recognize two categories of minors, namely 'mature minors' and 'emancipated minors'. 'Mature minor' is the term used for older teenagers who understand the risks and benefits of medical care and can give informed consent. The term 'emancipated minor' generally refers to teenagers who are free from parental control: married, members of armed forces, pregnant, or living away from home.

Legal systems tend to recognize that mature minors, and emancipated minors to the extent of their emancipation, may give legally effective consent to medical care without their parents' approval, or knowledge. That is, their consent prevents medical examinations and treatment from amounting in law to an assault. Legal recognition may be based on Ministry of Health regulations, legislation, or court decisions. Moreover, the law requires that these adolescent patients are entitled to confidentiality in the care they receive.

Laws exist in some countries that make consensual sexual intercourse with adolescents below a given age, such as 16, a criminal offence, sometimes described as 'statutory rape' because underage consent is legally ineffective. Such laws, however, do not make offenders of the adolescents themselves, but only of those who have intercourse with them. Therefore, health service providers who afford underage adolescents protection against pregnancy and STDs are not parties to any offence. Providers may be at legal risk, however, if they counsel and equip adolescents' sexual partners to have relations with them safely. Education and information given to adolescent males of a general nature is legally appropriate, for instance, for their own protection against STDs. However, giving advice on safety in intercourse with particular adolescent partners may implicate providers in the offence the males may commit.

5. Human Rights Aspects

The Children's Convention provides in Article 24(1) that states shall strive to ensure that no child is deprived of access to health care services. This means that parents cannot veto such services that are appropriate in an adolescent's circumstances. The Convention requires respect for parents' rights, but Article 14(2) requires that parental rights be exercised 'in a manner consistent with the evolving capacities of the child'.

The Cairo Plus Five Report echoed the central role of families, parents, and other legal guardians to educate their children about sexual and reproductive health, consistently with the 'evolving capacities of adolescents'.[11] These provisions embody the legal consent of the mature minor, who is capable of enjoying the rights, and of bearing the responsibilities, of an adult. They give effect to the transcending human rights principle that, when adolescents are capable of adult judgement and responsibility, they should not suffer discrimination on grounds of their chronological age.[12]

In addition, the adolescent has a right to health information, education, and services, and has a right to privacy and confidentiality. Governments have adopted the following provisions of the Programme of Action at the United Nations International Conference on Population and Development (ICPD), held in Cairo in 1994:[13]

Countries should, where appropriate, remove legal, regulatory and social barriers to reproductive health information and care for adolescents. (para. 7.45)

Countries must ensure that the programmes and attitudes of health-care providers do not restrict the access of adolescents to appropriate services and the information they need, including on sexually-transmitted diseases and sexual abuse. . . . These services must safeguard the rights of adolescents to privacy, confidentiality, respect and informed consent. (para. 7.45)

Countries with the support of the international community, should protect and promote the rights of adolescents to reproductive health education, information and care and greatly reduce the number of adolescent pregnancies. (para. 7.46)

Governments, in collaboration with non-governmental organizations, are urged to meet the special needs of adolescents and to establish appropriate programmes to

---

[11] UN, General Assembly, *Report of the Ad Hoc Committee of the Whole of the Twenty-First Special Session of the General Assembly: Overall Review and Appraisal of the Implementation of the Programme of Action of the International Conference on Population and Development*, A/S-21/5/Add.1 (New York: UN, 1999) (hereinafter Cairo+5), para. 73(*d*).

[12] R. J. Cook and B. M. Dickens, 'Recognizing Adolescents' "Evolving Capacities" to Exercise Choice in Reproductive Healthcare', *Int. J. Gynecol. Obstet.* 70 (2000), 13–21.

[13] UN, *Population and Development*, i. *Programme of Action Adopted at the International Conference on Population and Development, Cairo, 5–13 September 1994* (New York: UN, Department for Economic and Social Information and Policy Analysis, 1994), ST/ESA/SER.A/149.

respond to those needs. Such programmes should include support mechanisms for the education and counselling of adolescents in the areas of gender relations and equality, violence against adolescents, responsible sexual behaviour, responsible family planning practice, family life, reproductive health, sexually-transmitted diseases, HIV infection and AIDS prevention. Sexually active adolescents will require special family planning information, counselling and services. (para. 7.47)

Youth should be actively involved in the planning, implementation and evaluation of development activities that have a direct impact on their daily lives. This is especially important with respect to information, education and communication activities and services concerning reproductive and sexual health. (para. 6.15)

The Cairo Plus Five Report amplified duties arising under these subparagraphs 7.45–7.47 of the Cairo Programme, and requires countries to 'ensure that programmes and attitudes of health-care providers do not restrict access of adolescents to appropriate services and the information they need . . . and . . . remove legal, regulatory and social barriers to reproductive health information and care for adolescents'.[14]

6. *Approaches*

6.1. *Clinical duty*

Dr CD must speak to Miss B in order to assess her capacity to maintain a sexual relationship, and to protect her emotions in forming a romantic attachment to her partner. In the event of uncertainty, Dr CD should have Miss B speak to a colleague as well, to obtain a second assessment, or seek guidance on indicators of Miss B's maturity. Miss B should be advised about the available options for the contraceptive service she has requested, and also about protection against STDs. She should also be advised to request her partner to ensure his own reproductive health, and to use condoms at least until he tests negative for STDs, including HIV infection, and perhaps thereafter until he is prepared for the responsibilities of fatherhood. Dr CD should encourage Miss B to ensure her partner's education regarding sexual and reproductive health. If there is a risk of legal liability due to Miss B's age, Dr CD should not undertake that education of the male partner, but facilitate his receiving independent reproductive health counselling from another source. Miss B should be encouraged, in any event, to be self-reliant in her protection against unplanned pregnancy.

Dr CD should ensure that Miss B's confidentiality is protected by all physicians and office staff aware of her identity and care. If Miss B's parents will learn of Dr CD's care of Miss B because of payment for services and products

---

[14]   Cairo+5, para. 73(*f*).

she requires, Dr CD should nevertheless not present detailed information to them, but give only a generalized description of care of a gynaecological condition. If police or other such authorities seek access to Miss B's medical record in investigating her partner's possible offence, Dr CD should invoke medical confidentiality to refuse disclosure, and consult with appropriate professional and clinical licensing authorities and professional associations if pressed.

6.2. *Health care systems obligations*

The General Recommendation 24 on Women's Health of the Committee on the Elimination of Discrimination against Women (CEDAW) states that:

the obligation to respect rights requires states parties to refrain from obstructing action taken by women in pursuit of their health care . . . states parties should not restrict women's access to health services or to the clinics that provide those services on the grounds that women do not have the authorization of husbands, partners, parents or health authorities, because they are unmarried or because they are women. (para. 14)

The CEDAW General Recommendation 24 also states that: 'in particular, states parties should ensure the rights of female and male adolescents to sexual and reproductive health education by properly trained personnel in specially designed programmes that respect their rights to privacy and confidentiality' (para. 18).

General Comment 14 on the right to the highest attainable standard of health, of the Committee on Economic, Social and Cultural Rights, states that: 'the realization of the right to health of adolescents is dependent on the development of youth-friendly health care, which respects confidentiality and privacy and includes appropriate sexual and reproductive health services' (para. 23).

Dr CD should ask what reproductive and sexual health education Miss B has had, including during her schooling and, through her, what education her partner has received. Dr CD should also investigate how effectively general and specialist medical practitioners and other health care providers are organized, and collaborate with governmental and non-governmental agencies to provide necessary adolescent counselling and services. Dr CD should also consider whether to present information on the adequacy or inadequacy of services at the next meeting of the national or regional society of obstetrician/gynaecologists. Dr CD probably knows whether colleagues have faced similar issues in the provision of care to adolescents and whether there might be interest in developing professional guidelines on adolescent reproductive and sexual health care. Dr CD should also consider whether development of such guidelines would provide valuable opportunities to assess how principles such as respect for the evolving capacities of adolescents could be adopted through national or regional policies.

The calibre of preventive reproductive and sexual health care services should be assessed. Dr CD should pay regard to public tolerance and intolerance of adolescent sexual expression and the balance between social, including religious, restraints that emphasize sexual abstinence before marriage and the practical burden of unplanned adolescent pregnancy, childbirth, abortion, and STD infection.

6.3. *Social action for underlying conditions*

Dr CD should reflect on family and social determinants of Miss B's request, and identify whether she is exercising mature prudence against untimely pregnancy and STD, or is fearful that disclosure of her sexual activity would jeopardize her and her family's social standing, her physical security, or her very life. Dr CD should also address whether provision of medical advice and services to Miss B would be regarded in the community as conscientious routine care, or misunderstood as immoral complicity in a young couple's misconduct. Social leaders sometimes believe that education in sexual health and hygiene itself promotes adolescent sexual curiosity and misconduct. Dr CD should collaborate with health care colleagues and associations and governmental and non-governmental organizations to show the dysfunction of adolescent ignorance about sex, sexuality, and preventive health care. They could demonstrate that professional reproductive and sexual health education and services are compatible with parents' concerns for their adolescent children's best health care and interests.

4

Sexual Assault and Emergency Contraception

Case Study

Dr R is called down to the hospital emergency department to examine Ms S, who complains that she has been sexually assaulted. She says that her boyfriend raped her and that she wants to avoid pregnancy because she is not ready to bear its consequences. The local law permits abortion in the case of rape, when a complaint is filed with the police, and they conclude their inquiries into the circumstances. Ms S says her boyfriend has denied raping her, and Dr R knows police inquiries are often prolonged. What are Dr R's obligations in light of medical, ethical, legal, and human rights considerations?

1. Background

Violence against women is increasingly recognized as a serious public health problem.[1] Women have always been vulnerable to the horrendous crime of rape. Reliable data on the incidence of rape are not available, as it tends to be hidden and under-reported. Surveys in some countries have shown that between 10 and 20 per cent of young women had been raped.[2] The majority of perpetrators, contrary to common belief, are not strangers, but people known to the victim. A substantial group of victims are very young girls. For example, in one Latin American country, it is estimated that only seventy-two cases of sexual assault are reported of the 360 that happen each day, and that 60 per cent of pregnancies among 12- to 14-year-old girls result from rape by family members or persons close to the victims.[3]

Rape and sexual assaults, more than other types of injuries, cause both physical and profound emotional trauma. Victims also face the risk of unwanted pregnancy and sexually transmitted diseases (STDs), including HIV

---

[1] L. Heise, M. Ellsberg, and M. Gottemoeller, 'Ending Violence against Women', *Population Reports, Series L*, 11 (1999).

[2] Ibid.

[3] S. Tuesta, *The Search for Justice* (Lima: Movimiento Manuela Ramos, 2000), 5.

infection, and in many societies a social stigma. Psychological healing after rape takes a long time, particularly if the woman was raped by someone she trusted in a place that was 'safe' to her. She feels she has no safe place left as a refuge for her. One victim remarked that the body mends soon enough. Only the scars remain. But the wounds inflicted upon the soul take much longer to heal. And each time the victim relives these moments, the wounds start bleeding all over again. The broken spirit takes longest to mend; the damage to the personality may be the most difficult to overcome.

Women at all ages are vulnerable to sexual abuse. Child prostitution and sexual abuse have received recent international attention. Sex may also be economically coerced on adolescent girls, as in the case of African schoolgirls having to take up with 'sugar daddies' to afford school.[4] Sexual harassment is a reality that many women face in their communities, in the workplace and in various institutional settings, including those designed for their safety, and sometimes in their own homes, and that has received attention only recently.

Women do not usually wage war but they suffer more from the consequences. Women are often displaced as refugees and face sexual abuse by refugee camp guards and security patrols.[5] Forced prostitution and sexual exploitation by military forces is an enduring violation. In the Second World War, thousands of Korean, Philippino, and Indonesian women were forced into sexual slavery for Japanese troops in East and South-East Asia.[6] Rape and forced pregnancy were used as instruments of war in the more recent conflicts in the Former Yugoslavia[7] and, for example, in Rwanda.[8] Even though rape and other acts of sexual violence were formally recognized as international crimes, they were not prosecuted as such until the creation of the International Criminal Tribunal for the Former Yugoslavia (ICTY) in 1993 and the International Criminal Tribunal for Rwanda (ICTR) in 1994. The ICTR found that the accused ordered, instigated, and otherwise aided and abetted sexual violence,[9] and the ICTY found that rape can amount to a form of

---

[4] G. S. Mpangile, M. T. Leshabari, and D. J. Kihwele, 'Induced Abortion in Dar Es Salaam, Tanzania: The Plight of Adolescents', in A. I. Mundigo and C. Indriso (eds.), *Abortion in the Developing World* (New Dehli: Vistaar Publications, 1999).

[5] Human Rights Watch, *Seeking Refuge, Finding Terror: The Widespread Rape of Somali Women Refugees in North Eastern Kenya* (New York: Human Rights Watch, 1993); Human Rights Watch, *Seeking Protection: Addressing Sexual and Domestic Violence in Tanzania's Refugee Camp* (New York: Human Rights Watch, 2000).

[6] U. Dolgopol and S. Paranjape, *Comfort Women—An Unfinished Ordeal: A Report of a Mission* (Geneva: International Commission of Jurists, 1994).

[7] UN, *Report on the Situation of Human Rights in the Territory of the Former Yugoslavia* (New York: UN, 1993), UN Doc. E/CN.4/1993/50, at 19–20, 63–4, 67–73.

[8] Human Rights Watch, *Shattered Lives: Sexual Violence during the Rwandan Genocide and its Aftermath* (New York: Human Rights Watch, 1996).

[9] *Prosecutor v. Akayesu*, Judgment, ICTR-96-4-T (2 Sept. 1998) (International Criminal Tribunal for Rwanda).

torture when it is used during the interrogation as means of intimidating the victim.[10]

2. *Medical Aspects*

Victimization by sexual assault is multidimensional. Many health care providers, especially physicians, may feel best able to treat the presenting physical results of assault, and the risk of infection to which the victim has been exposed. It is clearly important that treatment be delivered as promptly as possible. Assault has wider consequences, however, because it has psychological effects that may be long-term, affecting a woman's self-esteem and self-confidence, in dealing with particular men and with how they believe they are perceived in their societies.[11] Accordingly, medical responses to sexual assault must be based on the immediate trauma, the risk of pregnancy, the possibility of STD infection, and the immediate and longer term psychological injury the victim may suffer.

If the woman reports early for treatment, emergency contraception may save her from the risk of an imposed pregnancy. Emergency contraception (EC) refers to contraceptive methods that can be used by women in the first few days following unprotected intercourse to prevent an unwanted pregnancy. Emergency contraceptive methods are effective and safe for the majority of women who may need them, as well as being simple to use.[12]

Two emergency hormonal contraceptive pill regimens can be used. The standard regimen consists of the combined oral contraceptive pills containing both oestrogen and progestagen in relatively high doses. This regimen is known as the 'Yuzpe method', named after Dr Yuzpe who developed the regimen. Two pills should be taken as the first dose as soon as convenient but no later than seventy-two hours after unprotected intercourse. These should be followed by two other pills twelve hours later. A new alternative is the levonorgestrel-only pill (with no oestrogen) containing 0.75 mgm. One pill is taken as the first dose, followed by another pill twelve hours later. It is equally effective as the Yuzpe method and has fewer side effects.[13]

The mechanism of action of emergency contraceptive pills has not been clearly established. Several studies have shown that they can inhibit or delay

---

[10] *Prosecutor v. Furundzija*, Judgment, IT-95-17/1, para. 163 (10 Dec. 1998) (International Criminal Tribunal for the Former Yugoslavia).

[11] WHO, *Women's Mental Health: An Evidence Based Review* (Geneva: WHO, 2000), WHO/MSD/MHP/00.1, Part 4: Violence Against Women.

[12] WHO, *Emergency Contraception: A Guide for Service Delivery* (Geneva: WHO, 1998), WHO/FRH/FPP/98.19.

[13] Task Force on Postovulatory Methods of Fertility Regulation, 'Randomized Controlled Trial of Levonorgestrel versus the Yuzpe Regimen of Combined Oral Contraceptives for Emergency Contraception', *Lancet*, 352 (1998), 428–33.

ovulation. It has also been suggested, but not proven, that they may prevent implantation, fertilization, or transport of sperm or ova. What is definitely known is that they are effective only within three days of unprotected sexual intercourse, that is, before implantation takes place, and therefore do not interrupt pregnancy. Thus, they are not medically considered to be a form of abortion.[14]

The failure rate of emergency contraception is about 2 per cent after a single act of unprotected sexual intercourse. Emergency contraception is not a substitute for regular contraceptive use. Moreover, emergency contraceptive pills offer no protection against sexually transmitted infection, including HIV. Psychological counselling on this topic should be provided along with diagnostic services and referral as needed.

A less commonly used method for emergency contraception is the insertion of a copper-releasing intra-uterine device within five days of unprotected sexual intercourse.[15] The available evidence is that it acts by interference with fertilization rather than implantation. It is not a suitable method if the woman is at risk of sexually transmitted infection.

3. *Ethical Aspects*

The microethical duties in cases of sexual assault are to address the gynaecological condition of the woman, to consider her request for maximum protection against pregnancy, to protect her as far as possible against suffering any sexually transmitted infection, and to address her psychological needs following the sexual assault. A wider duty is preservation of evidence that may confirm an assault, perhaps including semen and other tissue samples that may be relevant to subsequent enquiries. This duty is not contingent on being satisfied that an assault occurred, but arises out of respect for the explanation a woman gives of her request for care, and forensic requirements of legally admissible evidence.

The ethical right to autonomy that the woman enjoys entitles her to obtain protection against pregnancy. Not all practitioners who object to participation in abortion procedures are equally opposed to contraception. In any event, the health care provider is ethically obliged to ensure that the victim has access to the medical care indicated for her. Treatment is not dependent on police enquiries into the rape allegation, since emergency contraception may avoid the need for legal abortion. Indeed, the ethical duty to do no harm requires the doctor to act promptly in order to prevent unintended pregnancy and any of its consequences. This is so whether or not the sexual act amounted

---

[14] WHO, *Emergency Contraception*.   [15] Ibid.

in law to an assault, since the key issue is that the woman was involved in unprotected intercourse. The first ethical response owed to the woman, in accordance with her request, is to prevent any risk of pregnancy. Subsequent responses should address protection against risks that she has suffered transmission of infection, and against psychological injury.

4. *Legal Aspects*

The law reflects the medical distinction between contraception and abortion. In many countries legal controls over abortion have remained more rigid than over use of contraceptive means, so the critical legal distinction is between medical use of abortifacient and non-abortifacient means. Emergency contraception is non-abortifacient, since it is intended to prevent pregnancy, not to terminate pregnancy. Legal analysis has responded to the practice of *in vitro* fertilization, where achievement of ovum fertilization in a petri dish does not constitute the ovum donor's (or any other woman's) pregnancy. It is usually accepted in law that only when the fertilized ovum is embedded in a woman's uterus has her pregnancy begun.[16]

The legal definition of pregnancy follows the medical definition. A WHO Technical Report considered that pregnancy begins when implantation is complete, and that implantation is the process that starts with the attachment of the zona-free blastocyst to the uterine wall (days 5–6 post-fertilization); the blastocyst then penetrates the uterine epithelium and invades the stroma. The process is complete when the blastocyst develops primary villi and the surface defect on the epithelium is closed (days 13–14 post-fertilization).[17] In its 1998 definition of pregnancy, the FIGO Committee for the Ethical Aspects of Human Reproduction and Women's Health stated that pregnancy is that part of the process of human reproduction 'that commences with the implantation of the conceptus in a woman'.[18]

A practitioner who, on grounds of conscience, will not provide emergency contraception where it is the standard of care[19] is legally obliged to refer

[16] R. J. Cook, B. M. Dickens, C. Ngwena, and M. I. Plata, 'The Legal Status of Emergency Contraception', *Int. J. Gynecol. Obstet.* 75 (2001), 185–91.

[17] WHO, *Mechanism of Action, Safety and Efficacy of Intrauterine Devices: Report of a WHO Scientific Group. Technical Report Series 753* (Geneva: WHO, 1987), 12.

[18] International Federation of Gynecology and Obstetrics (FIGO) Committee for the Ethical Aspects of Human Reproduction and Women's Health, *Definition of Pregnancy, Recommendations on Ethical Issues in Obstetrics and Gynecology* (London: FIGO, 2000), 38, available at http://www.figo.org/default.asp?id=6082, last accessed 6 May 2002; repr. in *Int. J. Gynecol. Obstet.* 64 (1999), 317.

[19] American College of Obstetricians and Gynecologists (ACOG), *Practice Bulletin, Clinical Management Guidelines for Obstetrician-Gynecologists No. 25 (Emergency Oral Contraception)* (Washington, DC: ACOG, 2001); repr. in *Int. J. Gynecol. Obstet.* 78 (2002), 191.

women eligible to receive it to alternative practitioners or facilities where it will be available. Refusal or failure of appropriate referral constitutes legally actionable negligence through abandonment. Further, the practitioner who continues patient care without disclosure of the option lacks patients' adequately informed consent, possibly rendering the care an assault and childbirth that emergency contraception would have prevented an injury to patients, compensation for which could include costs of child support.

Many abortion laws make it an offence to act, as the widely followed English law of 1861 provided, 'with intent to procure the miscarriage of any woman whether she be or be not with child'. This language was designed to punish acts intended to induce abortion even when a prosecutor could not show biological evidence that the woman was actually pregnant by implantation of a fertilized ovum in her uterus. The law accordingly recognizes three conditions, namely pregnancy, possible pregnancy, and non-pregnancy. An act intended to terminate pregnancy or possible pregnancy will be governed by the abortion law, but an act intended to preserve non-pregnancy is not so governed. Emergency contraception, which is only effective if undertaken within seventy-two hours or three days of unprotected intercourse, is accordingly non-abortifacient.

As the time since intercourse grows, the possibility of pregnancy increases. That is, as time widens between unprotected intercourse and the medical intervention, the easier it is for a prosecutor to show that the initiator of the intervention must have been aware of the possibility of pregnancy, and had the intention to terminate it had it occurred. Accordingly, the sooner action is undertaken, the more secure is its legal status as non-abortifacient.

Laws concerning evidence necessary to convict men of rape have in the past been gendered. Evidence was usually required at least of women being injured in ways to which women would not normally consent, and of ejaculation. Accordingly, forensic inquiries had to show evidence of bruising and/or tearing, and semen had to be recovered from inside the woman's body, through invasive techniques.

Laws in many countries have evolved, however, to recognize that women can be terrified into passive submission to unwanted intercourse, and that some women's counsellors have advised women's passive submission in order to minimize risk of serious injury, as a preferable alternative to subjection to violent rape. Further, laws have evolved to be satisfied with evidence of forceful penetration without ejaculation, and to accept penetration by objects as constituting rape. Modern criminal investigations of allegations of rape recognize that men, including in positions in authority over women, based for instance, on their social status, can take sexual advantage of women in ways that the law should prohibit.

Advanced laws no longer include a category of 'rape', but differentially punish assaults by distinguishing among sexual assaults, aggravated sexual assaults, sexual assaults by persons in authority, and, for instance, sexual assaults by threats or use of weapons. Accordingly, for purposes of criminal prosecution, evidence of semen, bruising, or sexual penetration is not required, and distinctions are not drawn among proven victims of sexual assault between those who suffered sexual penetration and those who did not. This reduces the need for invasive examination of women to acquire forensic evidence.

5. *Human Rights Aspects*

States commit themselves to address and eliminate all forms of violence against women through general international human rights conventions, conventions specific to women, such as the Convention on the Elimination of All Forms of Discrimination against Women, and more focused conventions, such as the Inter-American Convention on the Prohibition of Violence against Women. These conventions are increasingly applied to require states effectively to enforce laws against women's victimization by violence. General Recommendation 19 on Violence against Women of the Committee on the Elimination of Discrimination against Women (CEDAW) explains that discrimination against women 'includes gender-based violence, that is, violence that is directed against a woman because she is a woman or that affects women disproportionately. It includes acts that inflict physical, mental or sexual harm or suffering, threats of such acts, coercion and other deprivations of liberty' (see Pt. III, Ch. 6, Sect. 1, para. 6). Significantly, this General Recommendation explains that gender-based violence breaches specific human rights, regardless of whether those provisions expressly mention violence. The rights include: the right to life, the right not to be subject to torture or to cruel, inhuman, or degrading treatment or punishment, the right to liberty and security of the person, the right to equality within the family, the right to just and favourable working conditions, and the right to the highest attainable standard of health.

CEDAW General Recommendation 24 on Women and Health places violence in the context of women's health by requiring states to address distinctive features and factors which differ for women in comparison to men, such as biological, socio-economic, and psycho-social factors, including postpartum depression (see Pt. III, Ch. 6, Sect. 2, para. 12). Human rights issues concern prevention of unplanned pregnancy, protection against sexually transmissible infection, and safeguarding of the victim's mental health. The transcending concern, conditioning responses to immediate pressing concerns, is that women complaining of assault be treated with respect for their human dignity, and not be subject to condemnatory, impersonal, or indifferent care that constitutes inhuman and degrading treatment.

The human rights violations of rape go beyond the danger to health from sexual assault because it places in peril women's control of their fertility, pregnancy, childbearing, and family building. The right to found a family includes a woman's right not to have a pregnancy imposed upon her by violence. Accordingly, the human right to physical and mental health and the right to found a family of her choice entitle a woman to emergency contraception to avoid unplanned pregnancy by rape.

Additional rights may be invoked in support of a woman's right to health and family integrity. A woman's right to the highest attainable standard of health justifies health care providers' treatment, and her rights to the benefits of scientific progress justify employment of the most effective, least invasive means for this purpose, including emergency contraception.

The human rights context of respect for a woman's personal dignity and protection from inhuman and degrading treatment require the woman to be in charge of the context of her care. Even where emergency interventions are medically justified, they cannot be imposed over the woman's objections, based for instance on her religious or other convictions. Similarly, she should not be subject to the religious objections others may have to providing indicated treatment for the conditions she presents. Accordingly, health care providers who consider emergency contraception to constitute abortion may invoke conscientious objection, but cannot refuse promptly to refer patients to providers who do not share this conviction. Laws that deny emergency contraception as constituting abortion are questionable under human rights provisions, for instance on inhuman and degrading treatment and, depending on the context, perhaps on torture.

Human rights provisions also address the longer term mental impact on women of sexual assault.[20] Mental health treatment may be indicated in itself, and processes of medical investigation, forensic testing, police inquiry, and, for instance, criminal trial, should be such as not to obstruct a woman's physical or mental health recovery, and not to aggravate her victimization. The traditional legal approach to rape is to treat accusations conservatively and sceptically because accusations of rape are easily made and difficult to defend, especially when made against male friends. This traditional approach is yielding to recognition of the frequency of rape, and that women can be so deterred and intimidated by processes of legal inquiry as to withhold complaints, and thereby afford assailants legal immunity. Women's human rights protections from inhuman and degrading treatment extend beyond the duties owed by health care providers to those binding police and judicial officers. It may fall to health care providers to protect women against insensitivity and inhumanity from these officers.

[20] L. Gulcur, 'Evaluating the Role of Gender Inequalities and Rights Violations in Women's Mental Health', *Health and Human Rights*, 5 (2000), 46–67.

6. *Approaches*

6.1. *Clinical duty*

Dr R should provide Ms S with emergency contraception, and manage this case of post-coital contraception like a request for pre-coital contraception. In addition, responses to rape should be initiated such as sexually transmitted disease (STD) protection, although more invasive techniques should be avoided, such as to recover semen samples for forensic purposes, because there is no need to identify an unknown assailant, unless local law still requires proof of ejaculation. The boyfriend's denial of rape may consist in denial of intercourse, but he is as likely to deny that admitted intercourse with Ms S was non-consensual. In either case, recovery of semen samples will usually be unnecessary, since most legal systems' definitions of rape are met by evidence only of sexual penetration. A wider concern is the boyfriend's HIV status, since Ms S may require treatment for exposure to HIV infection and appropriate counselling. Some legal systems mandate HIV testing of men accused of rape or sexual assault.

The psychological sequelae need careful attention, and proper counselling. In many industrialized and some developing countries, support groups play an integral role in healing and consciousness raising. Where such groups are available, Dr R should refer Ms S. In a support group, she will be able to communicate with women who have been through similar experiences and who have recovered from them. She will get hope that she can also recover.

6.2. *Health care systems obligations*

If modern means of emergency contraception are unfamiliar to Dr R's hospital, it may be necessary to confirm their clinical propriety, and to make clear that they do not involve abortion. Some agencies hostile to inducement of abortion are equally hostile to artificial contraception, and equate the latter with the former, but Dr R may have to show that medically, ethically, and legally, emergency contraception is not abortion, but like pre-coital contraception, is intended to prevent pregnancy, not terminate it. The FIGO Committee for the Ethical Aspects of Human Reproduction and Women's Health in its Guidelines in Emergency Contraception explained that 'emergency contraception is highly effective in diminishing the number of unwanted pregnancies without the need of an abortion . . . [and recommended] that the medical professional should advocate that emergency contraception be easily available and accessible at all times to women'.[21]

---

[21] FIGO Committee for the Ethical Aspects of Human Reproduction and Women's Health, 'Guidelines on Emergency Contraception', *Int. J. Gynecol. Obstet.* 77 (2002), 174.

Dr R might also address how sensitively the hospital examines victims of rape, because examinations may be unduly invasive, to the extent of being experienced as 'a second rape'. The risk may be greater where forensic evidence is sought for police enquiries, and to establish legal grounds for pregnancy termination. Proof beyond reasonable doubt is required before an alleged rapist can be criminally convicted, but proof of rape to this level is not necessarily required to justify emergency contraception or even termination of pregnancy on this ground. The woman's authentic sense of being violated justifies the procedure, even if adequate proof for legal conviction is not obtainable, for instance because an assailant cannot be found or identified or is mentally disordered and so cannot stand trial or be convicted.

Practitioners in hospital emergency departments and those responsible for training and equipping emergency care workers may consider contraception to be a preventive service or a part of family rather than emergency medicine. The service of emergency contraception should be available within family practice medicine, of course, but emergency personnel should also be encouraged, educated, and equipped to see emergency contraception as analogous to other forms of post-traumatic care for women who have been sexually violated. Further, emergency services should make this care available as a community service, not dependent on evidence of rape. That is, women who believe their contraceptive precautions to have failed should have prompt access to emergency contraception, delivered in the same conscientious, non-judgemental way as any other medical service. Such women's request and receipt of care should provide an occasion for their counselling on general pre-coital contraception, so that emergency contraception serves only as a fail-safe or back-up method, and does not become a means of primary contraception.

CEDAW's General Recommendation 24 on Women and Health calls on governments and those acting under the authority of government, such as hospitals, to develop treatment protocols for the care of victims of violence (see Pt. III, Ch. 6, Sect. 2, para. 15). Guidelines and protocols do exist,[22] and need to be reviewed for their applicability in different settings and how they guide the health care provider in the delivery of emergency contraception.

To ensure wide availability of emergency contraception, Dr R might explore with the health ministry switching emergency contraception from prescription only to over-the-counter distribution. Medical evidence indicates that emergency contraception is safe for self-medication, its inappropriate use does not cause serious harm, it has no documented medical contraindications, and no

---

[22] Brazil, Ministry of Health, *Prevention and Treatment of Harms Resulting from Sexual Violence against Women and Adolescent Girls* (Brazilia: Ministry of Health, 1999); S. MacDonald, J. Wyman, and M. Addision, *Guidelines and Protocols for the Sexual Assault Nurse Examiner* (Toronto: Sexual Assault Care Centre, Women's College Hospital, 1995).

medical intermediary is needed for its distribution. Moreover, it is in the public health interest because it will prevent abortion.[23]

6.3. *Social action for underlying conditions*

Societies' image of women may need to be corrected. There is sometimes a tendency to blame the victim. During a debate on the reform of rape law, one parliamentarian once commented that women should wear purdah (head-to-toe covering) to ensure that innocent men do not get unnecessarily excited by women's bodies and are not unconsciously forced into becoming rapists. If women do not want to fall prey to such men, he said, they should take the necessary precautions instead of forever blaming the men.[24] When a nursing student in a Latin American country reported being sexually molested by police officers while in custody, the response by the assistant to the public prosecutor was: 'Are you a virgin? If you are not a virgin, why do you complain?' In some Latin American countries—for example, Brazil, Costa Rica, Ecuador, and Guatemala—the law defines certain sexual offences as crimes only if they are committed against 'honest'—that is, virginal—women or girls.[25]

The International Federation of Gynecology and Obstetrics (FIGO) General Assembly in 1997 recommended that obstetricians and gynaecologists work with others to gain insight into the causes of the problem, and assist in the legal prosecution of cases of sexual abuse and rape by careful and sensitive documentation of the evidence.[26] Some societies of obstetricians and gynaecologists have taken initiatives to address the problem in comprehensive ways.[27]

---

[23] D. Grimes, 'Switching Emergency Contraception to Over-the-Counter Status', *New England Journal of Medicine*, 347 (2002), 846–9.

[24] H. Epstein, *The Intimate Enemy: Gender Violence and Reproductive Health. Panos Briefing No. 27* (London: Panos Institute, 1998), 6.

[25] L. L. Heise, J. Pitanguy, and A. Germain, *Violence against Women: The Hidden Health Burden. World Bank Discussion Paper*, 255 (Washington, DC: World Bank, 1994), 31.

[26] WHO, *FIGO General Assembly Resolution on Violence against Women, FIGO/WHO, Pre-Congress Workshop on Violence against Women: In Search of Solutions* (Geneva: WHO, 1998), WHO/FRH/WHD/97.38, at 33–4.

[27] R. F. Jones and D. L. Horan, 'The American College of Obstetricians and Gynecologists: A Decade of Responding to Violence against Women', *Int. J. Gynecol. Obstet.* 58 (1997), 43–50.

5

Hymen Reconstruction

Case Study

Two years ago when military conflict engulfed her village, Ms D, an unmarried young woman then aged 16, was raped by an invading soldier. Villagers know of the violence the community suffered, but not how severely individuals were victimized. Ms D is now engaged to be married, and her prospective husband and his family expect his bride to be a virgin. Ms D asks Dr E to undertake hymen reconstruction so that her marriage will not be impaired. Taking account of medical, ethical, legal, and human rights considerations, what should Dr E do?

1. *Background*

The hymen is the thin piece of tissue that partially blocks the entrance to the vagina. It is named after the Greek god of marriage and has no known biological function. The hymen does not cover the entire vaginal opening, allowing the menstrual blood to leave the body.

The hymen has historically been a marker of a woman's virginity. In cultures where a woman's virginity is highly valued, the belief is that it should remain intact until the woman is married. In certain traditional communities, it is the custom that defloration is performed manually on the wedding night to demonstrate and to celebrate the bride's virginity. If no bleeding occurs, she will be subject to public humiliation, will be considered a disgrace to her parents, and in some cultures may be killed to save the honour of the family.

In these cultures, women, understandably, will go to great lengths to get their hymens reconstructed before the wedding if the membrane has been torn. Even though many immigrants from African, Middle Eastern, and Asian countries have moved to northern countries, these immigrant groups still hold to the tradition that girls must be virgins when they marry.

The procedure of hymen reconstruction is relatively simple. However, it raises ethical, legal, human rights, and social concerns.

2. *Medical Aspects*

The hymen varies greatly in shape, size, and consistency. It may be elastic enough to allow penetrative sexual intercourse without being torn. It may be thick enough to hinder intercourse and may need to be excised to allow intercourse to take place. It may be torn completely only during labour. The hymen may be torn without intercourse, by a fall, vigorous sporting activities, or insertion of tampons during menstruation.[1] A woman can become pregnant even if the hymen is intact, and no penetration has occurred. Sperm deposited on the vulva may find their way to the vagina.

Reconstruction of the hymen (hymenorrhaphy) may be performed simply, as a temporary procedure, by using catgut (absorbable) sutures to approximate hymen remnants. This is done a few days before the wedding, and with the occasional incorporation of a gelatin capsule containing a blood-like substance, which bursts during intercourse. Alternatively, a more definitive procedure is performed in which hymen remnants are carefully approximated after refreshing their edges. Where hymeneal remnants are insufficient, a narrow strip of the posterior wall of the vagina is dissected for reconstruction. The operation is carried out as an outpatient procedure, and the notes are commonly not entered in the patient's medical record.

3. *Ethical Aspects*

The central ethical aspects Dr E must resolve are whether this procedure may ever be performed,[2] and if it may be, whether the circumstances in which rupture of a hymen has occurred may govern or influence whether the procedure should be performed. The initial question arises from the deception inherent in allowing a woman who is not a virgin to present herself as if she is.[3] This deception may be an injustice done to those who are induced to become falsely assured that their expectations or requirements of virginity have been met. The falsehood that Dr E would facilitate by complying with Ms D's request, were her prospective husband not informed of the procedure before marriage, raises ethical concerns not only of justice and truth-telling, but also of disrespect of his autonomous choice of marriage partner, and breach of the duty to do no harm or wrong.

---

[1] S. J. Eman, E. R. Wood, E. N. Allred, and E. Grace, 'Hymeneal Findings in Adolescent Women: The Impact of Tampon Use and Consensual Sexual Activity', *Journal of Pediatrics*, 125 (1994), 153–60.

[2] S. Paterson-Brown, 'Should Doctors Reconstruct the Vaginal Introitus of Adolescent Girls to Mimic the Virginal State?', *British Medical Journal*, 316 (1998), 461.

[3] D. D. Raphael, 'The Ethical Issue is Deceit', *British Medical Journal*, 316 (1998), 460.

This approach to the inherent ethical issue is, however, seriously incomplete. The principle of justice requires that an assessment of the prospective bride's purposes be matched by an assessment of those of the prospective husband and his family. In that the husband's family may require not only a different but a higher standard of purity of one partner to a marriage than of the other, they may seem to be acting unjustly. Their culture may ostensibly require virginity in both partners, but inequality remains in that only one is required to offer convincing proof. Since, for anatomical reasons, the husband can provide no more than his spoken assurance, it is unjust to require a higher standard of the wife. A medical procedure that reinforces any assurance she gives of necessary virtue is ethically defensible.

It is no ethical defence of the procedure, of course, that it equips both marriage partners to be equally deceptive. A defence may be made, however, by recognition that the requirement of a bride's virginity is discriminatory against women, and perpetuates oppressive control of women's sexuality. The requirement of brides' virginity may itself appear unethical. Further, Dr E has no ethical duty to comply with a prospective husband's unethical practice, or to monitor or enforce the duties that prospective marriage partners owe each other. Dr E may conscientiously object to perform the procedure on personal grounds, or decline on the professional ground that it is not indicated on medical grounds, but then must refer Ms D to another physician.

Relevance of the circumstances in which hymen rupture occurred relates to a contrast between virginity and chastity. The two words often appear synonymous, but, while the former refers to a biological or physiological condition, the latter refers to an ethical or moral status. A rape victim has not been immoral or acted unchastely or unlawfully. Similarly, a girl experiencing traumatic or accidental rupture is guiltless, and bears no taint that can ethically be stigmatizing. Performance of a medical procedure that brings a person's physiological condition into accordance with her moral status is not unethical, and is beneficent when it facilitates justified satisfaction of her husband's moral expectations of her in marriage, ethically suspect though those expectations may be. The ethical challenge this approach presents, however, is whether it is offensively judgemental and discriminatory to deny the procedure to a prospective bride who has freely indulged in the same sexual licence as their culture leaves available to her prospective groom.[4]

4. *Legal Aspects*

In the absence of legislation, such as may limit abortion, there is no general legal barrier to performance of a consensual but medically unnecessary

---

[4] E. Webb, 'Cultural Complexities should Not be Ignored', *British Medical Journal*, 316 (1998), 462.

procedure on a social indication, or simply on request of a mentally competent patient. Much cosmetic medicine is lawfully practised on this basis, such as inserting breast implants, to which hymen reconstruction to create a patient's preferred appearance is sometimes analogized. Ms D's physician bears her prospective husband and his family no legal duty of care or disclosure, nor a legal duty to enforce truthfulness of his prospective wife. Indeed, the legal duty of confidentiality may exceed usual limits in that, with due counselling on its implications, physicians may exclude reference to performance of the procedures from patients' medical records.

A physician usually risks legal liability, particularly for negligence, in omitting information of a medical procedure from a patient's record. The record is the instrument through which health care professionals share information among themselves concerning a patient, and, in the patient's interests, information should be identical among different users and complete. Informed consent to exclusion of medical information may be questionable when a patient cannot clearly understand the implications of the omission. However, hymen reconstruction is a relatively trivial, medically inconsequential procedure, often undertaken on an outpatient basis, with no drug treatment but only local anaesthetic. The benefit of inclusion of the procedure in the medical record is so minor and the risk to a patient may be so great, including in some instances physical violence approaching murder, and abandonment, that compliance with a patient's request, and offering her the opportunity for exclusion of reference to performance of the procedure from her medical record is legally justifiable.

Many adolescents explain their request for hymen reconstruction by their subjection to unwanted sexual intercourse they were physically or socially unable to resist. In many countries, physicians have legally enforceable duties to notify child protection agencies of their reasonable suspicions of child abuse and of children's liability to abuse. If, for instance, an adolescent of adult years discloses abuse, and a younger girl appears to be vulnerable to similar victimization by living in or near the abuser's residence, a legal duty to report the actual or anticipated abuse may arise. Where there is no duty to report, a power to report will often be legally recognized, provided that it is exercised without negligence and in good faith.

5. *Human Rights Aspects*

When health is understood as a state of physical, mental, and social well-being, hymen reconstruction can be seen to serve the rights to health of women whose social well-being depends on the appearance of virginity. Nevertheless, where it is required to evidence this condition in women but not in men, it is a form of discrimination against women and a denial of their right to equality in the family. Women who lack appropriate evidence will be placed at serious disadvantage, for instance in marriage, their societies, and their very survival against the menace of 'honour killing'. Any requirement of evidence of virginity therefore constitutes a gross form of discrimination against women on grounds of sex. The Convention on the Elimination of All Forms of Discrimination against Women (the Women's Convention) provides in Article 5(*a*) that States Parties shall take all appropriate measures to modify social and cultural patterns of conduct in order to eliminate customary and all other practices, which are based on stereotyped roles for men and women. Until such modification occurs, hymen reconstruction can protect women's human rights to life, to freedom from violence and from inhuman and degrading treatment, to marry, and, for instance, to the highest attainable standard of health, in addition to the underlying right to non-discrimination.

Women's role as virgins is particularly oppressive where women have no control over their sexual availability to men, not only in conditions of military conflict but in times of routine civil order when women cannot resist authoritative men, in their families and outside. The requirement of virginity as a symbol of virtue is an oppressive denial of human rights where women are powerless to protect their physical integrity. The Committee on the Elimination of Discrimination against Women (CEDAW) General Recommendation 19, on Violence against Women, focuses on women's need of protection against physical depredations. In addition, this General Recommendation requires states to report on how they have applied human rights to afford women protection against the social violence of denying them opportunities in life, including marriage, entrance to education and comparable programmes and career opportunities, unless they can satisfy examination of their virginity. Hymen reconstruction that protects women against the injustice of such examination promotes their human rights.

6. *Approaches*

6.1. *Clinical duty*

Dr E has no clinical duty to comply with Ms D's request, but, if refusing, should refer her to another physician, since the request is not unlawful and Ms D is entitled to assistance. Whether or not Dr E performs the procedure, Ms D's confidentiality in having or requesting the procedure must be protected. If Dr E declines the procedure on the suspicion that hymen rupture occurred in less compelling or sympathetic circumstances than Ms D explained, she should honestly be so informed, and be given an opportunity to reinforce her explanation in discussion with Dr E or another physician.

Further, Dr E should not risk future compromise of Ms D's medical care by writing negative remarks in her medical record, unless believing that her explanation has pathological implications such as paranoia or cognitive impairment.

If Ms D identifies or indicates a person who imposed sexual intercourse or like interference without her consent, Dr E must comply with applicable legal reporting duties, and discuss with Ms D available powers to inform third parties. Where no duty to report exists, Dr E may defer to Ms D's preference on exercise of the power of disclosure, recognizing that reporting may expose Ms D to further violence.

6.2. *Health care systems obligations*

Particularly for adolescent girls, physicians require better education in understanding the physical characteristics of the hymen, and the psychological impact of its rupture by personal violence, trauma, or other undesired circumstance. Education should also address failure to rupture on forced intercourse, as well as rupture, in order to offer necessary assistance and counselling when a woman cannot provide this evidence of the assault of which she complains.

6.3. *Social action for underlying conditions*

The conditions underlying the request for hymen reconstruction are the unjust and oppressively gendered social expectations to which Ms D is subject. They include requirements of women's virginity at marriage, women's vulnerability to disadvantage and violence, sometimes approaching a lethal level, on proof or just suspicion of premarital loss of virginity, and their liability to involuntary examination for 'proof' of their maintenance or loss of virginity.[5] Social action must be directed towards equality of the sexes and release of women's sexuality from social, communal, and parental oppression. This is not to argue for sexual licentiousness or licence, but only for women's relief from expectations of sexual virtue that are measured by unscientific and socially unrealistic standards to which men are not subject.

Cultures in which 'honour killings' of young women suspected of unchastity are allowed or only lightly punished, committed by brothers or parents, illustrate one end of the spectrum of oppression from which women require protection and relief by social action. Less lethal but equally unjust is a woman's loss of prospects of marriage and social status within her community on evidence that she has been victimized by rape. Similarly oppressive is the

---

[5] M. W. Frank, H. M. Bauer, N. Arican, S. K. Fincanci, and V. Iacopino, 'Virgin Examinations in Turkey', *Journal of the American Medical Association*, 282 (1999), 485–90.

requirement of public demonstration of blood on the sheet of her marriage bed, not least since medical evidence shows that women do not invariably bleed on their first sexual intercourse. Physicians should collaborate in, and instigate, social education to overcome ill-informed conventional beliefs of this nature, to promote sexual equality on eligibility for marriage, and for communal esteem of women not dependent on different criteria than affect men.

6

A Request for Medically Assisted Reproduction

Case Study

Mr and Mrs F have been married for ten years and have no children. Medical investigation showed that the husband is subfertile, with no motile sperm production by the testes. They are happy in their marital relationship, but Mrs F is keen to have a child of her own. They have ruled out the choice of adoption, and are considering resort to an artificial insemination donor. However, they worry about the right of the child to have a 'natural' father (that is, the wife's husband), or not to know its biological father. They ask Dr R for advice and possible assistance in arranging artificial insemination by donor. What should Dr R advise and assist, in light of relevant medical, ethical, legal, and human rights considerations?

1. Background

Infertility may result from disease, but is not necessarily a disease. In fact, in many cases of infertility, no evidence of any disease may be found. Infertility *per se* does not threaten life or endanger physical health. However, we define health as more than physical capacity. Health, as defined in the constitution of the World Health Organization, is not merely the absence of disease or infirmity, but a state of complete physical, mental, and social well-being. Patients do perceive the suffering from infertility as very real, and as compromising their health.

To some people, it may seem odd that we talk about infertility as a public health problem when the world urgently needs capacity for self-control of fertility. With the population problem at hand, is it appropriate that we continue to worry about the problem of infertility? The answer is that we should worry even more. The adoption of a small family norm, through voluntary infertility, which is a desired target at country and at global levels, makes the issue of involuntary infertility more pressing. If couples are urged to postpone and to widely space pregnancies, it is imperative that they should be helped to achieve a pregnancy when they so decide, in the more limited time they have available.

Definitions of infertility widely vary; some measures are based on failure to conceive after twelve months of contraceptively unprotected intercourse, while others are based on twenty-four months of failure to conceive. A general estimate is that between 8 and 12 per cent of couples experience some form of involuntary infertility during their reproductive lives. When extrapolated to the global population, this means that 50 to 80 million people may be suffering from some infertility problem.[1]

There would probably always be a certain percentage of couples who would be infertile, because of reasons we cannot prevent, we cannot treat, or we do not know. This is what is referred to as core infertility, the percentage of which is probably not more than 5 per cent, and could be much less. A prevalence of infertility higher than that is considered as acquired infertility, which generally indicates that there are causes in the community for adding a new layer of infertile couples. In certain parts of sub-Saharan Africa, the prevalence of infertility may be as high as 30 per cent or more.[2] The most important cause of acquired infertility is pelvic infection as a result of sexually transmitted diseases (such as chlamydia or gonorrhea), unsafe abortion, or puerperal (after delivery) infection.

2. *Medical Aspects*

New advances in reproductive technologies have opened new frontiers in medically assisted reproduction, where one of the four main requisites for conception (sperm, ovum, meeting of ovum and sperm, and implantation) is *completely* missing.[3] For such cases, the prognosis was previously almost hopeless.

- *Sperm.* The oldest technique of medically-assisted conception is artificial insemination by husband or artificial insemination by donor.
- *Meeting the ovum and sperm.* In the late 1970s the technique of human *in vitro* fertilization (IVF) had its first success. This involves three basic steps: picking up mature ova from the ovary, fertilization with the sperm in a culture medium outside the body, and embryo transfer to the uterus.
- *Ovum.* Ovum donation can allow a woman who does not ovulate to get pregnant. Even a post-menopausal woman can now be helped to get

---

[1] WHO, *Infertility: A Tabulation of Available Data on Prevalence of Primary and Secondary Infertility* (Geneva: WHO, 1991), WHO/MCH/91.9, at 2.
[2] M. F. Fathalla, *From Obstetrics and Gynecology to Women's Health: The Road Ahead* (New York and London: Parthenon, 1997), 49–60.
[3] Ibid.

pregnant. The woman will be the biological mother but not the genetic mother.
- *Implantation.* A surrogate mother can carry the fertilized ovum of another woman.

By medically assisted reproduction (MAR), it is now possible for a child to have up to five parents: a genetic father, a rearing father, a genetic mother, a gestating mother, and a rearing mother. There are concerns about the nature of medical practice, since the demarcation between experimental and established procedures is not always clear. The quality assurance of services in many countries leaves something to be desired. Cost is a major consideration, but additional concerns are about future research, and the potential for abuse for instance in embryo selection.

Modern practice is that fresh sperm not be used except when a husband is to be the father. Third-party donors have HIV tests, and their donations are frozen. If they test negative, they are retested six or more months later and, if they still test negative, the donation given earlier may be thawed and used in MAR. Ovum freezing and thawing are more challenging, but an embryo created from untested gametes may be frozen, and thawed after the gamete donors are shown to have been HIV negative at donation.

Among practical concerns raised by IVF which have ethical and legal implications are disposal of surplus embryos created *in vitro* that prove unnecessary or unsuitable for a couple's reproductive requirements, implantation of several embryos that results in high, multiple pregnancy, and creation of the same result by natural conception following medically induced superovulation, and the option of so-called 'selective reduction' to reduce multiple pregnancy. Multiple pregnancy involves health care of mothers, foetuses *in utero*, and newborn children, possibly born prematurely with low birth weight and risk of associated complications.

The issue of multi-foetal pregnancy reduction, and in some countries of disposal of surplus embryos *in vitro* or in cryopreservation, raises questions of how local abortion law is worded and applied. The challenge is to consider multi-foetal pregnancy reduction not as abortion *per se*, which ends pregnancy, but as a means of preserving pregnancy against the danger of spontaneous abortion of all embryos or foetuses *in utero*.[4]

3. *Ethical Aspects*

Ethical issues raised by MAR have been considered so profound that several countries, particularly those where the more advanced reproductive

---

[4] B. M. Dickens and R. J. Cook, 'Some Ethical and Legal Issues in Assisted Reproductive Technology', *Int. J. Gynecol. Obstet.* 66 (1999), 55–61.

technologies are applied, have created national commissions to address them and propose legal regulatory and other responses. The International Federation of Gynecology and Obstetrics (FIGO) Committee for Ethical Aspects of Human Reproduction and Women's Health has made statements and recommendations, notably on Ethical Guidelines on the Sale of Gametes and Embryos (1996), Donation of Genetic Material for Human Reproduction (1994), and Ethical Aspects of Gamete Donation from Known Donors (Directed Donations) (2000).

Procedures collectively referred to as medically assisted reproduction range from simple artificial insemination, by husband or donor, to technologically sophisticated intra-cytoplasmic sperm injection (ICSI) and surrogate motherhood. In many countries, indeed, attention to ethical implications of advanced reproductive technologies vastly overwhelms attention to ethical issues of natural reproduction, safe motherhood, and prevention of infertility. National and other public commissions tend in general to address MAR at the macroethical rather than the microethical level, considering the impact for instance of gamete and embryo transfer and surrogate motherhood in terms of social policy rather than of overcoming childlessness in particular patients. With regard to children produced by MAR technologies, however, commissions often come to the microethical level to consider the experience of children who are the genetic offspring of only one, or neither, of their social parents.

Approaches to availability of MAR based on assessment of 'the best interests of the child' are confounded by the consideration that prohibiting availability of MAR results in such children not being born. This raises the ethical concern of whether it can be in the best interests of particular children that they not be conceived. It may be considered to be in the interests of particular societies that children not be conceived by certain methods of MAR, but the claim that it is in particular children's interests not to be conceived and born is often resisted, for instance, on the ethical principle of beneficence, that it is better to be born than not to be.[5] This principle is often relied upon by opponents of choice of abortion. The issue exposes ethical conflicts of interest, such as between perceived macroethical interests of societies and of future children, and microethical interests of women to have the children they want and of children to be reared by or at least to know both of their biological parents.

Infertility raises different ethical implications in different societies, although it is more uniformly a source of emotional distress to people who want to be parents. In some societies, male-factor infertility in a couple is denied, and women bear blame for not conceiving their husband's children, at times to the point of their divorce, shame, and destitution. Ethical duties of respect for

---

[5] J. Harris, 'Rights and Reproductive Choice', in J. Harris and S. Holm (eds.), *The Future of Human Reproduction: Ethics, Choice and Regulation* (Oxford: Clarendon Press, 1998), 5–37.

individuals' reproductive autonomy and of beneficence, which support med- ically assisted reproduction, are limited in societies where third-party sperm donation is unacceptable, and considered as adultery. In the Islamic world, for instance, couples are encouraged to have the children they can support, but the integrity of family lineage is an important value, and third-party sperm donation is unacceptable. [6]

Where sperm donation is acceptable, ethical concerns include medical and social criteria of eligibility to donate, requirements of anonymity to recipients or allowance of designated donors, and subsequent identification of donors to their biological children. Donation should be altruistic rather than for profit, although costs of donation are recoverable, including both HIV tests. The number of uses of an individual donation should be limited to reduce the risk of different children of the same donor meeting and unknowingly considering marriage. Donation records should be kept so that resulting children's genetic heritage can be known, but, unless laws provide otherwise, donors and chil- dren should become identifiable to each other only with mutual consent. In rare cases, directed donation is acceptable.

4. *Legal Aspects*

Central legal issues in MAR are the consent of both members of an infertile couple, consent of gamete or embryo donors, and the legal status of a resulting child. A husband's consent to his wife's insemination by donor is usually required, in order that any legal presumption of his fatherhood be maintained. His objection would render the child not his legal responsibility, and he may disclaim paternity if the wife is serving as a surrogate mother to another man's child. Sperm or ovum donors must consent for lawful donation, but recovery of sperm from unconscious and recently deceased men raises concerns where not legally prohibited, such as how consent should be evidenced. [7] Legal ques- tions that are also unresolved in many countries arise when donation of a couple's cryopreserved embryo is possible, but only one member of the couple consents.

Laws differ on the status of children born by gamete and embryo donation. Where laws focus on children's welfare and avoidance of the stigma of illegiti- macy, strong presumptions are that children born during marriage, or within some generous time after it ends by the husband's death or divorce, such as

---

[6] G. I. Serour and B. M. Dickens, 'Assisted Reproduction Developments in the Islamic World', *Int. J. Gynecol. Obstet.* 74 (2001), 187–93.

[7] *R. v. Human Fertilisation and Embryology Authority, ex p. Blood*, [1997] 2 All ER 687 (Court of Appeal, England).

300 days, are the husband's legitimate children, unless he actively denies this. Similarly, where women gestate and deliver children, the children are presumed to be theirs, even if ovum or embryo donation occurred. In partial surrogate motherhood, where women are inseminated, usually artificially, with men's sperm and gestate their own fertilized ova for surrender of children to the men and their wives, the surrogates are the true biological mothers. Where full surrogate motherhood is involved, however, meaning that a woman gestates another woman's ovum that was fertilized *in vitro* and transferred to her for gestation, some legal systems will apply a test of genetic parenthood and recognize the ovum donor as the legal mother of the child. Where legal systems focus on integrity of the male genetic line for purposes of legitimacy and inheritance, sperm donation is unacceptable as constituting adultery. A husband presenting another man's child as his own, particularly a son, may face claims of misrepresentation and fraud against society, unless he can initiate some legally available procedure of legitimation or adoption.

Physicians and their associates must observe local laws regarding, for instance, medical consent and confidentiality in general, and medical assistance in reproduction in particular. More specific laws may concern such matters as spousal consent, gamete acquisition and donation, and disclosure among themselves of identities of different participants. In addition, medical licensing authorities and professional associations may adopt practices that practitioners are required to observe, such as on age limits beyond which motherhood should not be assisted, and limiting numbers of *in vitro* fertilized embryos that may be placed *in utero* in a single treatment cycle. Disregard of such practice guidelines may attract legally enforceable professional disciplinary sanctions.

The law on medical negligence applies to health assessments of women for pregnancy and to the screening of sperm donors regarding their genetic health and freedom from STDs, including HIV infection. It may also apply where physicians undertake to select donors of specific ethnic origins or body build and complexion, such as to match women's husbands. In addition, requirements of competent record keeping and identification of preserved gametes and embryos are expected to be met. Where advanced techniques of gamete or embryo screening are available, such as preimplantation genetic diagnosis, practitioners are obliged to discuss them with patients unless these procedures are obviously beyond patients' financial means. Damages awarded on birth of a disabled child may be substantial, but may be more modest when healthy but ethnically or otherwise mismatched children are born. In addition to their legal accountability to patients, practitioners are legally accountable to professional licensing bodies and medical associations for incompetent and unethical practice, such as deceptively inseminating patients with their own or otherwise unapproved sperm.

5. *Human Rights Aspects*

Some opponents of human reproductive technologies equate them with practices pioneered in veterinary medicine, and claim that they offend collective
rights to human dignity. Some international documents opposing reproductive cloning invoke the same concept. As against this, however, the right under
the International Covenant on Economic, Social and Cultural Rights (the
Economic Covenant) to the benefits of scientific progress supports resort to
new reproductive technologies. The general right to found a family, recognized
in many national constitutions and in many of the leading human rights conventions, supports medical assistance to prevent and to overcome effects of
infertility, whether or not scientific technology is applied. The right to private
and family life may show that enactment of intrusive legislation to prohibit or
monitor MAR on moral grounds is a human rights violation. Reinforcing
these human rights of resort to MAR is the right to the highest attainable standard of health. Health has physical, mental, and social dimensions, and infertility
among those who want children diminishes their mental and social well-being,
and may have physical health repercussions. The objection that many techniques of MAR do not cure medical infertility is correct, but they may overcome involuntary childlessness, and so serve human rights to health services.

Human rights claims indirectly relevant to MAR include the right to receive
and impart information. This right may be offended by laws or practices to
prohibit publicity of where MAR services may be obtained, including in other
countries, and also by laws that require or support confidentiality of gamete
donors' or recipients' identities. Children of gamete donors have a right to
information of donors' genetic characteristics, and they may seek to compel
disclosure of records of their biological parents' identities. A limit may be that,
while this right may require disclosure of an available record, it may not require
that information of a donor's personal identity initially be recorded. Similarly,
it may not require a possible donor to submit to involuntary DNA testing to
show genetic parenthood. Donors' rights to physical integrity protect them
against forced donation of samples for DNA testing. However, their rights to
private life may not prevail over children's rights to receive information so as
to prevent DNA testing of donors' samples legally acquired for other purposes.

Because couples seeking recourse to MAR are unable to conceive in the
course of nature, or want to avoid the risk of naturally conceiving a child of
their own that would be genetically compromised by use instead of third-party
gamete or embryo donation, they may claim a reproductive health disability,
and the human right not to suffer discrimination on that basis. Since married
couples are not subject to public monitoring or regulation in their natural
conception of children, a reproductively disabled couple may claim that any

burdens imposed upon their use of MAR, such as that they must satisfy criteria applied to select adoptive parents, amount to discrimination, and violate human rights. Their claim to reproduce as freely as non-disabled couples may, however, have a negative aspect for them. Couples who conceive in the course of nature may receive state-funded services in gestation and delivery, but may receive little if any state support for purposes of conception.

Publicly funded health care may entitle all women to routine gynaecological examinations and infertility preventive care, and women in reproductively impaired marriages will enjoy this same right. No state funding supports natural conception, however, and states may accordingly decline funding of MAR, since this would not deny services to women in infertile relationships that are available to women in fertile relationships. Recognition that non-funding of MAR does not discriminate against reproductively compromised couples indicates that human rights of access to MAR are only negative rights. Couples may claim unimpaired access to MAR services they can afford, but not require that the state provide them with access to services, which, like cosmetic medicine, fall into a category of 'luxury medicine'.[8]

6. *Approaches*

6.1. *Clinical duty*

Even if Mr and Mrs F came to request advice and assistance together, Dr R should consult with them separately to ensure that they freely share the same desire for donor insemination of Mrs F, and are not yielding to undue pressure or threat from the other. Dr R may also review whether they want to pursue any available options by which Mrs F may attempt to conceive Mr F's own child, such as ICSI. If local custom prohibits donor insemination, and in law it is considered to be adultery, Mr and Mrs F should be asked how they react to this, and to implications for legitimacy of the child. Similarly, Dr R should disclose any personal conscientious objections the doctor has to undertaking the procedure, and whether clinic colleagues will object to collaboration. Dr R should counsel Mrs F regarding possibilities and risks of multiple pregnancy, and options for management should it occur naturally or as a result of treatment to promote her fertility. Particular care should be given if Mrs F is approaching menopause.

If these matters are satisfactorily resolved, Dr R may seek to identify and approach a suitable sperm donor, or seek an appropriate sample from an accessible sperm bank. Issues of the donor's comparable ethnicity and

---

[8] *Cameron v. Nova Scotia (Attorney General)* (1999), 177 DLR (4th) 513 (Nova Scotia Court of Appeal, Canada).

matching of Mr F's colouring and stature may be relevant, in addition to ensuring the donor's genetic and other material characteristics, and of course his consent. A further factor may be a prospective donor's willingness to be identified to a child that biologically he fathered, subject to any local law that prohibits or compels disclosure of his identity. Dr R should preserve genetic and other information of the donor, in case it is relevant to the well-being or treatment of a subsequently conceived child.

If Dr R attends the birth of a child, no false information may be offered for purposes of birth registration, but local law will often permit Mr F to be registered as the father, unless he objects, where legal presumptions favour a child's legitimacy. Dr R cannot insist that Mrs F remain in the doctor's care throughout pregnancy, since a woman assisted to conceive may prefer to present herself to her general medical practitioner simply as a married, pregnant patient. However, Dr R should share information about Mrs F with the general practitioner, unless Mrs F explicitly refuses consent, and provide as much accurate information as is necessary for care of the child to be born.

6.2. *Health care systems obligations*

A primary goal of reproductive health care is prevention, rather than the cure or overcoming, of infertility. Accordingly, the origin of Mr F's reproductive impairment warrants study, and assistance to Mrs F should not compromise availability of resources needed to diagnose Mr F's condition.

Dr R should consider how accessible patients like Mrs F find MAR services to be, and how equitably they are available at local, regional, and national levels. The standard of services should also be addressed, with regard to screening of gamete donors, proficiency of services, skills of specialist and support personnel, the standard and maintenance of equipment including for preservation of gametes and embryos, and, for instance, accuracy and adequacy of data. Information of treatment outcomes for different procedures should be available, including of monozygotic and other multiple pregnancies and how they are managed. Information should also be available on cost-effectiveness of different treatment options, and of waiting lists in different centres. Dr R should be aware of the emotional as well as the financial costs of treatment, and consider how, for instance through counselling and Mrs F's involvement in an infertility support group, the emotional burden can be relieved.

As recommended by a WHO Scientific Group, respect for the principle of the quality of services requires:

- the initiation and promotion of professional self-regulation early in the development of new techniques so as to contribute to the development of a national policy;
- the integration of the procedure into the health care system;

- the auditing and accreditation of such services in order to ensure that they are of the necessary quality and that proper records are kept;
- the availability of the procedure to the population requiring such services;
- the education of both health workers and the general population in the techniques and role of MAR in the treatment of infertility;
- the promotion of international exchange of data.[9]

6.3. *Social action for underlying conditions*

Dr R should contribute to infertility prevention by seeking an understanding of the origin of Mr F's condition, such as due to disease, inheritance, occupational or environmental causes. Infertility in women may similarly be due to sexually transmitted infections, and to infections after labour or unsafe abortion.

On behalf of the profession, Dr R should publicize experiences in order to improve the law by exposing legal provisions that perpetuate sources of infertility, obstruct preventive efforts, or deny treatments to infertile patients. Dr R should also participate in professional activities aimed to improve standards of scientific and sensitively sympathetic care, and support laws and professional codes of conduct to advance the practice of MAR. Similarly, Dr R should contribute to professional and public debate, and consult with governmental and non-governmental agencies, to improve attitudes to infertile patients, and public confidence in the integrity of MAR practices and practitioners.

---

[9] WHO, *Recent Advances in Medically-Assisted Conception: Report of a WHO Scientific Group. WHO Technical Report Series 820* (Geneva: WHO, 1992).

7

Involuntary Female Sterilization

Case Study

Dr T is employed in a government-run hospital that treats an impoverished community. Dr T has grown up in that community, is dedicated
to its welfare, and intends a career in advancing the hospital's capacity
to care for local residents. There is concern in the country about the
high rate of population growth. The community in which Dr T is practising has a high birth rate, and the health care system is under pressure
from the government to increase contraceptive use and to decrease
fertility. The board of the hospital is proposing to introduce a hospital
regulation that any women who have four or more children can have
hospital delivery free of charge only if they agree to be sterilized after
delivery. How should Dr T respond, given relevant medical, ethical,
legal, and human rights factors?

1. Background

It is legitimate for a country to be concerned about population growth and its
impact on socio-economic development. But measures taken to influence the
number of a woman's pregnancies, whether for an increase or decrease, fall in
a wide spectrum, from the desirable to the acceptable to the objectionable.
Provision of family planning services, including education and information on
voluntary sterilization,[1] is a desirable social measure on its own. Maternity or
paternity benefits and family allowances, as measures intended to increase fertility, can also be considered desirable social policies on their own. Promotion
of public awareness of such social policies is acceptable, whether it is intended
to decrease or increase fertility. It is, however, at the borderline, as it can easily
slip into the objectionable if it results in undue psychological pressure on

---

[1] C. A. Church and J. S. Geller, 'Voluntary Female Sterilization: Number One and Growing',
Population Reports, C10 (1990), 1–23. J. A. Ross, 'Sterilization: Past, Present and Future', *Studies
in Family Planning*, 23 (1992), 187–98. EngenderHealth, *Voluntary Sterilization: Policies and
Perspectives* (New York: EngenderHealth, 1999).

individuals. In the category of the objectionable are incentives/disincentives/ coercion to decrease fertility, and restriction of access to family planning/abortion to increase fertility. Such strong-handed measures can impact adversely on the health of women, and are equally objectionable whether meant to decrease or increase a woman's fertility.

As far as the health of women is concerned, there is little to choose between *coerced contraception, sterilization,* or *abortion,* because society does not want the child, and *coerced motherhood,* because society wants the child. Both interventions deny women the dignity of making a choice in their reproductive lives.

The Programme of Action of the International Conference on Population and Development, Cairo, 1994, emphasized that: 'The aim of family-planning programs must be to enable couples and individuals to decide freely and responsibly the number and spacing of their children and to have the information and means to do so and to ensure informed choices and make available a full range of safe and effective methods', and that 'demographic goals, while legitimately the subject of government development strategies, should not be imposed on family-planning providers in the form of targets or quotas for the recruitment of clients'.[2] Female contraceptives are meant to empower women, to maximize their choices, and to give them control over their fertility, and thus their lives. The convenience of long-acting and permanent methods is welcomed by many women. These methods, however, can be used and have been used by governments and others to control rather than to empower women.

2. *Medical Aspects*

Female sterilization is a safe, simple, and very effective surgical procedure. It can usually be done under local anaesthesia and light sedation. Post-partum sterilization is done by minilaparotomy (a small abdominal incision).

Surgery to reverse sterilization is possible only for some women. The procedure is difficult, expensive, not widely available, and has a low success rate. When pregnancy occurs, there is an increased risk of ectopic pregnancy that is a life-threatening condition. Medically assisted reproduction remains a possibility, but procedures are neither generally available nor generally affordable, and success rates are not high. Sterilization, therefore, should be considered permanent.

---

[2] United Nations, *Population and Development,* i. *Programme of Action Adopted at the International Conference on Population and Development, Cairo, 5–13 September 1994* (New York: UN, Department for Economic and Social Information and Policy Analysis, ST/ESA/SER.A/149, 1994), para. 7.12.

Because female sterilization is permanent, the decision made by the woman should be based on voluntary informed choice and should not be made under stress or duress. Other methods of contraception should be explained and offered, to allow the woman to make a choice. The intra-uterine device is a good alternative for women who want long-term contraception, but are not sure that they will not want another child in the future. Modern intra-uterine devices are very effective and provide protection against unwanted pregnancy for up to ten years or more.

3. *Ethical Aspects*

Adherents to many religious and other duty-based ethical orientations consider voluntary sterilization to be morally unacceptable. Their objections of principle should be taken into consideration. A hospital board may claim that its policy does not compel sterilization, but only requires women with four or more children to pay for delivery at the hospital. This claim can be countered by pointing to the proposed policy's unethical discrimination against poor families, and against women whose religious convictions make sterilization wrongful for them. These arguments reinforce such a policy's violation of the ethical duties of respect for autonomy, beneficence, non-maleficence, and justice.

A policy of this nature will deny the only childbirth care to which poor women have access, aggravating problems of maternal mortality and morbidity, and of the related deaths and disadvantages of orphaned children. This utilitarian argument against such a proposed policy can be reinforced by the claim that a hospital publicly funded as a gesture of social solidarity should not be divisive in discriminating against poor families. An additional argument against the proposed policy is that women whose pregnancies are likely to be of greater risk due to their relatively high parity should not be offered care only on unacceptable conditions, and so be compelled to seek care from unqualified attendants, including those whose treatments include unsafe procedures.

The International Federation of Gynecology and Obstetrics (FIGO) Committee for the Ethical Aspects of Human Reproduction and Women's Health, in outlining ethical considerations in sterilization, stated in 2000 that 'no incentives should be given or coercion applied to promote or discourage any particular decision regarding sterilization. In particular, withholding other medical care by linking it to sterilization is unacceptable.'[3]

---

[3] FIGO Committee for the Ethical Aspects of Human Reproduction and Women's Health, 'Ethical Considerations in Sterilization', in *Recommendations on Ethical Issues in Obstetrics and Gynecology* (London: FIGO, 2000), para. 7 at 53. Available at website: http://www.figo.org/default.asp?id=6097, last accessed 2 May 2002.

4. *Legal Aspects*

The proposed policy is designed to deny unpaid services to women who belong to an impoverished community, some of whom may have religious objections to acceptance of sterilization the policy is intended to induce them to have. The policy amounts to discrimination on the grounds of poverty or religion, which might render the policy void on constitutional or other legal grounds that prohibit discrimination of this nature.

In the field of more private law, women who receive free services do not usually obtain them on a contractual basis, and are not then legally bound by any agreements they make as a condition of receiving them. Even if a contract exists, refusal of post-partum sterilization renders its imposition a serious criminal assault and a civil (i.e. non-criminal) battery by any doctor who performs it, and by the hospital itself. A woman's repudiation of a contractual agreement to be sterilized may be compensable, notably by requiring her to pay for services rendered without charge in exchange for her agreement, but legal proceedings for compensation brought against an impoverished woman would be futile. Any agreement a woman would make under this proposed policy would be unenforceable either by imposition of a sterilization procedure, or by attempted enforcement through the hospital's suit for compensation. Even a case initiated primarily to make a public example might additionally demonstrate its unenforceability. Courts often refuse to allow claims by more powerful parties based on an unconscionable agreement, and a court might declare any woman's promise and the proposed policy void due to a woman's dependency on the hospital's care and powerlessness to resist the oppressive condition of sterilization.

Hospitals do not have legal duties of medical care to persons they decline to admit as patients, but publicly funded hospitals are often legally obliged to admit indigent patients who live in their catchment areas. Once patients are admitted, they are protected by laws that prohibit their abandonment. They may be involuntarily discharged for persistent non-compliance with a treatment regimen, but cannot be discharged for refusal of conditions unrelated to their care. Sterilization is unrelated to delivery. Therefore, the hospital may be legally obliged to admit indigent pregnant women of the area as patients for delivery, and be unable to discharge them for refusing to be sterilized at or after delivery.

The board may have wide administrative powers under hospital by-laws, but courts will not allow such powers to subvert a central purpose for which the hospital exists, namely to provide necessary care without charge to those who require health services. The proposed policy may therefore be challenged on grounds of administrative law, as an abuse of board powers. The proposed by-law can be claimed as void as against public policy, since it would require doctors to perform invasive non-therapeutic procedures to which the patients did not freely consent, constituting criminal assaults and civil batteries. The board and by-laws cannot authorize violations of patients' protections under criminal or civil law.

5. *Human Rights Aspects*

The argument on behalf of the hospital board that the proposed policy does not compel sterilization, but only requires that women with four or more children pay for services can be dismissed as unconvincing, because the women in question lack means of payment. The policy would effectively deny delivery of care to women whose relatively high parity makes their pregnancies of higher risk, and therefore deny them their right to security of the person. Denying women the only skilled care to which they have practical access also constitutes inhuman and degrading treatment, even amounting to denial of their right to life or to the highest attainable standard of health. Among women who would accept such a policy of sterilization, there would be compromise of their right to decide on the number of their children and more broadly their right to private and family life. Accordingly, the policy can be shown to constitute a denial of many of the rights that cumulatively were recognized by the UN Cairo and Beijing conferences as necessary to protect reproductive health.

A number of professional agencies have proposed formulae for the appropriate offering of sterilization services sensitive to human rights.[4] In the UK, for instance, the Royal College of Obstetricians and Gynaecologists has issued good medical practice guidelines for contraceptive sterilization, applicable to both sexes. These provide that

there are no absolute contra-indications to sterilisation of men or women provided they make the request themselves, are of sound mind and are not acting under external duress. As a precaution against the risk of later regret, additional care must be taken when counseling those under the age of 25 or those without children. Care should also be exercised in discussions with those taking decisions during pregnancy, or in reaction to a loss of relationship, or who may be at risk of coercion by their partner or family or health or social welfare professionals . . . Counselors and advisers should also be aware and take account of cultural, religious, psychosocial, psychosexual and other psychological issues, some of which may have implications beyond fertility . . . [P]rior sanction by a high court judge should be sought in all cases of sterilisation where there is doubt over mental capacity to consent.[5]

⁴ R. J. Cook and B. M. Dickens, 'Voluntary and Involuntary Sterilization: Denials and Abuses of Rights', *Int. J. Gynecol. Obstet.* 68 (2000), 61–7.
⁵ 26 Oct. 1999, http://www.rcog.org.uk/guidelines.asp?PageID=108&GuidelineID=30, last accessed 6 May 2002.

The Committee on Ethics of the American College of Obstetricians and Gynecologists (ACOG) issued a Committee Opinion that: 'The physician's values, sense of societal goals, and racial, ethnic, or socioeconomic issues should not be the basis of a recommendation to undergo sterilization.'[6] Where resort to judicial authorization is not feasible, for economic or other reasons, practitioners may respect the human rights of person of questionable mental capacity to consent, by consultation with independent persons who know them and appear respectful of their interests, integrity, and dignity.

6. *Approaches*

6.1. *Clinical duty*

Dr T should make clear to the hospital board that, on ethical and legal grounds, including physicians' and patients' human rights, the proposed policy cannot be implemented at the clinical level. Dr T and colleagues can invoke their ethical duty of respect for patients' autonomy not to require pregnant women unable to pay for their services to agree in advance to sterilization as a condition of receiving free care. They could also use the same autonomy principle to explain why they will not undertake post-partum sterilization on women who have received free services if the women do not voluntarily agree at the time of delivery or later.

Further, any board attempt at implementation by disciplinary action against non-compliant physicians or other hospital staff for their refusal to enforce a discriminatory by-law would constitute a violation of national and international human rights law, for which the hospital, government, and country would bear legal liability and suffer international condemnation. While condemning this approach, Dr T and colleagues should continue to promote family planning services in the community, made available on the basis of recipients' freely made and informed choice.

6.2. *Health care systems obligations*

Dr T could collaborate with health care professional colleagues and associations to oppose any discriminatory and punitive policy that would condemn impoverished women to forgo the only safe delivery services to which they have access, or else to receive care conditioned on coerced acceptance of an

---

[6] ACOG Committee on Ethics, 'Sterilization of Women, Including Those with Mental Disabilities. Committee Opinion 216, April 1999', in ACOG, *Ethics in Obstetrics and Gynecology* (Washington, DC: ACOG, 2002), 92–5; repr. in *Int. J. Gynecol. Obstet.* 65 (1999), 317–20.

irreversible procedure not indicated on therapeutic grounds. The board's intention to restrain the high birth rate in the community is not necessarily misguided, but its oppressive means are. The concept that reproductive discipline can be imposed from above on unempowered populations is offensive to the egalitarian and democratic spirit. Further, the board's proposal to control use of hospital services and the local fertility rate by economic sanctions is inappropriate for such necessary services as delivery care. It reflects a market-driven philosophy that equates health care services with commercial services and elective consumerism, but this is inconsistent with the operation of a publicly funded hospital that provides necessary care for recipients lacking personal means of purchase. The board should be encouraged and facilitated to advance its purposes through legitimate inducements rather than illegitimate sanctions, and to apply a philosophy in harmony rather than in conflict with the community the hospital serves, including consultation with community members perhaps through their freely chosen leaders.

Alternative means could be proposed to the board by which an intention to reduce high parity rates in the community could be advanced consistently with patients' free choice. Broadening contraceptive choices and improving the access and quality of contraceptive services will increase the acceptance and continuation of contraceptive use.

6.3. *Social action for underlying conditions*

Dr T, as a responsible citizen, should join non-governmental organizations, active in the community, to advocate for social action to address the underlying conditions for high fertility, rather than try to deal with it with heavy-handed coercive measures. Among these underlying conditions, the most important is the status of women. Girls' education and empowerment of women are desirable social goals on their own, and are associated with low fertility. Women have more at stake in fertility control than anyone else. Governments would be short-sighted not to see that when women are given a real choice, and the information and means to implement their choice, they will make the most rational decision for themselves, for their communities, and ultimately for the world at large. Members of the health profession should stand beside women and behind women in their struggle to protect their human rights and due status in their communities.

The FIGO Committee for the Ethical Aspects of Human Reproduction and Women's Health, in a 1999 statement on the role of obstetricians/gynaecologists as advocates for women's health, advocated that the profession 'promote a wide debate in order to influence health practices and legislation favorable to women's reproductive health'. It observes that

[t]he debate should include a broad spectrum of society, such as other medical associations, women's organizations, legislators, educators, lawyers, social scientists and theologians. In addition, obstetrician-gynecologists are obligated to organise themselves and other professional groups to ensure that essential health services are available for disadvantaged and underprivileged women.[7]

In this spirit, Dr T should find support to oppose the proposed policy and urge its replacement by a policy agreeable to the women the hospital aims to serve.

---

[7] See FIGO Committee, 'Ethical Considerations', 'The Role of the Ob/Gyn as Advocates for Women's Health', London 1999, para. 6, in *Recommendations on Ethical Issues in Obstetrics and Gynecology* (London: FIGO, 2000) at 7. Available at website: http://www.figo.org/default.asp?id=6087, last accessed 2 May 2002.

8

Counselling and Caring for an HIV-Positive Woman

Case Study

Dr GH finds that a clinic patient, Mrs JK, who is eight weeks pregnant, tested HIV positive. Her husband also tested positive. The pregnancy is Mrs JK's first. She asks Dr GH about the risk to herself and her child, because she wants the pregnancy to continue, and whether she can have treatment that will protect the child before birth. What medical, ethical, legal, and human rights considerations should guide Dr GH's response?

1. *Background*

Twenty years after the first clinical evidence of acquired immunodeficiency syndrome was reported, AIDS has become the most devastating disease humankind has ever faced. Since the epidemic began, more than 60 million people have been infected with the virus. HIV/AIDS is now the leading cause of death in sub-Saharan Africa. Worldwide, it is the fourth-biggest killer. At the end of 2001, an estimated 40 million people globally were living with HIV. In many parts of the developing world, the majority of new infections occurs in young adults, with young women especially vulnerable. About one-third of those currently living with HIV/AIDS are aged 15–24. Most of them do not know they carry the virus. Many millions more know nothing or too little about HIV to protect themselves against it.[1]

   HIV infections are concentrated in the developing world, mostly in countries least able to afford to care for infected people. Of the 40 million estimated to be living with HIV/AIDS as at the end of 2001, 28.1 million are in sub-Saharan Africa and 6.1 million are in South-East Asia (see Table III.1.1 for country data on prevalence of HIV/AIDS among pregnant women).

---

[1] UNAIDS, *AIDS Epidemic Update: December 2001* (Geneva: UNAIDS, 2001), UNAIDS/01.74E-WHO/CDS/CSR/NCS/2001.2, at 1–2.

2. *Medical Aspects*

No established guidelines exist for defining access to fertility care for individuals infected with HIV. However, UNAIDS and the World Health Organization published a review of what is known about HIV in pregnancy, providing suggestions on the appropriate management of HIV-positive women during pregnancy, delivery, and post-partum care, breastfeeding and infection control and safe working conditions with regard to HIV in pregnancy.[2] The United States Centers for Disease Control have issued Revised Recommendations for HIV Screening of Pregnant Women.[3]

The WHO report explains that most studies show that pregnancy does not have a major adverse effect on the evolution of HIV. However, a number of African studies have reported adverse pregnancy outcomes for HIV-infected women, and studies from some Central African countries show AIDS has become a leading cause of maternal mortality.[4]

A primary concern for this patient is her life expectancy and the risk of viral transmission to the offspring. Depending on Mrs JK's nutritional status and concurrent infections, pre-term delivery and low birth weight might be factors for consideration. Combination anti-retroviral therapy has produced radical improvements in life expectancy and quality of life for both children and adults infected with HIV in developed countries.[5] Current estimates suggest that a disease previously associated with certain death is compatible with a life expectancy of at least twenty years from time of diagnosis, if one has access to anti-retroviral therapy.

In the overwhelming majority of cases, children acquire the HIV infection from their mothers before or around the time of birth, or through breast milk. An equally great majority lives in the developing world. The gap between rich and poor countries in terms of transmission of HIV from mother to child has been growing. In France and the USA, for instance, fewer than 5 per cent of children born to HIV-positive women in 1997 were infected with the virus.[6] In developing countries, the average was between 25 and 35 per cent. Judicious use of combination anti-retroviral therapy during pregnancy and labour,

[2] J. McIntyre and P. Brocklehurst, *HIV in Pregnancy: A Review* (Geneva: UNAIDS and WHO, 1999), WHO/CHS/RHR/99.15; UNAIDS/99.35E.

[3] Centers for Disease Control and Prevention, 'Revised Guidelines for HIV Counselling, Testing, and Referral and Revised Recommendations for HIV Screening of Pregnant Women', *Morbidity and Mortality Weekly Report*, 50 (2001), No. RR-19, 1–85. Also available at www.cdc.gov/hiv/ctr, last accessed 6 May 2002.

[4] McIntyre and Brocklehurst, *HIV in Pregnancy*, 7.

[5] D. H. Watts and R. C. Brunham, 'Sexually Transmitted Diseases, Including HIV Infection in Pregnancy', in K. K. Holmes, P. F. Sparling, P. Mardh, P. Piot, and J. N. Wasserheit (eds.), *Sexually Transmitted Diseases* (New York: McGraw-Hill, 3rd edn., 1999), ch. 80, 1089–1132.

[6] UNAIDS/WHO, *Report on the Global HIV/AIDS Epidemic—June 1998* (Geneva: UNAIDS, 1998), UNAIDS/98.10-WHO/EMC/VIR/98.2-WHO/ASDF/98.2, at 48.

delivery by Caesarean section, and avoidance of breastfeeding are proven measures which have potential to reduce the risk of vertical transmission to less than 2 per cent.[7] Potential teratogenic effects of anti-retroviral drugs taken during pregnancy remain an unresolved issue. Serious adverse effects appear rare, although damage to intercellular cytoplasmic components, particularly mitochondria leading to neonatal death, has been documented.[8]

In developing countries, it is estimated that between one-third and a half of all HIV infections in young children are acquired through breast milk. According to UNAIDS, more than nine out of ten HIV-positive women in developing countries have no idea that they are infected.[9] Breastfeeding protects the infant against a range of other infections. In many developing countries, a year's supply of artificial milk for the infant will cost more than the country's per capita gross domestic product (GDP).

Reproductive assistance to HIV discordant couples can make a significant impact in preventing viral transmission. The female partner of an HIV-positive man runs a 0.1–0.2 per cent risk of acquiring HIV in an act of unprotected intercourse, and attempting to conceive naturally carries a serious risk to the uninfected woman and her child.[10] Where artificial insemination is feasible, a highly significant reduction in the risk of viral transmission is achieved if spermatozoa are first washed free of seminal plasma and non-sperm cells before insemination into the woman during the time of ovulation. Prevention of viral transmission from an infected woman to an uninfected man is less sophisticated and relies on timed artificial insemination by husband.[11]

3. *Ethical Aspects*

The International Federation of Gynecology and Obstetrics (FIGO) Committee for the Ethical Aspects of Human Reproduction and Women's Health issued a statement on Ethical Aspects of HIV Infection and Reproduction noting that HIV infection has 'profound social and psychological implications for the woman, her partner and her family as well as for the health care team and society'.[12] An HIV-positive woman is entitled to the full ethical respect due to all patients, including her right to refuse testing and to appropriate care without discrimination due to her HIV-positive status. She is accordingly entitled to autonomous choice of available medical care.

---

[7] C. Gilling-Smith, jun., and A. E. Semprini, 'Editorial. HIV and Infertility: Time to Treat', *British Medical Journal*, 322 (2001), 566–7.
  [8] Ibid.   [9] UNAIDS/WHO, *Report*, 48.
  [10] Gilling-Smith and Semprini, 'Editorial'.   [11] Ibid.
  [12] FIGO Committee for the Ethical Aspects of Human Reproduction and Women's Health, *Recommendations on Ethical Issues in Obstetrics and Gynecology* (London: FIGO, 2000), 33.

Counselling must be non-directive as to pregnancy continuation or termination when lawful. If she decides to continue a pregnancy, the ethical entitlements of the child she intends to deliver must be considered. The WHO Report identified the following issues in counselling HIV-positive pregnant women in order that they can make informed decisions about their pregnancy.

- the effect of pregnancy on HIV infection;
- the effect of HIV infection on pregnancy: risks of adverse pregnancy events;
- the risks of coitus during pregnancy and the particular risks of STDs acquired during pregnancy;
- the risk of transmission to the foetus during pregnancy, delivery, and breastfeeding;
- termination of pregnancy options;
- treatment options during pregnancy;
- interventions available to attempt to prevent mother-to-child transmission;
- infant feeding options: the advantages and disadvantages of breastfeeding;
- disclosure of results to male partners and/or to other significant family or community members: advantages and risks;
- the need for follow-up of both mother and child;
- future fertility and contraceptive options.[13]

Although foetuses as such are not usually considered in law to be persons, ethical responsibilities apply to future persons, whether or not they are yet conceived. The prospect of the child to be HIV infected at birth, and to succumb to AIDS shortly afterwards, must therefore be included in the information given, together with the implications of continuation of pregnancy for a woman's own health and care. Information and counselling should also address the advantages and disadvantages of breastfeeding for the woman and her infant, given the resources available to Mrs JK. The FIGO Ethics Committee notes that: 'In societies where safe, affordable alternative methods of infant feeding are available, it may be unethical for an HIV infected mother to breastfeed her child. Where the risks of alternative infant feeding are high, the balance of risk to the infant may favor making breastfeeding ethically justified.'[14]

Ethical and legal challenges can arise for the health care provider regarding the patient's serostatus. Cases may arise where health care providers have competing obligations: on the one hand to protect the patient's confidentiality and on the other hand to disclose test results in order to prevent substantial harm to third parties. The FIGO Ethics Committee has explained that:

---

[13] McIntyre and Brocklehurst, *HIV in Pregnancy*, 31.
[14] FIGO Ethics Committee, *Recommendations*, 34.

Every effort should be made through counselling to convince individual patients of their responsibility to others including the importance of allowing such information to be used to protect sexual partners and health care workers. If in spite of every effort, consent [to release of information] is not obtained and the risk of transmission is high in certain circumstances, with consultation, it may be justified to override patient confidentiality.[15]

The American College of Obstetricians and Gynecologists (ACOG), in a Committee Opinion, explained that 'a breach of confidentiality may be ethically justified for purposes of partner notification when 1. there is a high probability of harm to the partner, 2. the potential harm is a serious one, 3. the information communicated can be used to prevent harm, and 4. greater good will result from breaking confidentiality rather than maintaining it'.[16] This Committee Opinion explains that, when a breach of confidentiality is contemplated, the negative consequences of breaking confidentiality need to be carefully weighed. The Committee Opinion explains that these consequences may include:

- Personal risks to the individual whose confidence is breached such as serious implications for the person's relationship with family and friends, the threat of discrimination in employment and housing, domestic violence, and the impact on family members
- Loss of patient trust, which may reduce the physician's ability to communicate effectively and provide services
- A ripple effect among cohorts of women that may deter other women at risk from accepting testing and have a serious negative impact on the educational efforts that lie at the heart of attempts to reduce the spread of disease.[17]

The facts of Mrs JK's case explain that her husband has tested positive, so the health care provider will not have competing obligations regarding whether to notify him, but the issue of confidentiality regarding Mrs JK's serostatus might arise regarding health care workers. As a general matter, the ACOG Committee explains that 'Confidentiality should not be breached solely because of perceived risk to health care workers. Health care workers should rely on strict observance of standard precautions to minimize risk. The patients' HIV serostatus, however, should be transmitted to other health care professionals to ensure optimal medical management.'[18] Of course, health care workers to whom information of a patient's HIV-positive status is disclosed

[15] Ibid. 33–4.
[16] American College of Obstetricians and Gynecologists (ACOG), 'Human Immunodeficiency Virus Infection: Physician's Responsibilities. Committee Opinion Number 255, April 2001', in *Ethics in Obstetrics and* Gynecology (Washington, DC: ACOG, 2002), 43–7 at 45.
[17] Ibid.   [18] Ibid.

for their own protection are bound by the ordinary duties of confidentiality not to disclose the patient's status to anyone else who is not at direct risk of exposure to the patient's body fluids.

4. *Legal Aspects*

When an HIV-positive woman decides to continue her pregnancy, she is entitled to the legal standard of care in prenatal care and childbirth. She must also be advised on breastfeeding and alternative options, including whether local law and child welfare agencies regard breastfeeding by HIV-positive mothers to present an unacceptable risk to the child, constituting child abuse.

Neither the woman nor her child should suffer discrimination on the ground of their HIV-positive status, although transfer to a conveniently accessible birthing centre that is specially equipped for HIV-positive patients will not be discriminatory. Legal duties are owed to the mother, and to her child once it is born alive, including for the quality of prenatal, delivery, and postnatal care and advice given.

Under occupational health and safety laws, health care facilities owe duties of care to staff members. For instance, a doctor must ensure that colleagues delivering prenatal, childbirth, or postnatal care to an HIV-positive woman and her baby are informed of and adequately safeguarded against the risks to them due to her HIV infection. Staff members have no legal right of conscientious objection to involvement in care of the woman or her child, but any who can show unreasonable risk to themselves or others, perhaps such as a pregnant nurse at risk of needle-prick exposure, might be excluded from duties of care if safely replaceable.

The treating physician bears no legal liability if anti-retroviral drugs or other necessary or desirable products for the care of the woman and her baby are unavailable due to causes outside the physician's control. Doctors may have a legal duty of reasonable advocacy, however, to request that others who control access to such products make them available in such cases.

5. *Human Rights Aspects*

An HIV-positive woman's rights to life and survival, under the International Covenant on Civil and Political Rights (the Political Covenant), and to the highest attainable standard of health, under the International Covenant on Economic, Social and Cultural Rights (the Economic Covenant), which includes her physical, mental, and social well-being, reinforce her legal rights to continue or terminate her pregnancy. If the choice is continuation of pregnancy, her human right to anti-retroviral medication is protected by the Convention on the Elimination of All Forms of Discrimination against Women (the Women's Convention), which requires the provision of 'appropriate services in connexion with pregnancy, confinement and the postnatal period, granting free services where necessary' (Article 12(2)). The right of the woman to appropriate services is reinforced by the child's right to appropriate care. The Convention on the Rights of the Child (the Children's Convention) requires states to ensure the provision of 'appropriate pre-natal and post-natal health care for women' (Article 24(2)). National courts and human rights tribunals have ruled that denial of medically indicated resources and care for those infected with HIV violates the right to life, the right to security of the person, and the right to health,[19] and the right to be free from inhuman and degrading treatment.[20]

In some communities, there can be subtle and not so subtle inducements for a pregnant woman with HIV/AIDS to have an abortion. Such inducements, even if indicated on medical grounds, might be a violation of Mrs JK's right to found a family, her right to decide the number and spacing of her children, and more broadly her rights to privacy and to liberty and security of her person.[21] Alternatively, where a pregnant woman with HIV/AIDS has chosen to terminate her pregnancy, she is legally entitled to do so in countries where abortion is permitted for reasons of preservation of health or where it is permitted for reasons of HIV/AIDS status.

6. *Approaches*

6.1. *Clinical duty*

Medical care of Mrs JK, and the well-being of a child she intends to deliver, will be affected by her access to short-course anti-retroviral drugs that reduce the risk of vertical HIV transmission. Dr GH should know or discover whether such drugs can be obtained through an agency, such as a Ministry of Health, that will bear the cost or reduce it sufficiently to ensure Mrs JK's treatment at

---

[19] *Cruz Bermudez, et al.* v. *Ministerio de Sanidad y Asistencia Social (MSAS)*, Case No. 15789 (1999) (Supreme Court of Venezuela), http://www.tsj.gov.ve/, last accessed 6 Sept. 2001); R. J. Cook and B. M. Dickens, 'Human Rights and HIV-Positive Women', *Int. J. Gynecol. Obstet.* 77 (2002), 55–63.

[20] *D. v. United Kingdom* (1997) 24 EHRR 423 (European Court of Human Rights).

[21] United Nations, *HIV/AIDS and Human Rights: International Guidelines: The Results of the Second International Consultation on HIV/AIDS and Human Rights, 23–25 Sept. 1996* (Geneva: UN, 1998), HR/PUB/98/1, 47; for summary see Pt. III, Ch. 7. Reprinted in UNAIDS and Inter-Parliamentary Union (IPU), *Handbook for Legislators on HIV/AIDS and Human Rights* (Geneva: UNAIDS/IPU, 1999). Available at: http://www.unaids.org/publications/documents/human/index.html, last accessed 6 May 2002.

least in late pregnancy. Dr GH has an ethical and legal duty of reasonable advocacy on behalf of Mrs JK if she cannot afford and has no assured access to such drugs.

Mrs JK should be informed of the duties that Dr GH owes to the health care team members attending her, and that they have to be aware of her HIV-positive status. That is, Mrs JK must be informed that Dr GH's colleagues must know her HIV status in order to take universal precautions to protect themselves and other patients who may be at risk, but also that they will protect her confidentiality to the maximum extent possible. 'Universal precautions' are not uniform, but are related to the degree of risk of exposure. For instance, those exposed to spurting blood require masks and eye protection, whereas those only handling tubes of body samples require little more than gloves. In this case, precautions will be needed to prevent, for instance, contamination of equipment used in the patient's care, such as for natural or Caesarean delivery.

Dr GH should review the capacity of the clinic to treat an HIV-positive patient to ensure the safe care of Mrs JK, of clinic staff, and of the baby Mrs JK will deliver. If a clinic to which Mrs JK has convenient access has been specially equipped and staffed to care for HIV-infected patients, Dr GH may offer her the option to be transferred there. If Mrs JK remains Dr GH's patient, Dr GH should provide her with information and counselling relevant to her choice to continue the pregnancy. Dr GH should address means to provide Mrs JK with at least a short course of anti-retroviral medication in late pregnancy and around delivery, and counsel her regarding breastfeeding and alternatives to be considered following childbirth. Dr GH should also counsel Mrs JK regarding her future contraceptive care.[22]

Mrs JK should be advised of the advantages to herself and to the child of finding alternatives to breastfeeding. While further research is needed, concerns about the effect of breastfeeding on maternal health in HIV-positive women include the potential effects of breastfeeding and resultant weight loss on the immunity and long-term prognosis of the mother.[23] Given the increased risk of HIV transmission through breastfeeding, the feasibility of potential modifications of infant feeding practices should be discussed with Mrs JK. They include complete avoidance of breastfeeding, early cessation, pasteurization of breast milk, and avoiding breastfeeding in the presence of breast abscesses or cracked nipples.[24]

There might be social pressures on Mrs JK to breastfeed because, in many communities, if women do not breastfeed, they are suspected of having

---

[22] W. Cates, 'Use of Contraception by HIV-Infected Women', *International Planned Parenthood Federation (IPPF) Medical Bulletin*, 35 (2001), 1–2.
[23] McIntyre and Brocklehurst, *HIV in Pregnancy*, 26.   [24] Ibid.

HIV/AIDS. If Mrs JK decides to be open about her HIV status, and for example decides not to breastfeed, she should be encouraged to find the support she needs, through AIDS networks, in dealing with the stigma of being HIV positive.

6.2. *Health care systems obligations*

Dr GH should treat the access that Mrs JK and her baby have to necessary resources, including anti-retroviral drugs and safe alternatives to hazardous breast milk, as representative of how the health system responds to pregnancy among women with HIV/AIDS. If resources are adequate, Dr GH's effort is to maintain them. If they are not, effort, energy, and advocacy must be directed to influence the personnel and agencies able to bring them to the necessary level favourably, in order to maximize Mrs JK's potentials for survival and health, and the similar potentials of her child. Dr GH must consider how such influence can be generated and maintained, including by collaboration with colleagues, medical associations, HIV-advocacy groups, and comparable non-governmental agencies.

Laws that prohibit discrimination on grounds of disability require that Mrs JK be treated even though she is HIV positive. However, Dr GH and colleagues involved in her care should be appropriately educated and equipped for their own protection against exposure to her body fluids in her prenatal care and in continuation of her pregnancy leading to childbirth. If the local health care system concentrates treatment of HIV-positive patients in centres where universal precautions are provided, Dr GH may refer Mrs JK to the centre most conveniently available to her.

In addition to ensuring that Mrs JK has access to appropriate services to prevent the development of complications and sequelae, Dr GH might join with other colleagues to review how the national STD/HIV/AIDS prevention and control programme might be improved to ensure that women in Mrs JK's situation do not contract HIV/AIDS. They might start by examining whether their national programme is widely supported by the national leadership and wide spectrum of civil society and whether it meets the guidelines for comprehensive national STD programmes developed and revised regularly by the World Health Organization and UNAIDS.[25] A comprehensive public health package includes the following:

- health promotion to reduce risk of exposure to infection and adoption of safer sex practices, including the use of condoms and the maintenance of safe behaviours;

[25] WHO, *Management of Sexually Transmitted Diseases* (Geneva: WHO, 1994), WHO/GPA/TEM/94.1; WHO, *Policies and Principles for Prevention and Care of Sexually Transmitted Diseases* (Geneva: WHO, 1996); UN, *HIV/AIDS and Human Rights*.

- adequate management of patients with STD and their partners;
- intensified interventions in population groups with highest rates of risk behaviours;
- case finding and treatment of syphilis in antenatal populations;
- treatment to prevent eye infection in newborns.[26]

If the national programme does not meet these guidelines, Dr GH might work with other colleagues and the Ministry of Health to ensure the development, dissemination, and implementation of new guidelines.

6.3. *Social action for underlying conditions*

Dr GH may face the greatest professional challenge in resolving the obstacles to Mrs JK and her baby having access to the quality of products and care enjoyed by families in the best of developed countries. Dr GH must be engaged with medical and associated professional bodies, even at national and international levels, and with governmental and comparable agencies, to gain patients' access to affordable drugs. Collective approaches may be made to commercial and generic drug manufacturers to determine how patent laws and enlightened commercial practices can stimulate innovation in drug and vaccine therapies, and ensure affordable and equitable access to patients in need. Dr GH may focus initially on how the national government and commercial institutions in the country in which Dr GH practises can be mobilized in this effort, and how they may be inspired to international efforts to provide relief in addition to other countries and populations affected by HIV infection.

Dr GH might also explore working with women's health advocacy groups to:

- decrease the risk of contracting HIV/AIDS;
- decrease the vulnerability to contracting HIV/AIDS;
- decrease the impact of HIV/AIDS.[27]

Risk reduction strategies focus on particular behaviours and their modifications, and the remedy of situations where there is risk of HIV infection. Behaviour modification includes abstinence, partner reduction, mutual monogamy, male and female condom use, and the avoidance of high-risk sexual practices, such as anal sex and reduction of use of infected injecting equipment. Improvements in situations focus on where there is a risk of HIV infection,

[26] C. Johannes van Dam, G. Dallabetta, and P. Piot, 'Prevention and Control of Sexually Transmitted Diseases in Developing Countries and Resource Poor Settings in Industrialized Countries', in Holmes *et al.* (eds.), *Sexually Transmitted Diseases*, ch. 100, pp. 1381–90.

[27] UNAIDS, Programme Coordinating Board, *Framework for Global Leadership on HIV/AIDS* (Geneva: UNAIDS, 2000), UNAIDS/PCB(10)00.3.

such as the prevention of HIV transmission through blood and blood products, and prevention or reduction of situations where anyone is forced or induced into having unsafe sex.

An individual's or a community's vulnerability to HIV/AIDS is a measure of the ability to control the risk of infection. Factors that influence individual vulnerability include:

- particular characteristics and the overall empowerment of the individual (negotiation and refusal skills, avoidance of sexual abuse in childhood, knowledge and information),
- design and implementation of essential health services (the degree of availability of and access to services and their acceptability) for those who are most vulnerable to HIV/AIDS, including groups marginalized by such factors as stigma, poverty, race and ethnicity, and age,
- social and legal norms, such as the ability of individuals to talk frankly about sex and their ability to negotiate safe sex,[28] the degree of condemnation, acceptance, and practice of abusive or coerced sex, extra-marital sexual practices and unions, equality of men and women especially in family life, such as the legality of polygamy, and the degree of respect and protection of human rights.[29]

Individuals, families, communities and nations face the challenge of decreasing the impact of the HIV/AIDS epidemic. Impact mitigation strategies at the individual and family level include increased support for children orphaned by AIDS, and improved access to treatment for those living with HIV/AIDS, including legal services for the protection of their human rights. Impact mitigation strategies at the community level include the improvement of the capacity of organizations to carry out their activities, including outreach and the provision of care and social support to affected families. Strategies to mitigate impact at the national level include strengthening national AIDS programming and coordination across all sectors of government, external investments in health, education, and social services, and improved access to essential drugs and commodities through price or trade concessions.

The particular design of these strategies, whether aimed at the reduction of risk, vulnerability, or impact, will vary according to local and national circumstances, and will need to be tailored to particular groups, whether they

---

[28] G. R. Gupta, E. Weiss, and P. Mane, 'Talking about Sex: A Prerequisite for AIDS Prevention', in L. D. Long and E. M. Ankrah (eds.), *Women's Experiences with HIV/AIDS: An International Perspective* (New York: Columbia University Press, 1996), 333–50.

[29] S. Gruskin and D. Tarantola, 'HIV/AIDS, Health and Human Rights', in P. Lamptey, H. Gayle, and P. Mane (eds.), *HIV/AIDS Prevention and Care Programs in Resource-Constrained Settings: A Handbook for the Design and Management of Programs* (Washington, DC: Family Health International, 2001).

be women or men, adolescents, groups marginalized by race, ethnicity, income, or stigma. For example, care and thought are needed in understanding how social constructions of gender and sexuality affect HIV/AIDS strategies. Gender is not the same as sex. Gender refers to the widely shared expectations and norms within a society about appropriate male and female behaviour, characteristics, and roles. Understanding how gender attitudes are specifically constructed by a culture is also important, as there can be significant differences in what women and men can or cannot do in one culture in contrast to another.[30]

Understanding the pervasive and distinct nature of gender differences, how sexuality is constructed, and how gender and sexuality interact with poverty in a community is essential in tailoring any intervention strategy to ensure the highest probability of effectiveness.[31] Gender differences exist, for example, in sexual behaviour, communication, and negotiation skills, and in partner management, in susceptibility and transmission of STDs/HIV/AIDS, in health care-seeking behaviour and access to health services, and in detection of, and in adverse health outcomes of, STDs/HIV/AIDS.[32]

Sexuality is distinct from gender yet intimately linked to it. Sexuality is the social construction of a biological drive. An individual's sexuality is defined by whom one has sex with, in what ways, why, under what circumstances, and with what outcomes. It is more than sexual behaviour; it is a multidimensional and dynamic concept. Implicit and explicit social rules, influenced by one's gender, power differences between the sexes, age, social demands for procreation often influenced by economic and social status, can influence an individual's sexuality.[33]

Constructions of women as 'good women' who are expected to be ignorant about sex and passive in sexual interactions make it more difficult for women to learn about sex and develop refusal and negotiation skills. Constructions of men assume they are knowledgeable about sex, making it more difficult for men to admit their lack of knowledge and to obtain essential information. Moreover, social norms that require men to have multiple sex partners make it more difficult for them to have monogamous relationships.[34]

Programme strategies that address gender imbalances in sexual interactions include:

[30] G. R. Gupta, *Gender, Sexuality and HIV/AIDS: The What, the Why, and the How, Plenary Address XIIIth International AIDS Conference, Durban, South Africa* (Washington, DC: International Center for Research on Women, 2000).

[31] P. Farmer, M. Connors, and J. Simmons (eds.), *Women, Poverty and AIDS: Sex, Drugs and Structural Violence* (Monroe, Me.: Common Courage Press, 1996).

[32] G. Bolan, A. A. Ehrhardt, and J. Wasserheit, 'Gender Perspectives and STDs', in Holmes *et al.*, *Sexually Transmitted Diseases*, ch. 8, pp. 117–27.

[33] Gupta, *Gender*.   [34] Ibid.

- gender-neutral approaches that promote messages such as 'be faithful' or 'keep to one partner'—these are helpful because they do not reinforce gender stereotypes like using macho images to sell condoms;
- gender-sensitive approaches that begin to respond to the gender-specific needs of men and women, for example, by promoting female condoms and in so doing recognize that many women cannot require that their partners use a male condom;
- approaches, such as games, role plays, and group discussions, that attempt to transform gender roles to facilitate healthy, respectful sexuality among young men;
- empowerment approaches that try to free individuals from the effects of destructive gender and sexual norms. Examples of such approaches include empowering women with information, skills, and services relevant to sexual protection and to encourage their participation in group decision-making that fosters group identity and empowerment.[35]

---

[35] Ibid.

9

HIV Drug Research and Testing

Case Study

An HIV test six months ago showed Ms P, an unmarried young woman aged 21 living in a country with few health care resources, that she had contracted the virus. She has been informed that a new drug combination to control the infection is being tested in the area, and that she is eligible to be a subject in the study. She asks Dr Q, who serves in a reproductive health clinic in the town and is actively involved in the study, whether she should participate. How should Dr Q reply, in light of medical, ethical, legal, and human rights considerations?

1. Background

Until recently, the widespread perception of AIDS was as a hopeless, untreatable disease. It was only around 1995 that highly active therapy (anti-retroviral drugs) became available. Before then, it seemed that one could do very little about HIV infection.

Currently available drugs are too expensive, have to be taken continuously for years, and are beyond the reach of most populations in developing countries. Usually, three such drugs have to be taken simultaneously, to overcome virus resistance.

Search continues for other anti-retroviral drugs that are more effective, more easy for compliance, and associated with fewer side effects. Since populations with high rates of infection are needed to conduct clinical trials in a timely manner, large pharmaceutical companies look for trial sites in developing countries where the disease is highly endemic. This raises ethical, legal, and human rights issues, not the least of which is whether the drug, if the trial is successful, will be made available at an affordable cost to the population on whom it has been tested.

2. Medical Aspects

HIV is a slow-acting virus that usually takes years to produce illness in an infected person. Over a decade or so, the immune defences become gradually undermined, and various pathogenic organisms (viruses, bacteria, fungi, and parasites) take advantage of the lowered resistance in the body and cause serious illnesses. Effective therapies exist to prevent, treat, or even cure many of these opportunistic diseases, thus easing the suffering of the patient and prolonging life.

Effective anti-retroviral therapy is now available, though at high cost. The virus can easily mutate to develop resistance to any one drug. Hence, it is recommended to give a combination of drugs, to attack the virus from different vulnerable mechanisms. There is good evidence that treatment of asymptomatic patients can delay the onset of the disease, though cure has not been demonstrated.

HIV-infected people do not need drugs only. They also need psychological and social support to cope with the implications, for themselves and for their families, of having a life-threatening and often stigmatizing disease.

3. Ethical Aspects

The ethics of research with human subjects has been a focus of profound debate and contention for four or more decades, and has produced a voluminous literature. In more recent years, the focus has been on research, sponsored by commercial or governmental interests in economically developed countries or by intergovernmental agencies, that is to be conducted in economically developing countries and countries in economic transition. The ethical issues that dominate research in developed countries, such as subjects' informed, voluntary consent, confidentiality, favourable benefit-to-risk ratio, and management of conflict of interest, also apply in research hosted in a developing country. They often have a sharper focus, however, since, even when each individual is to be properly recruited and the microethics of a study are in good repair, the macroethics may be suspect due to a perception that it is exploitive, for instance of poverty and deprivation, for the study to be proposed in a developing country. If the scientific purposes of an investigation could be accomplished in a developed country, the intention to locate it in a developing country may require special ethical justification.

The apprehension may be, for instance, that the study sponsors believe the study will be less expensive to conduct there, that subjects will be less comprehending of study risks or more willing to take them out of desperation to acquire potential benefits, or that sponsors' and investigators' legal obligations will be less vigorously pursued there, or less costly to satisfy. Apprehension is magnified when the study concerns treatment for a condition more prevalent in developed countries than the developing country intended to host the study, or an equally prevalent condition but host country residents cannot afford to buy commercial products that result from studies, their government will not or cannot purchase supplies, and the sponsoring manufacturer does not propose free or low-cost supplies.

Caution must be exercised in responding negatively to this apprehension of exploitation, however, when responsible governmental, scientific, or other agencies in a developing proposed host country welcome a study, grant it approval under ethical guidelines, and complain of discrimination when studies are confined to developed world populations. Their urging that studies be conducted in their countries may be less convincing when the disorder under investigation is not prevalent there. A concern in HIV research is that it may be directed primarily towards viral strains prevalent in developed countries, but that do not exist, or are not significant, in the proposed host country. When a disorder or viral strain is proposed to be studied that is as prevalent in a proposed host country as elsewhere, local officers' claims that research would offer their populations opportunities for employment and training of specialized indigenous personnel who can develop and conduct studies from which their developing country would benefit have more ethical merit. Research can appear to bring capacity-building benefits to resource-poor countries that would advance their economies in general and their health care systems in particular.

Ethical dilemmas are most acute when ethical guidelines for research in study sponsors' or investigators' own countries seem to demand more from them than they might be required to provide in intended host countries. Internationally contentious are two relevant articles of the World Medical Association's Declaration of Helsinki on medical research involving human subjects, as amended in October 2000 (see Pt. III, Ch. 2). These are:

29. The benefits, risks, burdens and effectiveness of a new method should be tested against those of the best current prophylactic, diagnostic, and therapeutic methods. This does not exclude the use of placebo, or no treatment, in studies where no proven prophylactic, diagnostic or therapeutic method exists.

30. At the conclusion of the study, every patient entered into the study should be assured of access to the best proven prophylactic, diagnostic and therapeutic methods identified by the study.

Article 29 allows placebo or no treatment for affected patients in a control group where no proven treatment exists for a condition under investigation. If the reason why no proven treatment exists is that, although such treatment is available in an affluent developed country, patients in the impoverished developing country intended to host the study cannot afford it and are not given it, sponsors may economize by offering that the study be hosted there. Article 30 may be intended to prevent exploitive economy by providing that, at the conclusion of the study, both treated and untreated control group patients be assured of access to the best proven care. This may deter ethical sponsorship of studies to be conducted in developing countries that their leaders want them to host, since it may require commercial companies to assure therapies in developing countries that national health care infrastructures and public resources do not make available. Studies that sponsors support that conform to Article 29 may risk later violation of Article 30, unless a study identifies no best method of care. However, governments in possible host countries that would welcome studies under the condition of Article 30 may require more than commercial sponsors consider should ethically be required of them alone, and so potential sponsors may decline to undertake studies from which developing country populations would benefit.

4. *Legal Aspects*

Medical professional consideration of research proposals is overwhelmingly pitched at the ethical level, but proposals also raise several issues of legal concern. As for any proposed medical treatment, the legal requirement is that recruits' consent to participation be adequately informed, and be voluntary. Informed consent relates to the law on unauthorized touching, namely assault and battery, and to negligence law where due disclosure concerns discharge of the legal duty of care. Coerced consent is not considered in law to be consent at all, but the effect of inducement can be uncertain.

The inducement of contributing to the advance of science, particularly medical science and the relief of suffering, is precisely the inducement that legitimately inspires the altruism of participation in research. The inducement to obtain wealth at low risk, such as of mild discomfort or public ridicule, also suggests that consent to participation is genuine and sincere, even though primarily mercenary. The legal concern arises when consent is unduly induced. Undue inducement negates legally effective consent, and arises when an inducement is offered that unconscionably tempts a person to forgo customary self-protective caution, and take a significant physical risk, in the hope of gaining an actual, speculative, or illusory benefit.

In innovative therapy, undertaken not primarily for advance of generalizable knowledge but for instance in an attempt to prolong survival of an unavoidably dying patient, an inducement is not necessarily undue and invalidating. It may be acceptable when a dying patient gives consent to implantation of a theoretically credible but untested mechanical device, or to transplantation of a transgenically prepared organ from a non-human primate or, for instance, a pig. In contrast, however, an inducement may be undue when a person is invited to consume an unproven and potentially risk-laden product for a relatively sizeable money reward in the hope of finding relief from a relatively minor ailment, or when an existing product of a study sponsor's commercial competitor would offer comparable relief.

A growing area of legal concern arises when an investigator who invites a person to take some risk for the advance of therapeutic care or medical understanding, such as of an adverse health effect or discomfort, fails to disclose a conflict of interest. Courts are particularly aware that when sick patients are asked or recommended to undertake medical procedures by their own physicians or by physicians in facilities to which they have gone for help, they usually believe that its purpose is to be beneficial to them. They may fail to recognize that physicians, customarily serving their health care interests, are in this case acting instead as scientific investigators, and asking them to risk jeopardizing their interests for a purpose from which the investigators hope to benefit, indirectly or directly. Accordingly, courts expect researchers to disclose their own monetary and other interests in studies in which they invite patients and others to enter, and accept risks and discomforts. Failure to disclose the conflict negates participants' consent, and may afford them remedies, particularly for adverse effects.

5. *Human Rights Aspects*

The modern international human rights movement was largely a reaction to events leading to and during the Second World War, including revelations of research on vulnerable populations which the Universal Declaration of Human Rights of 1948 included in the description in its Preamble of 'barbarous acts which have outraged the conscience of mankind'. National and international statements provide protection against individuals' involuntary recruitment into projects of medical experimentation, either in explicit terms, or through guarantees of protection of the dignity and worth of human persons and against denials of security of the person. The International Covenant on Civil and Political Rights expresses this inspiration in Article 7, which provides that 'No one shall be subjected to torture or to cruel, inhuman or degrading treatment or punishment. In particular, no one shall be subjected without his free consent to medical or scientific experimentation.'

Even with potential participants' free consent, there are limits to research that individuals may be invited to enter. Human rights provisions specifically applicable to research involving human subjects set minimum standards, for instance of scientific merit, conduct, and monitoring, to which studies must conform. Research guidelines are frequently expressed in what are described as codes of ethics. However, where research addresses pandemics and other widely prevalent diseases, it may transcend clinical medicine to affect considerations of public health. It has been recognized that the role played by ethics in clinical medicine is played in public health initiatives by the concepts and language of human rights.[1] Accordingly, a considerable range of basic human rights, such as to life, liberty, and security of the person are available to provide protection against risks that are unavoidably present in research involving unproven medical products. Risks include physical injury and death, postponement or denial of routine effective treatment, psychological injury, and such 'harmless wrongs' as indignities.

As against this, however, such benefits have resulted from various forms of medical research, that it is being recognized as a human rights violation not to undertake studies to improve the care of those who suffer disease. The refusal or failure to undertake studies may constitute discrimination on grounds such as ethnicity, age, and sex. The women's health movement, for instance, has become insistent that research be undertaken into conditions that affect women as well as men, and that affect women in particular. In many regions of the world, HIV infection is as prevalent, or more prevalent, among women as among men. Accordingly, not only is there a human rights claim that research be conducted into HIV/AIDS, but also that such studies include women. This fits within human rights claims to non-discrimination, to the benefits of scientific progress, and to the highest attainable standard of health.

Research into HIV/AIDS is double-edged in the context of human rights. It presents risks of being undertaken in violation of human rights, such as without free and informed consent and in abuse of vulnerable populations. Equally, however, failure or refusal to undertake it, at all or involving particular populations, may itself be a human rights violation concerning, for instance, non-discrimination and access to benefits of scientific progress. Human rights require that such research be undertaken, but that it be undertaken ethically.

6. *Approaches*

6.1. *Clinical duty*

As an active investigator or organizer of the study, Dr Q should ensure familiarity with relevant ethical guidelines, and their enforcement. Although the study at hand concerns drugs, attention should be paid for instance to the

---

[1] J. H. Mann, 'Medicine and Public Health, Ethics and Human Rights', *Hastings Center Report*, 27/3 (1997), 6–13.

UNAIDS guidance document entitled 'Ethical Considerations in HIV Preventative Vaccine Research'.[2] Dr Q's first duty is to inform P of the doctor's status as an investigator or organizer of the study, and offer to refer her to another physician who can provide disinterested advice. Where such a physician is inaccessible to P, however, Dr Q may offer advice after declaring the interest. Indeed, if another physician is accessible, Dr Q may still declare the interest and then offer to advise P, on the basis of possessing best knowledge of what the study entails for her, its potential risks and benefits, and Dr Q's capacity to provoke and respond to P's questions. However, Dr Q could not ethically introduce the study to P and invite her to participate.

A bias that commonly arises is that, as a general rule outside high-risk studies, it is more in patients' interests to be in studies than not to be. That is, the care and attention that patients receive as subjects of studies is superior to what they would receive outside, since services can be supplied from the study budget more generously than from alternative sources, such as governmental or private funds. P's right to informed decision-making may require that she be given this information, unless Dr Q considers that it constitutes an undue inducement.

A concern with testing of HIV drugs and combination therapies is that, because they are unproven and often expensive, study sponsors have refused to make them available except in studies or other evaluative programmes. Sponsors sometimes react to accusations of unethically exploiting infected persons' fears and vulnerability that compel them to comply with the discipline of a study, by providing a limited supply of a test regime for open use outside the framework of a study. This raises a criticism, however, of confusing the distinction between a therapeutic and an unproven treatment regime. Dr Q must inform P of her access to treatment inside and outside the study, and the implications for her health and capacity for activities under each option. In particular, if the study design includes allocation of participants between groups that receive drug and placebo treatment, or among groups receiving, for instance, the test drug combination, routine drug treatment, and placebo, P must be informed that, if she participates in the study, she may nevertheless not receive any active medication.

6.2. *Health care systems obligations*

Any inducement to which P is susceptible to enter the study may arise from her sense of a lack of alternative means to maintain her health. The more the health care system can assist this goal, the less she may feel compelled to accept risks

[2] UNAIDS, *Ethical Considerations in HIV Preventive Vaccine Research: UNAIDS Guidance Document* (Geneva: UNAIDS, 2000).

of taking unproven treatment. Advice to P in particular, and to others infected with HIV in general, regarding lifestyle choices, nutrition, exercise, and health care monitoring, for instance, may facilitate her to maintain good health without turning to unproven products or drug regimens.

Advice may include sexual matters, marriage, and planned pregnancy, as well as conditions that may pose special risks to women whose immune reactions may be compromised by HIV infection. However, she may not be able to maintain long-term compliance with an experimental drug study protocol while pregnant. Advice from her health care services on HIV and pregnancy may leave her capable of planning for her future in confidence, without feeling the need to enter a study for her own advantage. Similarly, she can assess the implications for her of the altruistic gesture of complying with the study conditions in order to advance knowledge intended to be beneficial to others in her circumstances.

6.3. *Social action for underlying conditions*

The groundswell of ethical controversy that has arisen regarding studies conducted in developing countries that are sponsored particularly by commercial corporations based in developed countries involves conflicting views on the application of the principles of justice, particularly distributive justice. This requires an equitable balance between risks and benefits, which critics do not find when poor people in developing countries are induced by minor rewards to take, and may suffer from, risks, in order to provide commercial products whose profitable sale enriches corporate and private investors in developed countries. HIV/AIDS research has been particularly contentious in this regard.

Justice also requires that like cases be treated alike, and different cases differently. A basic conflict concerns compliance with ethical guidelines for protection of human subjects of research. The universalist view is that subjects in developed and developing countries are alike in their universal entitlement to protection, and should have the same protections in the application of international protective guidelines such as the Declaration of Helsinki. The relativist view is that subjects in the circumstances of developed and developing countries are different, and that each may be treated in relation to their own opportunities and expectations. It is accordingly unjust to condition studies welcomed in developing countries on sponsors in developed countries bringing subjects to the same standard of material or therapeutic provision as subjects in developed countries enjoy. Respect for persons in developing countries who seek to attract or who approve study proposals that accommodate different treatments for differently situated subjects requires that they be considered to know what is in their own countries' interests, and not to be ignorant, callous, self-interested, or otherwise corrupt.

   Proponents of these conflicting views on the propriety of different conditions for the conduct of research between developed and developing countries raise legitimate concerns. Medical professionals through national societies can contribute to educated debates and decisions on the circumstances under which research may properly be proposed, accepted, and undertaken, and to the advice it is appropriate for professionals to give patients who are considering personal participation.

10

Responding to a Request for Pregnancy Termination

Case Study

Mrs R, aged 36, has two children aged 10 and 3, and suffers from chronic active hepatitis that has persuaded her and Mr R, on her physician's advice, not to have another child. Mrs R's physician, Dr T, has now found her to be two months pregnant, and Mrs R has requested Dr T to terminate the pregnancy. The local legislation states only that 'Any person who unlawfully procures a woman's miscarriage commits an offence punishable with up to 14 years' imprisonment'. Taking account of medical, ethical, legal, and human rights considerations, how should Dr T respond?

1. *Background*

Women's ability to obtain abortion services is affected by the prevailing law in a particular country and how it is interpreted and applied. It is an over-simplification to classify abortion as legal or illegal. Many countries, even those that criminalize the procedure, permit abortion in some circumstances. However, the exceptions legally allowed to criminal prohibitions are frequently unwritten or ambiguously worded, and not easily understood by health care providers and women seeking services. As a result of this ambiguity, health care providers are reluctant to provide those services, even though women might be legally entitled to them.

A global trend towards liberalization of abortion laws has continued in recent years. Since 1985, nineteen nations have significantly liberalized their abortion laws; only one country has substantially curtailed legal access to abortion.[1] Currently, 61 per cent of the world's people live in countries where induced abortion is permitted either for a wide range of reasons or without

---

[1] A. Rahman, L. Katzive and S. K. Henshaw, 'A Global Review of Laws on Induced Abortion, 1985–1997', *International Family Planning Perspectives*, 24 (1998), 56–64.

restriction as to reason; in contrast, 25 per cent reside in nations where abortion is generally prohibited. However, even in countries with highly restrictive laws, induced abortion is usually permitted when the woman's life is endangered. In contrast, access is often limited in countries with liberal laws, because of lack of availability of reasonably priced services, limitations on the types of facilities that perform induced abortions, and, for example, third-party authorization requirements.[2]

Determining the legal status of abortion in any given country is a complex but necessary task. Laws regarding abortion are often addressed in multiple statutes, codes, and regulations, and often court decisions, all of which apply simultaneously. Where abortion is criminalized, it is addressed in the criminal code, usually in language that is understandable only to lawyers, and not easily operationalized by health care providers.

Countries agreed to address the public health consequences of unsafe abortion at two United Nations Conferences, one held in Cairo in 1994 on Population and Development, and the other held in Beijing in 1995 on women, and were further considered at their subsequent five-year reviews. Governments agreed at the 1994 Cairo Conference

to strengthen their commitment to women's health, to deal with the health impact of unsafe abortion as a major public health concern and to reduce the recourse to abortion through expanded and improved family-planning services. Prevention of unwanted pregnancies must always be given the highest priority and every attempt should be made to eliminate the need for abortion. Women who have unwanted pregnancies should have ready access to reliable information and compassionate counselling. Any measures or changes related to abortion within the health system can only be determined at the national or local level according to the national legislative process. In circumstances where abortion is not against the law, such abortion should be safe. In all cases, women should have access to quality services for the management of complications arising from abortion. Post-abortion counselling, education and family-planning services should be offered promptly, which will also help to avoid repeat abortions.[3]

A year later at the 1995 Beijing Conference, governments agreed to 'consider reviewing laws containing punitive measures against women who have undergone illegal abortions'.[4]

    [2] R. J. Cook, B. M. Dickens, and L. E. Bliss, 'International Developments in Abortion Law from 1988 to 1998', *American Journal of Public Health*, 89 (1999), 579–86.

    [3] UN, *Population and Development*, i. *Programme of Action Adopted at the International Conference on Population and Development, Cairo, 5–13 September 1994* (New York: UN, Department for Economic and Social Information and Policy Analysis, ST/ESA/SER.A/149, 1994), para. 8.25.

    [4] UN, Department of Public Information, *Platform for Action and Beijing Declaration: Fourth World Conference on Women, Beijing, China, 4–15 September 1995* (New York: UN, 1995) (hereinafter Beijing Platform), para. 106(k).

At the twenty-first special session of the United Nations General Assembly in July 1999, in order to further the implementation of the Cairo Programme of Action, governments agreed that in circumstances where abortion is not against the law 'such abortion should be safe'[5] and that 'health systems should train and equip health-service providers and should take other measures to ensure that such abortion is safe and accessible'.[6] In order to train health service providers and take measures to ensure that abortion is safe and accessible, health ministries will need to clarify the situations in which abortion is not against the law, through, for example, the development of regulations or treatment protocols.

2. *Medical Aspects*

Hepatitis means, literally, inflammation of the liver. This can have a multiplicity of causes but the most frequent hepatitis is due to viruses. There are a number of these viruses. The acute manifestations are more or less the same, but they differ in their propensity to lead to chronic hepatitis and liver cancer.

The significance of each virus is determined by two factors: the mode of transmission and the persistence of the infection. In public health terms, the viruses can be regarded as falling into two groups: (1) the viruses transmitted by the faecal-oral route, which cause acute hepatitis and no persistent infection; (2) the sexually and parenterally transmitted viruses, which lead to persistence and chronic liver disease. These two groups also have different geographical distributions. Hepatitis A and E are transmitted by a faecal-oral route and are common in developing countries with poor sanitary conditions. They can assume epidemic dimensions. Hepatitis B, C, and D are transmitted by the sexual route and parenteral routes, for instance by injection or blood transfusion. While Hepatitis B is quite rare in developed countries and most of Latin America, rates of infection are much higher in China and sub-Saharan Africa. Hepatitis B is particularly a problem for intravenous drug users. The Amazon basin is the area in which it represents the largest public health problem. Hepatitis C infection occurs in both developed and developing countries primarily in adult life.[7]

Pregnant women seem to be particularly vulnerable to hepatitis. Incidence rates as well as case fatality rates are higher than in non-pregnant women.

---

[5] UN, General Assembly, *Report of the Ad Hoc Committee of the Whole of the Twenty-First Special Session of the General Assembly: Overall Review and Appraisal of the Implementation of the Programme of Action of the International Conference on Population and Development*, A/S-21/5/ Add.1 (New York: UN, 1999), para. 63(i).

[6] Ibid., para. 63(iii).

[7] A. J. Hall, 'Viral Hepatitis', in K. S. Lankinen, S. Bergstrom, P. H. Makela, and M. Peltomaa (eds.), *Health and Disease in Developing Countries* (London: Macmillan, 1994), 239–46.

Pregnant women are particularly susceptible to acute Hepatitis E infection. In some epidemics, the case fatality rate in pregnant women has been as high as 25 per cent.[8] The outcome of pregnancy in women with chronic active hepatitis is related to the extent of the disease. In some countries, viral hepatitis ranks among the most important causes of maternal death. There is no effective treatment for the pregnant woman with chronic active hepatitis. Cure can occur only after acute hepatitis, if it does not turn chronic. The woman with chronic active hepatitis runs the risk of deterioration of the liver function, which can lead ultimately to death.

Perinatal loss rates are usually high in pregnant women with poor liver function. Premature birth is common. Foetal infection *in utero* is rare, but the neonate may be exposed to the virus at delivery and the virus may be transmitted by breastfeeding. Babies born to mothers with the disease may be saved if immunization is available and undertaken. Hepatitis virus immunoglobulin should be given to a baby within twelve hours after birth, and the hepatitis virus vaccine should be given in three doses: after birth, at one to two months, and at six months.

3. *Ethical Aspects*

The ethical challenge is aggravated by uncertainty in the meaning of the law, which is expressed in ambiguous yet commonly used language. Mrs R's life may not necessarily be endangered by continuation of her pregnancy, but it is likely that her health would be, including her ability to care for her growing children. Her interests and theirs would be served by pregnancy termination, which for her health should preferably be undertaken as soon as possible and preferably within the first trimester.

An obvious ethical issue in abortion concerns the moral status of the embryo/foetus. This is often a contentious issue. Some think that the ethical principle to do no harm requires that the interest of the embryo should prevail over the interest of the woman. Others think that the ethical principle of respect for persons requires that there is consideration and regard for women's autonomous choices. That is, respect for persons requires that we treat women not as instruments of governmental birth control policies, whether pro- or anti-natalist, but as their own moral agents. Moreover, the ethical principle of beneficence might well favour the woman taking critical decisions on behalf of her family and dependent children.

The ethical principle of justice would require an exploration of why women are being treated differently from men by the law with respect to their health

---

[8] A. J. Hall, 'Viral Hepatitis', in K. S. Lankinen, S. Bergstrom, P. H. Makela, and M. Peltomaa (eds.), *Health and Disease in Developing Countries* (London: Macmillan, 1994).

needs, the health system, and the larger society. Men can serve their health needs, regarding treatment for hepatitis and other health conditions, without fear of committing a criminal offence. Further, justice would require consideration of whether compelling women, such as Mrs R, to serve their unborn against their will is discriminatory on grounds of sex, reflecting a disrespectful attitude towards women. Neither women nor their husbands can be legally compelled to afford their born children necessary blood or, for instance, bone marrow transfusions or other resources available from their bodies.[9] Justice might also require accommodating the plurality of views on this issue by ensuring that the law respects those who conscientiously object to the procedure by not requiring their involvement, but also allows for the provision of services for those who have conscientiously decided that they need such services.

There are also microethical and macroethical perspectives that need exploration. Interests in prenatal life might best be respected in ways that are consistent with the interests of the woman. That is, a microethical approach is to look at the woman and her foetus as an interdependent unit, and not in adversarial terms where the interests of the woman are pitted against the interests of the foetus.[10] From a macro perspective, the ethical principle of beneficence requires an examination of what else needs to be done to ensure healthy pregnancies and childbirth for women whose pregnancies are wanted. This principle requires, for example, ensuring the provision of appropriate preventive care for women who might be at risk of hepatitis, such as hepatitis B vaccination, or appropriate treatment for excessive drug use to reduce the risk of contracting hepatitis. The American College of Obstetricians and Gynecologists (ACOG) has recommended universal vaccination against hepatitis B for all adolescents, to be given at age 11–12, with immunization for older adolescents based on risk status. ACOG notes that hepatitis B is the only sexually transmitted disease for which effective vaccination is now available.[11]

The ethical principle of respect for persons requires respect for Mrs R's religious convictions. In this case, her request for abortion indicates how she has resolved her responsibilities to her existing children, her family, her religious conscience, and to herself. Accordingly, if the doctor has no conscientious objections, there may be few ethical barriers to complying with the woman's request. If the doctor has conscientious objections, then the ethical duty would be for Dr T to refer her directly to an appropriate facility willing to end her pregnancy on health grounds.

---

[9] J. J. Thompson, 'A Defense of Abortion', *Philosophy and Public Affairs*, 1 (1971), 47–66.

[10] P. King, 'Helping Women Helping Children: Drug Policy and Future Generations', *Milbank Quarterly*, 69 (1991), 595–621.

[11] American College of Obstetricians and Gynecologists, *Hepatitis B Immunization for Adolescents. Committee Opinion Number 184, June 1997* (Washington, DC: ACOG, 1993); repr. in *Int. J. Gynecol. Obstet.* 58 (1997), 341.

The procedures the clinic has conducted, however, have been to preserve women's lives endangered by pregnancy. Many clinics do not characterize life-saving procedures that terminate pregnancies as constituting abortions. Under the concept of 'double effect', pursuit of a legitimate goal is not prohibited when a relatively minor result not permissible in itself is unavoidable. For instance, hospitals that decline to perform abortions as such will remove ectopic pregnancies or treat pregnant women with cervical cancer in order to save their lives. Treating a pregnant woman with cervical cancer may be incompatible with the continuation of pregnancy since removal of the uterus and radiation both require ending foetal life.

4. *Legal Aspects*

Critical to legality is the meaning of the language in the local legislation. This makes a person punishable who 'unlawfully' procures miscarriage. Widely followed court judgments have interpreted this language to show that there are circumstances in which the procedure may be undertaken lawfully. It is widely accepted that abortion is lawful when undertaken to save a pregnant woman's life. A leading judgment has further explained that saving 'life' includes not simply the fact of life, but also the quality of life, meaning physical and mental health, when pregnancy would cause it to be seriously and enduringly impaired.[12] Accordingly, courts interpreting this legislation may consider abortion lawful when undertaken to preserve a woman's health from prolonged, serious impairment.

A governing principle of criminal law is that, when the meaning or scope of the law is uncertain, it is to be interpreted in favour of a defendant. If the assessment of the woman's health condition and prognosis is made in good faith, confirmed perhaps by a concurrent second opinion, and acted upon non-secretively, the latitude of the law should protect the woman's request and the doctor's compliance. This might be equally so even if the word 'unlawfully' was not explicit in the legislation, because a court would be likely to find it implicit. Courts occasionally read legislation restrictively so as to minimize protections it affords criminal suspects, but are disinclined to do so when there is liability to heavy punishment.

Many court systems decline to give rulings on hypothetical facts, but require an actual dispute, so that it may not be possible to find in advance whether abortion governed by law of uncertain effect would be lawful in the circumstances of a certain case. It may be possible to initiate a dispute by seeking

---

[12] *R. v. Bourne*, [1939] 1 KB 687 (Central Criminal Court, London, England).

a judicial declaration, in an action against a government officer such as a Minister of Justice, or of Health, that the procedure requested would be lawful. However, it may be impossible to obtain such a ruling to accommodate Mrs R's request within the first trimester of her pregnancy. Prevailing uncertainty of the law's meaning therefore presents the doctor with the dilemma of either refusing a woman's legitimate request, and thereby risking her health, or complying with it and risking prosecution and conviction. That is, the doctor's legal, and ethical, choice is between serving this patient's needs or the physician's interests in remaining available for serving future patients.

5. *Human Rights Aspects*

National courts and international human rights tribunals considering women's claims to safe abortion have increasingly applied certain human rights provisions. International tribunals draw on an expanding body of decisions based on international human rights conventions, and national courts also draw on these, often to reinforce provisions in their own national laws, including constitutional laws. In addition, agencies that monitor international human rights conventions have become increasingly critical of countries whose restrictive laws, and restrictive enforcement of laws that could be interpreted more generously to women's interests, result in women's deaths and injuries to health resulting from unsafe pregnancies or abortions. The common theme in these human rights applications is that women's decisions to terminate unplanned and otherwise inappropriate pregnancies are not to be regarded as criminal defiance of laws, but as conscientious decisions made in the best interests of their own lives and health, and those of their families, that women should be allowed to make.

The human rights involved include women's rights to life not only against the significant threat of maternal mortality, but against conscientious resort to unskilled means of reproductive self-determination, and related rights to security and liberty of their persons. Depending on the level of state repression of women's choice, rights to be free from inhuman and degrading treatment may be involved, and even without repression, women's rights to private life and family life are necessarily implicated. Further, since men are free to have recourse to medical means to advance important interests in their lives, but women are denied this right to terminate inappropriate pregnancies, rights to sexual non-discrimination in access to health care are implicated. The human rights movement has been inspired by recognition that individuals should be free to make critical decisions in their lives by their own choice, and are not involuntarily at the disposal of governmental or religious policies or purposes. Nevertheless, human rights outrages are amplified when state laws and governments deny women safe abortion services when they are victims of rape and comparable sexual abuse.

As against the trend in favour of women's rights to free choice of maternity are constitutional court decisions and amendments to national constitutions that protect life from the moment of conception. These provisions are rarely written in absolute terms, since the same constitutions also claim to protect the lives, health, and dignity of all persons, including women. As a result, it is not clear whether these provisions prevail over women's rights to life, security, and liberty of the person, rights to private and family life, and to sexual non-discrimination in access to health services. It is also not clear whether provisions on respect for prenatal interests are intended only to prohibit abortions or would be applied consistently with women's rights to give birth to wanted children by requiring governments to provide more adequate prenatal services or emergency obstetric care to ensure safe delivery. Some governments invoking constitutional provisions to deny lawful abortion fail to provide women with prenatal care that evidences the entitlement to protection that governments claim to attribute to foetal life.

Human rights treaty bodies are increasingly concerned with high rates of preventable maternal death, and are characterizing governmental failures to address pregnancy related death as violations of women's rights to life.[13] Such bodies are additionally critical of national laws that are interpreted and applied to deny lawful abortion in cases of rape and sexual violence, finding that they amount to inhuman and degrading treatment of women.[14] The term 'forced pregnancy' has emerged as a way of describing how women view the denial of abortion services, equating such denial to the outrage of rape. Forced pregnancy was condemned by governments at the Beijing Fourth World Conference on Women as a violation of women's rights.[15] The Committee on the Elimination of Discrimination against Women (CEDAW) has issued a General Recommendation on Women and Health that addresses the discriminatory dimensions of denial of abortion by observing that: 'It is discriminatory for a State party to refuse to legally provide for the performance of certain reproductive health services for women' (see Pt. III, Ch. 6, Sect. 2, para. 11) and that the obligation to respect women's right to health requires that States

[13] UN, Report of the Committee on the Elimination of Discrimination against Women, 16th Session, Concluding Observations on the Report of Morocco (New York: UN, 1997), paras. 68 and 78, Doc A/52/38/Rev 0.1. Available at http://www.unhchr.ch/tbs/doc.nsf/(Symbol)/17345aada861de818025649d00322a05?Opendocument, last accessed 2 May 2002.

[14] UN, *High Commission for Human Rights, Concluding Observations on the Report of Peru* (New York: UN, 1995), paras. 15 and 22, CCPR/C/79/Add 0.72, available at http://www.unhchr.ch/tbs/doc.nsf/(Symbol)/6f1b83cb65d8071cc12563f400376673?Opendocument, last accessed 2 May 2002.

[15] UN, Department of Public Information, *Platform for Action and Beijing Declaration. Fourth World Conference on Women, Beijing, China, 4–15 September 1995* (New York: UN, 1995), paras. 114, 132, 135.

parties remove barriers to women's access to appropriate health care, which include laws that criminalize medical procedures only needed by women (see Pt. III, Ch. 6, Sect. 2, para. 14).

6. *Approaches*

6.1. *Clinical duty*

If Dr T determines that termination of pregnancy is in the patient's best health interests, and the best interests of her family, the law presents the challenge to conscience and courage of deciding whether to undertake the procedure. If Dr T conscientiously finds that continuation of pregnancy would endanger the patient's life, termination of her pregnancy would be non-contentious. However, if it is determined that the patient would most probably survive pregnancy but suffer seriously diminished health, Dr T must consider whether compliance with the law requires her to bear that consequence.

Codes of professional ethics usually provide that a conscientious physician will put the interests of a patient above those of the attending physician. However, other patients in addition to Mrs R may depend on Dr T's availability for their care. Dr T may legitimately consider that their interests also weigh in the balance, and would be prejudiced by Dr T's involvement in legal proceedings and imprisonment. Accordingly, the clinical response to Mrs R's request could be governed by non-clinical considerations unrelated to her care, including Dr T's confidence in legal advice on how broadly the local legislation is interpreted.

If Dr T decides to proceed with the termination of pregnancy, clinical guidelines on care of women requesting abortion might be useful in determining pre-abortion management and which procedures are appropriate for a woman in Mrs R's circumstances.[16] If no clinical guidelines exist in Dr T's country, Dr T might want to work with his or her professional colleagues on steps to develop them.

6.2. *Health care systems obligations*

Dr T may legitimately protest that uncertainty in the law should not distort professional capacity to exercise conscientious medical judgement in patients' health interests. Dr T might collaborate with professional, governmental, and

---

[16] See e.g. Royal College of Obstetrics and Gynaecologists (RCOG), *The Care of Women Requesting Induced Abortion: Evidence-Based Guideline No. 7* (London: RCOG, 2000). Available at http://www.rcog.org.uk/guidelines.asp?PageID=108&GuidelineID=31, last accessed 6 May 2002. National Abortion Federation, *Clinical Policy Guidelines* (Washington, DC: National Abortion Federation, 2002). Available at http://www.guidelines.gov, last accessed 7 Aug. 2002.

non-governmental agencies to provide technical and policy guidance for health systems.[17]

Clarification of the law might be needed to ensure that health care professionals can readily respond to the needs of patients, such as Mrs R, in accordance with the ethics of medical and related care. Dr T should face no conflict between serving the needs of one patient, such as Mrs R, and remaining at liberty to serve the interests of other patients. Similarly, Dr T should be free to render conscientious services to all patients without distraction by fear of legal proceedings or detention.

Through collective professional action, Dr T might join with colleagues to seek clarification of the law so as to enable health care providers to serve the health care needs of their community. A collective request may be made, perhaps through a general or specialized medical body, to the government's Minister of Justice, Attorney-General, or for instance Minister of Health, for clarification of the scope of the law. If the need for greater clarity remains unsatisfied, the medical body itself may set a protocol governing conditions in which abortion will be undertaken, and ask for a response from the government's chief legal officer.

If there is no adequate response within a predetermined time, the medical body, or an individual physician such as Dr T, may seek to initiate judicial proceedings against the government. These proceedings might seek a declaration that the legislation allows termination of pregnancy for preservation of women's lives, or of their health when medically considered to be in danger. Alternatively, a declaration might be sought that the legislation is void for vagueness, thus infringing upon the doctor's duty to provide necessary health services. They might also seek a declaration that the legislation violates women's human rights, including their right to life, their right to security and liberty of their person, their right to be free from inhuman and degrading treatment, and their right to sexual non-discrimination in access to health care.

6.3. *Social action for underlying conditions*

Abortion laws have historically been expressed only in prohibitive terms because they were designed against a background of unskilled and harmful practice, and were often reinforced by a religiously inspired moral agenda. Politicians, courts of law, social leaders, journalists, and others can be given case studies, perhaps modelled on the circumstances of Mrs R related anonymously, to demonstrate the need for clarification of laws in order to ensure access to services to which women are legally entitled.

There is a need for doctors, perhaps through their societies of obstetricians/ gynaecologists, to enter into a constructive dialogue with the legal profession

---

[17]   WHO, *Safe Abortion: Technical and Policy Guidance for Health Systems* (Geneva: WHO, 2002).

and other groups, including women's health advocates, to clarify the circumstances when abortion may not be against the law. This might include outlining the kinds of conditions that put a pregnant woman's life in danger or would damage her health. The indications for therapeutic abortion constitute a long list in textbooks of obstetrics and gynaecology and include certain diseases of almost all body systems, which may be aggravated by the pregnant condition and put the health or life of the pregnant woman at risk. They also include certain congenital anomalies of the foetus. Such conditions might vary in prevalence from country to country, and some may need to be clarified in a dialogue between the medical and legal professions. Some societies, for example, have been able to reach agreements with governments to clarify the fact that the life-saving indication for abortion would permit providing abortions to women with HIV/AIDS.

The World Health Organization/International Federation of Gynecology and Obstetrics (WHO/FIGO) Task Force, in collaboration with Centro de Pesquisas das Doencas Materno-Infantis de Campinas/Universidade Estadual de Campinas, convened a workshop in Campinas, São Paulo, Brazil, on the topic of 'Abortion—a Professional Responsibility for Obstetricians and Gynecologists'. The workshop highlighted that, although laws may differ, medical communities and societies in general in countries share a common handicap: lack of knowledge of the legislation. As a consequence, laws are not being applied to the extent they could be to benefit the health of women. The workshop recommended that societies of gynaecology and obstetrics

inform professionals on the legal status of abortion in the country, the procedures to be followed for a legal abortion, the interpretation of the laws being applied, and also on appropriate international legislation, and the impact of these legal contexts on maternal morbidity and mortality;

establish norms for performing abortions permitted by law, so that health care providers feel supported and authorized to carry out the procedure within the law. These norms should be the result of informed discussions of multidisciplinary teams including lawyers;

stimulate the establishment of legal abortion care services in university hospitals and other centers of excellence, as many of them have adequate technical-professional capacity and are responsible for training the new generation of health professionals; [and]

lead in the implementation of legal abortion care services in each hospital, and stimulate a wide discussion, including all the professionals who will be directly or indirectly involved in the legal abortion care process. Social scientists and representatives of women's groups should also participate in this process to present the user's point of view.[18]

---

[18] WHO/FIGO Task Force, *Abortion—A Professional Responsibility for Obstetricians and Gynecologists. Report of the WHO/FIGO Task Force, Campinas (Brazil) Workshop, 2–5 March 1997* (London: FIGO, 1997).

11

Prenatal and Pre-Implantation Genetic Diagnosis for Risk of Dysgenic Inheritance

Case Study

The second child of Mr and Mrs J, a son, died two years ago of Tay-Sachs disease. They inform Dr K, who works in a reasonably well-equipped modern facility, that they would like to have another child, but only if it will be certain not to inherit that condition, and ask Dr K for advice. What should Dr K advise, in light of relevant medical, ethical, legal, and human rights factors?

1. *Background*

The advances in our understanding of genetics, and the successful deciphering of the human genome, have opened a new chapter in medicine. With better understanding of the genetic basis of disease, there will be better possibilities for prevention, early detection, diagnosis, and therapy. This scientific breakthrough raises ethical, legal, human rights, and social implications. Tay-Sachs disease is a case in point.

Tay-Sachs disease is the most well-known Jewish genetic disease, potentially affecting one in every 2,500 Ashkenazi Jewish newborns. The disease is inherited in an autosomal recessive manner. The mutant gene has been located on chromosome number 15, and several specific mutations have been identified. A newborn has to have the mutant gene from both parents in order to have the disease. If the newborn inherits the mutant gene from only one parent, s/he becomes only a carrier of the disease. For each 'carrier couple', there is a one in four chance in each pregnancy to have an affected child. There is a one in two chance for the baby to be a carrier, and a one in four chance to be free of the mutant gene.[1]

---

[1] National Foundation for Jewish Genetic Diseases, *Tay Sachs Disease* (New York: National Foundation for Jewish Genetic Diseases, 2001), available at http://www.nfjgd.org/FactSheets/taysachs.htm, last accessed 2 May 2002; National Institute of Neurological Disorders and Stroke (NINDS), *Tay-Sachs Disease Information Page* (Bethesda, Md.: National Institute of Neurological Disorders and Stroke, 2001), available at http://www.ninds.nih.gov/health_and_medical/disorders/taysachs_doc.htm, last accessed 3 May 2002.

2. Medical Aspects

There are two forms of Tay-Sachs disease: the well-known infantile-onset form, and the more rare late-onset or adult form. The disease is an inherited metabolic disorder. The basic defect is the deficiency of the enzyme hexosaminidase A. The function of this enzyme is to break down a naturally occurring fatty substance called GM2-ganglioside. Gangliosides are made and biodegraded rapidly in early life as the brain develops. Deficiency of the enzyme leads to toxic accumulation in the cells of the nervous system. The condition progresses rapidly. Affected children become totally debilitated by 2–5 years of life. They become blind, deaf, and unable to swallow. Paralysis sets in, and epileptic seizures may occur. Presently there is no treatment for Tay-Sachs disease. Children usually die by age 5. Research, at an early stage, is ongoing for delivery of the corrective enzyme and the normal gene to the brain of a patient.[2]

The newborn child develops normally, with no evidence of the disease for the first few months. An early sign of the disease is an abnormal cherry red spot in the retina of the eye observed only by the use of an ophthalmoscope.

The carrier status can be identified by measurement of the enzyme hexosaminidase A activity in plasma or white blood cells, and can be confirmed by performing gene mutation analysis. The ability of screening programmes to identify carriers opens the way for possibilities to prevent the disease, for example by choice of a partner who is not a carrier. If the couple are carriers, they can resort to *in vitro* fertilization and pre-implantation genetic diagnosis. Alternatively, prenatal diagnosis is quite reliable, by performing either chorionic villus sampling early in the first trimester, or amniocentesis in the second trimester. If the foetus is affected, abortion is an option.

3. Ethical Aspects

In their intention not to take the risk of another child of theirs inheriting Tay-Sachs disease, Mr and Mrs J are ethically pursuing the principle of non-maleficence. However, ethical responses to their request for advice may present Dr K with some challenges, depending on the cultural background of the couple and Dr K, the resources of the facility, and local law. There can be no certainty that a child a couple conceives will not suffer an adverse genetic inheritance, but Dr K must inform them that the risk can be minimized. The least positive response Dr K can make is that Mr and Mrs J seek to avoid

[2] Ibid.

conception by contraceptive practice, and terminate any accidental pregnancy if local law, and their own values, permit. Other responses, if the couple's religious faith allows them, include seeking to adopt a child to which neither of them has a genetic link, and seeking to have Mrs J's child through a suitably screened sperm donor.

Risk of the genetic child of them both being born with the condition can be reduced by them undertaking normal conception, and obtaining prenatal diagnosis to determine the child's status. If it has the disease, termination of pregnancy may be conducted if local law allows and the couple finds this ethically acceptable. If Dr K objects to conducting a procedure the couple wants, their ethical (and legal) entitlement is that they be referred to another physician known not to object. If local technology allows the procedures, and the couple can and agree to cover the financial costs, the couple can also contribute gametes for *in vitro* fertilization (IVF) and pre-implantation genetic diagnosis (PGD) of resulting embryos, followed by attempted implantation of one or more not at risk of inheritance of the disease. This has the advantage of making abortion unnecessary, but will be expensive, uncertain as to outcome, including of successful IVF, conception of an unaffected embryo and successful implantation, and may waste any surplus embryos.

Dr K should conduct general discussion with the couple in order to determine the range of options that the couple finds ethically and financially acceptable. Among that range, Dr K must inform the couple of those that Dr K's facility can undertake, and where other acceptable options are accessible to them.

4. *Legal Aspects*

In law, physicians are not taken to guarantee or underwrite a prognosis or diagnosis, so Dr K incurs no risk of legal liability in diagnosing Mr and Mrs J, or in assessing their potential for conception of an unaffected child. This is provided Dr K does not give any specific guarantees of successful results and is not negligent in falling below the legally required standard of care. The standard applies to both conducting diagnostic and other procedures, and giving Mr and Mrs K the information they require for decision-making, including regarding natural and artificial conception and their practical and financial access to their options.

Where local legislation or binding judgments require Dr K to observe particular prohibitions, procedures, or, for instance, statistical or other reporting responsibilities, they must be followed. These may concern such matters as a maximum number of embryos created *in vitro* that may be placed *in utero* in a single cycle of treatment, disposal of preserved embryos, and informing a monitoring agency of treatments undertaken and their outcomes. Compliance with legal rules does not preclude the legal capacity to contest their authority on grounds, for instance, of violation of constitutional, human rights or other legal guarantees. Laws on termination of pregnancy must be observed, although when restrictive these often permit abortion for serious foetal impairments. Tay-Sachs disease is considered to be a serious disorder, although carrier status is not. Genetic diagnosis of an *in vitro* or *in utero* embryo or of a foetus will disclose its sex, and where patients have legal rights to inspect or gain information in their medical records, there may be no legal basis on which to deny them this information.

Should Mr and Mrs J conceive and give birth to an affected child, by natural or medically assisted conception, when exercising their choice based on advice and services that conform to legal requirements, neither they nor the child will have a legal claim against Dr K or others. Similarly, the child will have no legal claim against the parents, since they have a transcending legal right of parenthood. If legally substandard advice or services were given, however, the parents will usually be entitled to legal remedies, although jurisdictions differ on the financial and emotional costs that justify compensation. Whether a born child can recover compensation is more doubtful, since negligence did not cause its disease and the claim that he should not have been conceived or born is considered a 'wrongful life' claim, which several laws and courts have ruled should not be compensated, as a matter of public policy.

5. *Human Rights Aspects*

The most obvious human right implicated in access to IVF and PGD is the right to the benefits of scientific progress. This right serves goals, however, of other human rights such as the right to found a family and the right of a future child and of the parents themselves to the highest attainable standard of health; the right to health of the child would primarily concern its physical health, while the right to health of the parents would involve their rights to mental and social well-being. Observance of the rights of Mr and Mrs J and any future child would not compromise the right of Dr K to religious conscience, because the doctor would have to refer the couple to other practitioners if finding IVF, PGD, abortion, or subsequent embryo wastage through non-implantation conscientiously objectionable.

Many if not all of these procedures may not be funded by public health insurance programmes, and Mr and Mrs J may sense discrimination if people of means can avail themselves of these technologies while their income and resources place the use of such technologies beyond the couple's means. National courts have established limits on governmental duties to allocate costly care for purposes even of preserving human life,[3] and courts in affluent countries usually decline to require state-funded health services to cover high costs to address reproductive health impairments that are not life endangering.[4] The international human rights movement is moving towards recognition of the collective rights of impoverished populations, and towards narrowing the resource gap between developing and developed countries, but this has not been applied to address gaps between affluent and impoverished families at national levels. Accordingly, although Mr and Mrs J may be outraged and anguished that their limited resources preclude their access to reproductive technologies that would afford them the best chance to have a healthy infant, their distress on this ground does not necessarily constitute a human rights violation. Reproductive health falls within the right to health protected by many national constitutions and Article 12 of the International Covenant on Economic, Social and Cultural Rights (the Economic Covenant), but currently exists more as a negative than a positive right, so that reproductive technologies do not compel public funding.

6. *Approaches*

6.1. *Clinical duty*

The duties that Dr K bears, to gather genetic and personal information of patients, to advise them on medical options and their implications, and to provide approved procedures with legally required competence, must be directed to the disease in issue and its prevention in a future child, but are not otherwise distinctive. The distinguishing feature of Dr K's clinical duty may be that the patients' theoretical options for achieving their goal through advanced technologies are unavailable in practice.

If unavailability is due to lack of equipment, personnel, or other clinic resources, Dr K should make reasonable enquiries to inform the patients if they are accessible elsewhere. If unavailability is due to the patients' inadequate means to meet the costs, Dr K should be cautious in order not to distress them by tantalizing them with options of which they cannot avail themselves. That is, Dr K's duty to provide material information should be catered to options that are within patients' reasonable access. In order not to be paternalistic, Dr K may risk erring on the side of overinforming rather than underinforming, since the couple may be willing to make sacrifices Dr K does not

---

[3] *Soobramoney v. The Minister of Health, Kwazulu Natal*, 1998 (1) SA 776 (Constitutional Court of South Africa).

[4] *Cameron v. Nova Scotia (Attorney General)* (1999), 177 DLR (4th) 611 (Nova Scotia Court of Appeal).

consider possible or reasonable. There is no duty, however, to provide information of options in distant countries, or of unproven possibilities available only at immense cost, to which the patients have no practicable access, since that information, though of interest, is not material to the autonomous choices they can make.

6.2. *Health care systems obligations*

Publicly funded health care systems have tended to give low priority to services to overcome genetic hazards in reproduction by promoting births of unaffected children. There may be preventive programmes to promote, for instance, women's ingestion of sources of folic acid, and in some more developed countries, prenatal diagnosis of affected foetuses to facilitate lawful abortion. This may directly assist Mr and Mrs J, in that they may initiate normal pregnancy, when Mrs J may have prenatal genetic diagnosis such as by amniocentesis, and terminate an affected pregnancy. Mrs J has a relatively high percentage chance of conceiving an unaffected foetus, and her access to abortion is often considered macroethically tolerable, since it leads to children being conceived and born who otherwise would not be. The governmental inspiration of such programmes may be, however, their reduction of births of impaired children it will be costly for health care and social welfare systems to maintain.

The more costly assisted reproductive technologies tend to rank as 'luxury medicine'. Health care systems should therefore consider the proportion of scarce medical skills and resources they want to go to private services. They can increase the proportion by public-sector rationing of access to opportunities, and attempt to decrease it by inducement to practitioners to join public services or, more coercively, by licensing and other restraints on private services.

6.3. *Social action for underlying conditions*

It is not clear how the conditions underlying the couple's risk of adverse genetic transmission can be relieved. They are not infertile, but affected by a natural condition not itself amenable to therapy. Where particular genetic conditions affect a self-defining community, whose members identify themselves with each other, such as Tay-Sachs disease which disproportionately affects Ashkenazi Jewish communities, voluntary genetic testing may be made available in some communities to couples considering marriage, in order for them to anticipate reproductive implications. As genetic understanding expands, and individuals become more accustomed to management of their genetic characteristics and disabilities, impacts on prospective children may be factored into individuals' intentions for founding of their families. Similarly, with better communal education, innate genetic conditions may be less stigmatizing of affected individuals. Effective gene therapy appears too remote at present, but may offer some relief in time. While such developments are slow, however, the concern of Mr and Mrs J may be considered an individual misfortune to be addressed at a family rather than a communal or social level.

12

Sex-Selection Abortion

Case Study

Mrs M, a 34-year-old mother of three daughters aged 12, 10, and 5, lives in a modest home on the outskirts of a large city with her 40-year-old husband. He is often unemployed and in poor health. Mrs M is healthy enough to do part time work to support the older girls' schooling. The home has a small plot of land where vegetables are grown and a few chickens are kept. Mr and Mrs M strongly feel they need a son for support in old age. Mrs M's health and the family's poor economic circumstances convince the couple that she should not have more than one additional child. Health services are available at low cost at the local public hospital, where Mrs M arrives when she is about ten weeks pregnant. The law is liberal about abortion on socio-economic grounds. Mrs M asks Dr B whether she can have a test to determine if the foetus is male or female. Mrs M says that she would be willing to continue the pregnancy only if she would have a son. What responsibilities does Dr B have in this case, taking account of the key medical, ethical, legal, and human rights principles?

1. *Background*

Son preference is deeply seated in many cultures. A proverb from ancient China states that 'eighteen goddess-like daughters are not equal to one son with a hump'. This son preference is coupled with under-estimating the worth of the girl child. Son preference is manifested by a differential access to health care, an unequal share of nutrition from the small family plot, and possibly shorter durations of breastfeeding. The International Conference on Population and Development, convened in Cairo in September 1994, urged that 'leaders at all levels of the society must speak out and act forcefully against patterns of discrimination within the family, based on preference for sons'.[1]

---

[1] Cairo Programme, para. 4.17, 4.23.3.

The ancient practice of female infanticide has not been completely abolished. It has been brought earlier with the utilization of new 'medical' technologies for the selective abortion of the female foetus. Ultrasound, amniocentesis, and chorionic villus sampling have been abused for this purpose. Figures from China and South Korea about the trends in sex ratio at birth show how the ratio can be skewed with the use of selective abortion. For all births, there were 113 males for every 100 females. The figures are more striking when one looks at birth order. For the fourth child in Korea, there were two males born for every female; for China, the sex ratio was 130:100.[2]

In India, the sex bias against female children has contributed to India's declining proportion of females to males; the ratio dropped from 935:1,000 in 1981 to 927:1,000 in 1991.[3] Despite a 1994 law banning abuse of sex selection techniques in India,[4] the practice seems to have continued unabated. The latest census of India has put the national sex ratio as 933 females to 1,000 males. In the age group of 0–6 years, it was 927 females to 1,000 males. In the northern state of Haryana, the declining sex ratio is 861 girls to 1,000 boys, while in the neighbouring Punjab it is 874 females to 1,000 males. In the age group 0–6 years, the imbalance in the sex ratio is even more exaggerated. Haryana has 820 females per 1,000 males, while Punjab has 793 females.[5] In certain communities in the northern states of Bihar and Rajasthan the ratio has plummeted to 600:1,000, one of the lowest in the world.

2. *Medical Aspects*

Prenatal tests developed to detect abnormalities in the foetus have been misused as foetal sex tests. The procedures commonly used are referred to as amniocentesis, chorionic villus sampling, and ultrasound diagnosis. In amniocentesis, the doctor extracts cells from the amniotic fluid surrounding the foetus. It is normally performed when the pregnant uterus is accessible from the abdomen, commonly from the sixteenth to the seventeenth week. For chorionic villus sampling, the doctor uses a catheter inserted vaginally through the cervix to extract a few milligrams of placental tissue. It has the advantage

[2] Z. Yi, T. Ping, G. Baochang, X. Yi, L. Bohua, and L. Yongping, 'Causes and Implication of the Recent Increase in the Reported Sex Ratio at Birth in China', *Population and Development Review*, 19 (1993), 283–302.

[3] G. Mudur, 'Indian Medical Authorities Act on Antenatal Sex Selection', *British Medical Journal*, 319 (1999), 401.

[4] The Pre-natal Diagnostic Techniques (Regulation and Prevention of Misuse) Act, 1994, Indian Parliament Act No. 57 of 1994.

[5] Registrar General of India, *Provisional Population Totals, Census of India 2001* (New Delhi: Office of the Registrar General India, 2001). Available at http://www.censusindia.net/resultsmain. html, last accessed 25 Sept. 2002.

of being used at an earlier date in the pregnancy, but it carries more risk. Ultrasound diagnosis has the advantage of being non-invasive (done from the outside of the body) but it has the disadvantage of being accurate only later in the second trimester of pregnancy.

These tests are important in medical practice in providing valuable information about genetic abnormalities of the foetus. The diagnosis of foetal sex may be important if the genetic abnormality in question is sex-linked, that is it occurs only in males or females.

3. *Ethical Aspects*

The International Federation of Gynecology and Obstetrics (FIGO) Committee for the Ethical Aspects of Human Reproduction and Women's Health, in a 1994 Statement on Sex Selection, opened with the observation that 'The Committee deplored that deeply-rooted gender discrimination is still prevalent in many societies, and that selective abortion of the female fetus has recently emerged as another manifestation of this social injustice.'[6] There was disagreement, however, on the ethical response. Most Committee members adopted a macroethical perspective that addresses the social impact and significance of sex-based abortion, but others took the microethical approach of considering the burden that socially unfair attitudes, customs, and laws may have on families unable to influence repressive cultures.

The majority view, not distinguishing between male and female abortion, invoked the ethical principles of protection of the vulnerable and justice, concluding that 'no fetus should be sacrificed because of its sex alone'.[7] This left open ethical abortion of a foetus affected by a severe sex-linked genetic disorder, since the basis would then be severity of the disorder and not foetal sex alone. However, other committee members invoked the ethical principle of autonomy, which 'is violated by complete prohibition of sex selection abortion'.[8] The Committee also stated that preconceptional sex selection (if perfected and available) can be justified on medical grounds to avoid sex-linked genetic disorders, and can be justified on social grounds, in certain cases for the objective of allowing children of the two sexes to enjoy the love and care of parents. For this social indication to be justified, it must not conflict with other society values where it is practised.

---

[6] FIGO Committee for the Ethical Aspects of Human Reproduction and Women's Health, 'Sex Selection', in FIGO, *Recommendations on Ethical Issues in Obstetrics and Gynecology* (London: FIGO, 2000), 8. Available at http://www.figo.org/default.asp?id=6094, last accessed 2 May 2002.

[7] Ibid., para. 1.   [8] Ibid., para. 2.

The Ethics Committee of the American Society of Reproductive Medicine (formerly the American Fertility Society) maintains that couples should be free to use sex selection, but that providers should use 'moral suasion' to encourage couples to allow sex determination to be resolved by chance even when advanced reproductive technologies are used, and sex selection before pre-embryo transfer is therefore possible.[9] The Committee on Ethics of the American College of Obstetricians and Gynecologists (ACOG) accepts, as ethically permissible, the practice of sex selection to prevent sex-linked genetic disorders. The Committee opposes meeting requests for sex selection for personal and family reasons, due to the concern that such requests may ultimately support sexist practices.[10]

Many ethical statements on the issue lack a balance between a socially based and an individually based ethical approach. The former condemns abortion of foetuses simply because they are female as an offensive embodiment and perpetuation of women's inferiority to men, and a devaluation of the girl child. The latter, individually based approach is fearful of sacrificing a woman's autonomous choice because she is conditioned by cultural, economic, and legal influences she cannot quickly change. The former view is directed to social policy and legislative or regulatory reform, which has been achieved in some countries. The latter view is more engaged with the dilemma that doctors face. It concerns whether women may be allowed prenatal diagnosis of foetal sex, which is seen as potentially harmful and demeaning to womankind, and perhaps abort a female foetus, or be denied diagnosis, as an involuntary contribution to social equality of the sexes, and perhaps abort a male foetus.

The ethic of justice requires that circumstances that are significantly different not be treated without regard to that difference. In China, India, and many other countries, abortion of foetuses because of their sex has been common, but in other countries there is no marked preference leading to sex-based abortion. In Canada, for instance, a governmental Royal Commission of inquiry undertook a national survey of preferences regarding the sex of children. The Commission reported that 'The survey revealed that, contrary to what has been found in some other countries, a large majority of Canadians do not prefer children of one sex or the other. Many intervenors . . . assumed that Canadians have a pro-male bias with regard to family composition; we found that this assumption appears to be unfounded.'[11] Interest in prenatal sex

[9] American Fertility Society Ethics Committee, 'Ethical Considerations of Assisted Reproduction Technologies', *Fertil. Steril.* 62 (1994), 5(1 suppl.), 1S–126S.

[10] American College of Obstetricians and Gynecologists (ACOG) Committee on Ethics, 'Sex Selection. Committee Opinion Number 177, November 1996', in ACOG, *Ethics in Obstetrics and Gynecology* (Washington, DC: ACOG, 2002), 85–8; repr. in *Int. J. Gynecol. Obstet.* 56 (1997), 199–202.

[11] Royal Commission on New Reproductive Technologies, *Proceed with Care: Final Report of the Royal Commission* (Ottawa: Minister of Government Services Canada, 1993), 889.

determination was found to be very low, and concerned with family balancing. The Commission found that 'preferences were generally seen as unimportant, almost trivial. The survey showed that virtually all prospective parents want, and feel strongly about having, at least one child of each sex.'[12] In this environment of sex neutrality, where family balancing is strongly desired, application of severely restrictive policies on prenatal sex determination appears unnecessary, and therefore unjust and unethical.

4. *Legal Aspects*

The legal doctrine of informed consent to medical management may justify a woman's claim to information of the sex of the foetus she bears, when information is obtainable. However, the right to information relevant to medical choice of legally available care may go no further than to allow a woman to know whether her foetus is healthy or unhealthy, for genetic or congenital reasons. That is, a woman may have a legal right to information only of whether or not the foetus has a disorder, which, if it exists, may be sex-linked. As against this, however, many courts appear willing to hold that patients are entitled to inspect information in their medical records and to have their medical records interpreted to them, whether or not the contents may influence a future medical choice, because the information in their medical records is under their control and at their disposal.

Some countries have, or are considering introducing, laws to prohibit performance of the foetal sex test, unless it is indicated for the diagnosis of a severe sex-linked disorder, considerably more severe than carrier status. Such laws are designed to prevent women terminating pregnancies on grounds of foetal sex. It may be argued that these laws, though conscientiously intended to promote equality of children regardless of their sex, may violate human rights to receive and impart information. Human rights provisions, which have been amplified in judicial decisions on abortion, prohibit governments from controlling what individuals are allowed to know for fear that they may gain knowledge that inspires action of which governments disapprove.

This argument may not be valid, however, where the issue is not disclosure of available information, but performance of a medical test, often with an invasive procedure (if conducted early in pregnancy), for a non-medical indication. When ultrasound examination is performed later in pregnancy to assess the medical condition and well-being of the foetus, and if the sex of the foetus is apparent, it is current medical practice that this information is not withheld from the parents. Normally, however, this information becomes available in the third or late second trimester.

---

[12] Ibid. 890.

The Act passed by the legislature of India in 1994 bans sex determination, and imposes fines and imprisonment on doctors who reveal the sex of the foetus to parents. But there is consensus that the law has failed. Doctors and parents work in collusion, and sex determination involves only oral verdicts by doctors, such as by describing the foetus as 'he' or 'she' rather than, for instance, 'it'. Without written evidence of disclosure, law enforcement agencies cannot easily discharge the burden of proving beyond reasonable doubt that doctors provided prohibited information.

5. *Human Rights Aspects*

In common with ethical and legal aspects, human rights aspects of sex selection abortion show strong arguments both to permit and to prohibit this practice. The human rights most implicated to support legal and professional prohibition are based on the often justified perception that selection will prejudice births of girl children, and so violate the right to non-discrimination on grounds of sex. States' human rights duties for this purpose are contained principally in the Convention on the Elimination of All Forms of Discrimination against Women (the Women's Convention), Article 5(*a*) of which requires states to modify social and cultural patterns of conduct 'with a view to achieving the elimination of prejudices and customary . . . practices which are based on the idea of inferiority or the superiority of either of the sexes or on stereotyped roles for men and women'. The underlying cause of devaluation of girl children is often founded on economic burdens associated with their marriage, the dishonour that they risk their families by loss of virginity before marriage, their lack of employment and other economic opportunities to support elderly parents, and their departure from their families of birth on marriage. Many of such causes of devaluation are human rights violations in themselves.

To claim that prohibition of sex-based abortion is sufficient to remedy these human rights violations is unrealistic. Prohibition of sex-based abortion cannot serve as 'the tail that wags the dog'. On the contrary, reform of entrenched customs that prejudice economic and other capacities of women might so enhance the status of women that prejudice against girl children would be resolved. Even without reform of customs, gross imbalance in birth rates between male and female children might over a generation create a scarcity value in girl children as potential brides of sons and mothers of their children as to show prevailing sex-selection practices to be a short-lived phenomenon not justifying repressive laws.

The human rights arguments favouring tolerance of prenatal and pre-implantation sex diagnosis are comparable to human rights claims advanced in favour of a general right to choose whether or not to have an abortion. They are that individual women, who may already be oppressed by family and social cultures they are powerless to change, should not be burdened by continuation or initiation of pregnancies they do not want. Women are not the perpetrators of their devaluation, but the victims. Compelling their continuation of pregnancy risks further victimizing the victims, and an increase in female infanticide and death through neglect.

Modern human rights react against compulsion of women to maintain pregnancies against their free choice, and introduction of new barriers to women's reproductive choice run counter to this value. Reinforcing women's rights to select pregnancy continuation or termination are rights to found families of their choice, to information, and, for instance, to the benefits of scientific progress. Accordingly, the dilemma of sex-selection abortion is not soluble by a simple or direct application of a dominant human right. Although such abortion violates women's rights to non-discrimination, compulsion of women to continue pregnancies against their wishes is itself another instance of such discrimination. Approaches may be advanced through the application of human rights to advance the value of girl children in their families and communities to the same status as sons, so that the prejudice that results in sex-selection abortion of females disappears.

6. *Approaches*

6.1. *Clinical duty*

If local law, hospital regulations, or, for instance, Dr B's licensing authority so require, Dr B will have to inform Mrs M that prenatal diagnosis cannot be undertaken for the purpose only of telling her the sex of the foetus. Dr B should add that the 'sex test' cannot be performed unless a serious sex-linked genetic disorder is reasonably suspected.

If a test is indicated on suspicion of a sex-linked genetic disorder, Dr B may inform the patient whether the foetus is an affected foetus or if it is not, without distinguishing between a negative result showing a healthy male foetus and showing a female foetus. If the test result discloses the foetal sex, however, Dr B cannot deny the patient access to the information if she requests it. If the patient discovers that the foetus is female and requests abortion, Dr B cannot invoke conscientious objection to sex-based abortion to deny participation if willing to participate in abortions requested on other grounds.

If the local culture shows no preference for male children, and local law does not prohibit prenatal sex diagnosis, Dr B may grant the patient's request for testing in order to balance her family with children of both sexes, and follow her preference in light of the test result.

6.2. *Health care systems obligations*

Dr B should participate in information and education campaigns if they are needed to discourage the practice of sex-selection abortion. Professional societies have a duty to discourage the performance of the procedure, by persuasion or by disciplinary action, where sex-selection abortion is prevalent. If the local abortion law is liberal, however, the health care system will have to tackle the paradox that Mrs M may be able to terminate the pregnancy, for instance on socio-economic grounds, but not be encouraged to continue it by receiving information that the foetus is male, if it is shown to be.

In India, the Termination of Pregnancy Act, 1971, is relatively liberal. Nevertheless, the Indian Medical Association has recently circulated a set of directives to all its 1,700 branches across India asking doctors to stop offering sex determination services. Law enforcement agencies cannot easily act on complaints from individuals not involved in the sex determination procedure, but the Indian Supreme Court has directed federal and state governments to enforce prohibitive laws.[13] The Indian Medical Association announced that it will carry out independent investigations on the basis of even such 'third party' complaints. The Association has appealed to the Indian media to launch campaigns against female foeticide. The Medical Council has promised to revoke licences of doctors found guilty of wrongful disclosure of foetal sex. Social activists and legal experts, however, are sceptical that any short-term solutions will emerge while the social practices that led to preferences for sons remain. There is a feeling that this is a situation where there is social sanction to an outlawed practice. Until that situation changes, it will be difficult to convict doctors or parents.[14]

6.3. *Social action for underlying conditions*

None of the clinical or health systems approaches above addresses the background issue in the prevailing culture and/or law of Dr B's and Mrs M's community. This is that, if or when Mr M cannot support the family by working, or by farming the plot of land the family has, a son will be needed to support the parents, because none of the daughters can be relied upon for this purpose. The need is reinforced by laws of succession on death that preclude widows and daughters from land and perhaps other property inheritance. Where women suffer grossly disabling discrimination, having to abandon their parents on marriage and lacking means to support them by employment or property inheritance, a family's need for a son is clear. In non-discriminatory

---

[13] 'India to Crack Down on Sex Tests', *New York Times* (6 May 2001), sec. 1, p. 24.
[14] Mudur, 'Indian Medical Authorities'.

societies that lack government-sponsored social security systems, where daughters have the same economic, social, and other opportunities as sons, and the same responsibilities to their parents, the need to have a son is less pressing.

As an advocate for women's improved status in society, Dr B may demonstrate that laws or policies to prohibit sex-based abortion do not address the roots of the problem, and fail to remedy the injustice of pervasive discrimination against girl children and women.[15] The symbolism of the prohibitory gesture may be satisfying, but it may appear futile if it does not recognize that remedies to the injustice of women's inequality should be sought in other areas as well. When such remedies are achieved, future parents will not have the need for a son that Mr and Mrs M feel.

[15] B. M. Dickens, 'Can Sex Selection be Ethically Tolerated?' *Journal of Medical Ethics*, 28 (2002), 335–6 (Editorial).

13

Treating a Woman with Incomplete Abortion

Case Study

Mrs A, the 25-year-old mother of two children, is brought into the hospital emergency room suffering from bleeding from the vagina. On examination, she is diagnosed as having incomplete abortion. On questioning, Mrs A stated that the pregnancy was not wanted, but she did not admit that abortion was induced. Abortion is legally restricted in the country to conditions in which the life of the woman is endangered. Dr XY is brought in to care for Mrs A. How may Dr XY provide care, in accordance with medical, ethical, legal, and human rights considerations?

1. Background

Nature is very selective in establishing a pregnancy and in enabling it to continue.[1] It is estimated that 16 per cent of fertilized ova do not divide, 15 per cent are lost before implantation, and 27 per cent are lost during implantation. Approximately 50–75 per cent of pregnancies end in spontaneous abortion.[2] Most of these pregnancy losses are unrecognized because they occur before or at the time of the next expected menses. About 15 per cent of clinically recognized pregnancies are lost in the first trimester. An additional 5 per cent are lost in the second trimester.

Incomplete abortion is the situation when the abortion process has started spontaneously or has been induced, but the products of conception have not been completely expelled from the uterus. Abortion is only complete when the uterus has been completely emptied of all the products of conception. Until the abortion is complete, the woman continues to bleed, and the retained products of conception are liable to infection.

---

[1] M. F. Fathalla, *From Obstetrics and Gynecology to Women's Health: The Road Ahead* (New York and London: Parthenon, 1997).

[2] C. E. Boklage, 'Survival Probability of Human Conceptions from Fertilization to Term', *International Journal of Fertility*, 35 (1990), 75–94.

2. Medical Aspects

In a case of incomplete abortion, cramps are usually present but may not be severe; bleeding generally is persistent and is often severe enough to constitute life-threatening haemorrhage necessitating the need for blood transfusion and/or immediate surgical evacuation of the uterus to stop the bleeding. Sepsis may develop, particularly if the abortion has been induced under unsafe circumstances. Infection may spread to the pelvic structures, and septicemia may even develop. Anaerobic bacteria are frequently responsible and death may occur. Late sequelae include debility because of the blood loss, and consequences of infection including infertility.

Incomplete abortion is a clinically different condition from inevitable and missed abortion. Inevitable abortion is the term used to describe the condition in which the abortion process has already started with continuous and progressive dilatation of the cervix of the uterus, but without expulsion of the products of conception. Once the cervix has dilated and the process of inevitable abortion has started, nothing can be done medically to save the pregnancy. In order to protect the health and life of the woman, the practitioner must ensure that the contents of the uterus are completely evacuated. Otherwise the woman will continue to bleed, and the bleeding may be severe.

In missed abortion, the embryo or foetus dies *in utero* but the products of conception are still retained in the uterus. In order to protect the life and health of the woman, the practitioner must ensure that the process of expulsion of the dead embryo or foetus is not unduly delayed. There is a risk that fibrinogen levels in the blood may be depleted, interfering with the natural process of blood clotting, and can result in bleeding which is difficult to control. If the uterus is not evacuated once the diagnosis of missed abortion is made, fibrinogen levels in the blood should be monitored.

Incomplete, inevitable, and missed abortion can result from a spontaneous or induced abortion. All abortions not voluntarily induced are classified as spontaneous, even if an external cause such as trauma, accident, or disease is involved.[3] Induced abortion, in contrast to spontaneous abortion, is the deliberate termination of pregnancy before viability of the foetus. Where an induced abortion is performed by a trained provider, and in an adequate facility, it is usually completed in a safe and effective manner. Unsafe abortion, on the other hand, may be incomplete because, for example, products of conception might still remain in the uterus. It is not generally easy to decide whether an incomplete abortion is spontaneous or has been induced, unless the patient volunteers the information, or there are signs of interference, injury, or infection.

[3] E. Royston and S. Armstrong, *Preventing Maternal Death* (Geneva: WHO, 1989), 107.

3. *Ethical Aspects*

The primary motivation and vocation of medicine is to provide care to those in need with respect for their innate dignity. Accordingly, the ethical duty of beneficence that a doctor owes to a woman presenting with incomplete abortion is to provide medical care for her diagnosed condition, whatever its origins may have been. If the medically indicated care is safe completion of the diagnosed incomplete abortion, the ethical duty is to undertake completion and to ensure that this is done promptly, with appropriate safety and skill.

Questions regarding the legality of the woman's prior conduct are ethically as irrelevant to her care as are the reasons why, for instance, a patient with gunshot injuries was shot by a police officer. A professional physician must immediately treat the condition from which the patient suffers without regard to its legal, social, or other conditioning influences.

4. *Legal Aspects*

A country's abortion law, however framed, is not applicable to routine medical management of incomplete or inevitable spontaneous abortion. Health care professionals who deal with emergencies of this nature are not procuring abortion, and as a result are not regulated by the abortion law. In treating an incomplete abortion, they are treating an emergency condition. They have no right of conscientious objection to rendering due care indicated by the diagnosed emergency condition.

Treating such conditions is regulated like any other medical procedure. Accordingly, in treating incomplete abortions, practitioners have to meet the standard duty of care. If they refuse to deal properly with patients who present with this condition, they might well be liable for professional misconduct under the professional licensing code and be sanctioned accordingly. They might be liable for negligence through abandonment if the patient has been in their care for a period of time. Liability for negligence might also arise if the woman suffers from complications arising from the failure to treat, or for criminal negligence or manslaughter if the woman dies as a result of the failure to treat.

5. *Human Rights Aspects*

Since incomplete abortion presents a danger to women's lives, the human right to life compels health facilities to ensure prompt, proficient management of patients who present with this condition. Reinforcing the right to life are women's rights to security of the person, and to the highest attainable standard of health.

It is so self-evident from a human rights perspective that women presenting with the life-endangering emergency of incomplete abortion be appropriately treated, including with speed and efficiency, that governmental agencies responsible for protection of the health of the public come under severe scrutiny for their failures to make provisions. No religion objects to necessary treatment for this life and health endangering emergency, and health care practitioners have no grounds of conscientious objection to treatment. However, some governments, medical licensing authorities, and medical schools permit trainees with conscientious objections to performance of abortion to be trained and qualified to practise without knowledge of the process of abortion and management of induced abortion. This may leave them untrained and unprepared to manage incomplete abortion, whether of spontaneous or induced origin. Where training and skill are required to manage life and health endangering conditions affecting men, but not this condition affecting women, women's human rights to non-discrimination on grounds of sex are violated.

Further, women may risk exposure to the violation of suffering inhuman and degrading treatment if they are treated with suspicion and disrespect. Their right to security of the person is additionally jeopardized if local law or institutional or professional practice cause women presenting with incomplete abortion to be reported to police authorities on suspicion of involvement in unlawful behaviour.[4]

6. *Approaches*

6.1. *Clinical duty*

The distinction between spontaneous and incomplete abortion induced by unlawful means may not be self-evident. In either case, Dr XY is required to be non-judgemental in rendering prompt indicated medical care. For a physician to treat incomplete abortion by removal of the products of conception is lawful medical care, even when initiation of the abortion was by another's illegal act. If any illegality is attached to Mrs A's conduct, it does not implicate Dr XY. Any harmful distortion of Mrs A's indicated medical care that Dr XY were to introduce, such as delay in order to preserve evidence to assist a public prosecuting authority, would represent an unethical conflict of interest.

[4] *Insurralde, Mirta, Case T. 148 PS. 357/428.* Corte Suprema de la Provincia de Santa Fé, Argentina. 2 Aug. 1998; cited in B. M. Dickens and R. J. Cook, 'Law and Ethics in Conflict over Confidentiality?', *Int. J. Gynecol. Obstet.* 70 (2000), 385–91.

Moreover, refusal to treat an incomplete abortion is not protected by the right of conscientious objection.

A contemporaneous report in Mrs A's medical record following the medical care provided by Dr XY balances Mrs A's need of care against Dr XY's entitlement to security against suspicion of illegally initiating abortion. Any apprehension that Dr XY may have of becoming involved in completion of an unlawfully initiated procedure are ethically overcome by the writing of a reasonably contemporaneous report of Mrs A's presenting condition, its diagnosis, and delivery of an indicated treatment according to standard medical practice, with appropriate follow-up care.

Mrs A is entitled to treatment under the general conditions of medical confidentiality, so that no report of suspicions of illegal origins of the incomplete abortion should be volunteered to police or comparable authorities. If local legislation compels Dr XY to report such suspicions to law enforcement authorities, Dr XY should exercise greatest care against the risk to Mrs A of filing a report of mistaken suspicion. After providing Mrs A with indicated care, Dr XY may want to consult with colleagues about whether the circumstances fall within any legislated duty to report. In post-treatment discussion with Mrs A, Dr XY should enquire whether she practised contraception, and assist her with appropriate care.

6.2. *Health care systems obligations*

Dr XY does not practise in a vacuum, of course, and after providing the indicated care, Dr XY may reflect on how typical is Mrs A's case, how its occurrence can be prevented, and, for instance, how it is best managed. This raises issues of how well trained Dr XY is to deal with the case, and how well Dr XY trains junior colleagues and medical students in its management. Physicians have an ethical claim of conscientious objection to initiate any elective abortion, but cannot invoke this to refuse to be trained in or to undertake safe management of incomplete abortion, whether of spontaneous or induced origin.

Dr XY should be aware that hesitation in affording proper emergency care to Mrs A may harm not only her health, but also confidence among women who depend on the hospital for their own and their families' health care that they will be treated respectfully. Any intervention in the management of patients who suffer incomplete abortion that fractures the therapeutic relationship between patient and physician, such as police enquiries or legally mandatory reporting of possible criminal initiation of abortion, should be resisted.

Dr XY should act with colleagues, professional associations, and, for instance, governmental health authorities to explain that the physician's professional and social responsibility to patients in need cannot be discharged if a duty is imposed to become a police informant. Breach of confidentiality would inhibit patients from requesting medically necessary care, and impair their lives or health, and those of the children who depend on them. Mandatory reporting laws could be explained to be unethical in principle and dysfunctional in practice. In fact, the WHO/FIGO workshop in Campinas, Brazil, 1997, recommended the societies of gynaecology and obstetrics 'to advise their members to honour the code of professional ethics, observing medical confidentiality by not reporting women suspected of submitting themselves to any procedure for pregnancy termination'.[5]

6.3. *Social action for underlying conditions*

After Mrs A's condition has been treated, Dr XY should question whether she practised effective contraception, whether she was a victim of domestic or other sexual violence, and, for instance, whether she was eligible to terminate her pregnancy by lawful, safe means had she wished to do so. Answers to such questions should indicate what measures are appropriate to limit repetition of the emergency.

If women's lack of access to safe reproductive services was an aggravating factor in Mrs A's emergency, Dr XY should work with medical professional associations to develop treatment protocols or ethical and legal guidance for emergency responses to incomplete abortions. Legal guidance might be useful in clarifying the law for health care providers who are reluctant to treat incomplete abortions because they are intimidated by threats of sanctions or vigorous prosecution practices. Ethical guidance on the need to protect confidentiality to ensure respect for persons might be useful to health care providers if they are confused about whether they might be required to report suspected criminal activity. Such ethical guidance would also be useful support for health care providers in questioning 'laws and regulations, which force physicians to report women suspected of voluntary interruption of pregnancy, and require police presence in obstetric clinics and emergency services' as was encouraged by the WHO/FIGO Campinas workshop.[6]

---

[5] WHO/FIGO Task Force, *Abortion—A Professional Responsibility for Obstetricians and Gynecologists. Report of the WHO/FIGO Task Force, Campinas (Brazil) Workshop, 2–5 March 1997* (London: International Federation of Gynecology and Obstetrics, 1997), Recommendation 9.

[6] Ibid., Recommendation 8.

14

Confidentiality and Unsafe Abortion

Case Study

Three weeks ago in Dr G's public hospital department, Ms H was treated for serious injuries caused by unskilled abortion. Ms H came to Dr G's department from the hospital emergency department, where she had been admitted as an indigent (non-paying) patient unconscious and suffering heavy blood loss. When she regained consciousness under Dr G's care, she explained that she had sought abortion from a retired nurse she knew who occasionally helped women in difficulty. Ms H did not want to give her own full name for fear that she might lose her office cleaning job if her employer, a government agency, learned that she had obtained an abortion. Dr G treated Ms H as well as possible, but doubts that she will be able to bear a child in the future. Dr G has just been telephoned by a senior police officer to say that the officer wants to interview Dr G to find evidence against a resident of the area suspected of performing criminal abortions. The law has heavy penalties against abortion, and women are occasionally imprisoned for obtaining abortion. How should Dr G respond, in light of medical, ethical, legal, and human rights aspects of the case?

1. *Background*

It is estimated that between 36 million and 53 million induced abortions are performed in the world each year, an annual rate of 32 to 46 abortions per 1,000 women of reproductive age. Information on clandestine abortions is difficult to document. Combining various estimates yields an annual total of 15 million clandestine abortions. However, since these figures cannot be fully relied upon, the actual number may be as low as 10 million or as high as 22 million.[1] Contrary to common belief, most women seeking abortion are married or living in stable unions and already have several children. However, in all

---

[1] S. K. Henshaw, 'Induced Abortion: A World Review, 1990', *International Family Planning Perspectives*, 16 (1990), 59–65.

parts of the world, a small but increasing proportion of abortion seekers are unmarried adolescents; in some urban centres in Africa, they represent the majority.

Unsafe abortion and illegal abortion are not synonyms. Unsafe abortion is defined as a procedure for terminating an unwanted pregnancy performed either by persons lacking the necessary skills, or in an environment lacking minimal medical standards, or both.[2] Illegal abortion is terminating or attempting to terminate a pregnancy when it is against the law. Illegal abortion is commonly unsafe because it is performed in secret, and often by persons lacking the necessary skills or in an environment lacking the minimal standards of safe practice. In countries where abortion is illegal, physicians are usually not well trained to perform the procedure. This is, however, not always the case. In many countries where abortion is illegal, for example in Latin America, private physicians often perform safe abortions for relatively high medical fees, and the law is rarely enforced.

By the same token, not all legal abortions are safe. Medical graduating and licensing authorities may fail to ensure that practitioners have been adequately trained in initiating abortion and treating incomplete abortion. Some developing countries, for example India, have liberalized abortion law but their health care systems are inadequate to cope with the load of cases. Women in India who lack access to medically qualified providers of services have to go to medically unqualified abortionists lacking the skill and facilities to conduct safe procedures.

2. *Medical Aspects*

The moral and religious controversies about abortion tend to obscure its dimension as a clinical and public health problem. Where abortion is performed under safe conditions, the risk of the procedure is very low, averaging 0.6 deaths per 100,000 procedures.[3] When performed under unsafe conditions, the mortality can be as high as 1 in 150. Every year at least 70,000 women die from complications related to unsafe abortion, according to World Health Organization estimates. Worldwide, unsafe abortions account for 13 per cent of all maternal deaths, but in some countries up to 60 per cent of all maternal

---

[2] UN, *Population and Development*, i. *Programme of Action Adopted at the International Conference on Population and Development, Cairo, 5–13 September 1994* (New York: UN, Department for Economic and Social Information and Policy Analysis, ST/ESA/SER.A/149, 1994), n. 20, p. 85.

[3] WHO, *Unsafe Abortion—Global and Regional Estimates of Incidence of and Mortality Due to Unsafe Abortion with a Listing of Available Country Data* (Geneva: WHO, 3rd edn., 1997), 4. WHO/RHT/MSM/97.16.

deaths are due to unsafe abortion. These deaths represent only a fraction of the disease burden caused by unsafe abortion. Many more women survive, but suffer from acute and chronic morbidity. WHO estimates that more than half of the deaths caused by induced abortion occur in South and South-East Asia, followed by sub-Saharan Africa. WHO data show that the global case fatality rate associated with unsafe abortion is probably 700 times higher than the rate associated with legal induced abortion in the USA; in some regions it is well over 1,000 times higher. Even in developed regions, the fatality rate is eighty times higher for an unsafe abortion than for a legal abortion procedure (see Pt. I, Ch. 2, Sect. 8.3).

3. *Ethical Aspects*

Preservation of patients' confidentiality is a central principle of medical professionalism, with Hippocratic roots. Confidentiality is of major instrumental significance where sensitive issues of sexual and reproductive health arise, since sick and endangered people are liable to forgo necessary help rather than seek it from people and agencies that will not protect their identities and information. It is ethically objectionable that injured people can receive medical help only from people who are disposed or compelled to betray their confidentiality.[4] It is also ethically objectionable for a state to place health care providers in a conflict of interest in caring for patients by conscripting providers as police informants.

The ethical dilemma comes from the patient's disclosure of information that may identify an unskilled practitioner of unlawful abortion whose mistreatment has caused the patient considerable physical injury that is liable to have profound emotional or psychological repercussions for her, and that might have caused loss of her life. The ethical principles of beneficence, achieving the good of ending this person's misconduct, and of non-maleficence, avoiding the harm of shielding the person from discovery, seem to coincide in support of full collaboration in police enquiries.

Strongly and perhaps decisively countering the application of these principles at a macroethical or societal level is the microethical application of the autonomy principle. The patient wants skilled medical care with protection of her identity and confidentiality, and doctors cannot betray her expectations and expose her to the danger of prosecution and imprisonment. This would be an individual ethical wrong against the patient, and socially dysfunctional in deterring persons in need of help from seeking it, and deterring others capable

---

[4] B. M. Dickens and R. J. Cook, 'Law and Ethics in Conflict over Confidentiality?', *Int. J. Gynecol. Obstet.* 70 (2000), 385–91.

of leading persons in distress to sources of medical assistance from approaching hospitals.

4. *Legal Aspects*

Laws occasionally compel physicians to report suspected unlawful abortions, or to answer questions put to them in police enquiries with information of patients' identities. Such laws are ethically offensive and may be challenged, but cannot be ignored. Physicians have legal and ethical duties to be as protective of patients' identities as is possible, for instance by refusing disclosure of patients' identifiable information unless police obtain a judicially issued search warrant, and appealing against any that are judicially issued.

In most cases, there is no legal duty to report suspected crimes to police or other authorities, and questions police officers ask do not have to be answered in ways that violate confidentiality. Physicians and health care facilities must protect not only information of patients' medical conditions, but also the very identities of who their patients are. Refusal to provide patients' names or other identifying information to police officers does not constitute an offence of obstructing police officers in the execution of their duty. Their demands for access to documents must be supported by a judicially issued search warrant. A warrant cannot be comprehensive, allowing indiscriminate inspection of medical records, but must be specifically targeted to identifiable documents. However, police questions may voluntarily be answered as informatively as possible, provided that patient anonymity is preserved.

5. *Human Rights Aspects*

The human rights violations to which women are exposed in seeking care for injuries due to unskilled abortion stem primarily from the repressive nature of restrictive abortion laws. The claim that women would suffer no such violations if they complied with the law by not seeking illegal abortion ignores the common reality of human rights violations associated with legally compelled continuation of unwanted pregnancy, which is increasingly condemned as 'forced pregnancy'. Men are not legally compelled involuntarily to give the facilities of their bodies in the service of others, for instance as bone marrow or blood donors, and the legal requirement that women serve involuntarily for this purpose constitutes discrimination against women on grounds of sex.

Women's security of the person is violated not only because their pursuit of reproductive self-determination directs them to illegal practitioners, but also because their pursuit of conscientious goals in their lives may subject them to police investigations, court proceedings, and imprisonment. The denial of women's human rights to security of the person, to private life, and to freedom from the risk of inhuman and degrading treatment, is aggravated by women's pregnancies being caused by rape, other sexual violence, or exploitation, that they have no practical means to resist. Protection of women's human rights affords little scope for the enforcement of restrictive abortion laws. This is so, even if women are not liable to prosecution and imprisonment for involvement in illegal abortion when acting in pursuit of their interests in deciding whether, when, and in what circumstances to give birth to children. Their rights to pursue these interests are included within their right to reproductive health as protected by Article 12 of the Women's Convention.

6. *Approaches*

6.1. *Clinical duty*

The principal duty of Dr G is to the patient. If the police officer's questions concerning the suspected offender can be answered informatively without disclosure of Ms H's name or identifying details, they should be. However, Dr G's statement that an identified person performed an abortion on Dr G's patient is only hearsay, which many courts disallow prosecutors to introduce as evidence. Police may, therefore, insist on disclosure of patients' identities, in order to have them testify against alleged abortionists. Dr G is in no position to bargain for Ms H's immunity from prosecution in exchange for disclosure of her identity and her evidence, and should not attempt to do so. A lawyer instructed by Ms H may do this as part of 'plea bargaining', and prosecutors are often willing to assure immunity in exchange for a woman becoming a witness for the prosecution at an alleged abortionist's trial. Such an assurance cannot be guaranteed, however, and Dr G should not request it, nor give Ms H's name if it is offered. This is a matter for a lawyer acting on Ms H's behalf, and on her instruction, even though Ms H probably has no means to pay for legal services.

A consequence of Dr G telling the police officer that Dr G knows the name or identifying details of Ms H but will not disclose this information in questioning is that, if a trial proceeds on the basis of other police investigations, Dr G may receive a subpoena to attend the trial to testify regarding this information. The subpoena may be legally opposed, but cannot be ignored. If Dr G is called as a witness, questions are likely to be asked whose answers would reveal the name or identifying details of Ms H. Dr G should initially refuse to answer such questions, but request the trial judge to protect the patient's identity from disclosure, or at least to bar revelation in open court and in news media reports. Dr G is entitled to representation by a lawyer to protect Dr G from compulsion to violate a patient's confidentiality. If a medical defence association furnishes Dr G with a lawyer, that lawyer may also be able to represent the interests Ms H has in anonymity. Judges are frequently sympathetic to preservation of confidentiality, but Dr G must comply with any final judicial direction to give what is known of Ms H's name or identity.

6.2. *Health care systems obligations*

Medical librarians or record personnel may come under pressure to make medical information available to police, and may face threats of prosecution for obstructing police searches for evidence. There is usually no legal duty to collaborate in police investigations, however, and usually a duty not to if patients' medical confidentiality would be violated. Anonymous data can be given, and aggregated data can be publicized. For instance, it is appropriate for a facility to publicize the burden on its emergency and gynaecological services of unskilled abortion, and whether periodic rates are rising or falling. Personally identifying information can become available, however, only on presentation of a judicially approved search warrant, and any warrant issued can usually be appealed against to a higher court, by a lawyer instructed by a facility. Accordingly Dr G may inform the hospital medical record personnel of the pending police enquiries, and ensure that no identifying information is given without proper legal process.

The twenty-first special session of the United Nations General Assembly, in July 1999, approved the following key action: all governments and relevant intergovernmental and non-governmental organizations are urged to strengthen their commitment to women's health, to deal with the health impact of unsafe abortion as a major public health concern, and to reduce the recourse to abortion through expanded and improved family planning services.[5] In all cases, women should have access to quality services for the management of complications arising from abortion. Post-abortion counselling, education, and family planning services should be offered promptly, which will also help to avoid repeat abortions. Governments should take appropriate steps to help women avoid abortion, which in no case should be promoted as a method of family planning, and in all cases provide for the humane treatment and counselling of women who have recourse to abortion.

---

[5] UN, General Assembly, *Report of the Ad Hoc Committee of the Whole of the Twenty-First Special Session of the General Assembly: Overall Review and Appraisal of the Implementation of the Programme of Action of the International Conference on Population and Development*, A/S-21/5/ Add.1 (New York: UN, 1999).

6.3. *Social action for underlying conditions*

Women's resort to unskilled abortion practitioners is often an indicator of dysfunctional law. In many countries, restrictive abortion laws have been liberalized on the basis of narratives of experiences women have had to endure in order to achieve the reproductive freedom that human rights laws and conventions promise them. These real-life narratives, which tragically include real-death narratives, show the futility and dysfunction of repressive laws, including those under which women face imprisonment. Exposure to the actual consequences of repressive laws has moved some legislatures out of a 'crime and punishment' approach to abortion, and into a 'health and welfare' approach, particularly when the experiences concern women with whom legislators identify themselves, such as through their wives, daughters, and sisters.

Dr G may publicize anonymized case histories of patients, such as Ms H, and aggregated data of the prevalence of injuries due to unskilled abortion, to urge humanitarian laws and policies that would allow patients to achieve reproductive autonomy in safety and dignity. Similarly, Dr G may channel anonymized case histories through NGOs, particularly women's groups, to press governments and legislators for more humane, and more effective, laws, for instance on access to family planning services that reduce unplanned pregnancy and resort to abortion.

The International Federation of Gynecology and Obstetrics (FIGO) Committee for the Ethical Aspects of Human Reproduction and Women's Health recommended that 'after appropriate counselling, a woman had the right to have access to medical or surgical induced abortion, and that the health care service had an obligation to provide such services as safely as possible'.[6] The FIGO General Assembly in 2000 adopted the report of the Committee.[7]

---

[6] FIGO, 'Ethical Aspects of Induced Abortion for Non-Medical Reasons', in FIGO, *Recommendations on Ethical Issues in Obstetrics and Gynecology* (London: FIGO, 2000), 56–9 at 59. Available at http://www.figo.org/default.asp?id=6057, last accessed 2 May 2002.

[7] FIGO Committee for the Ethical Aspects of Human Reproduction and Women's Health, 'Ethical Aspects of Induced Abortion for Non-Medical Reasons', *Recommendations on Ethical Issues in Obstetrics and Gynecology* (London, FIGO 2000), 56–7, available at: www.figo.org/default.asp?id=/00000090.htm, last accessed 6 May 2002.

15

Domestic Violence

Case Study

In a prenatal examination of Mrs N, Dr O finds her to have chest and abdominal injuries that appear to have been caused by violence. Dr O asks Mrs N if she has been struck and she gives an evasive response, including an explanation of falling that is inconsistent with her injuries. Dr O knows of the high frequency of domestic violence in the community, and asks if her husband has attacked her. Mrs O replies that she does not want any investigations that may impair her husband from working, because the family, which includes three children, needs his income. What are the medical, ethical, legal, and human rights obligations of Dr O?

1. *Background*

The term 'violence against women' has been defined in the United Nations Declaration on the Elimination of Violence against Women, and adopted by the Fourth World Conference on Women in Beijing in its Platform for Action, as: 'any act of gender-based violence that results in, or is likely to result in, physical, sexual or psychological harm or suffering to women, including threats of such acts, coercion or arbitrary deprivation of liberty, whether occurring in public or private life'.[1] Accordingly, violence against women is understood to encompass, but is not limited to:

(a) physical, sexual and psychological violence occurring in the family, including battering, sexual abuse of female children in the household, dowry-related violence, marital rape, female genital mutilation and other traditional practices harmful to women, non-spousal violence, and violence related to exploitation;
(b) physical, sexual and psychological violence occurring within the general community, including rape, sexual abuse, sexual harassment and intimidation at

---

[1] UN, Declaration on Violence against Women, UN General Assembly Resolution, 48/104, 20 Dec. 1993. Art. 1.

work, in educational institutions and elsewhere, trafficking in women and forced prostitution;

(c) physical, sexual and psychological violence perpetrated or condoned by the State, wherever it occurs.[2]

The Report of the Fourth World Conference on Women states that 'in all societies, to a greater or lesser degree, women and girls are subjected to physical, sexual and psychological abuse that cuts across lines of income, class and culture'.[3]

The most pervasive form of gender violence is abuse of women by intimate male partners. Surveys now available from a wide range of countries show that between one-tenth to over one-half of women interviewed have been beaten by a male partner, the majority being beaten at least three times a year.[4] Intimate partner abuse, often referred to as domestic violence, wife beating, and wife battering, is usually part of a pattern of abusive behaviour and control, rather than an isolated act of violence, and is often associated with psychological abuse.

National reports show how societies have required women's social subordination and their subjection within their own homes in ways that conceal and so facilitate domestic violence, and what positive steps have been taken through the different social, health, and legal sectors to address domestic violence.[5]

2. Medical Aspects

Violence has serious adverse consequences for the physical, mental, and reproductive health of women, and can also have serious effects on the health of their infants and children (particularly when they are also victims, or in the case of children, witnesses). Violence against women in families does not abate during pregnancy. In fact, pregnancy makes women more vulnerable. Pregnant women may miscarry as a result of violence.

The most important consequence, and one that characterizes gender-based violence, is its impact on mental health.[6] This is particularly noticeable with sexual violence and domestic violence. Sexual violence violates the integrity of

---

[2] UN, Declaration on Violence against Women, UN General Assembly Resolution, 48/104, 20 Dec. 1993, Art. 2.

[3] UN, Department of Public Information, *Platform for Action and Beijing Declaration: Fourth World Conference on Women, Beijing, China, 4–15 September 1995* (New York: UN, 1995), para. 112.

[4] L. Heise, M. Ellsberg, and M. Gottemoeller, 'Ending Violence against Women', *Population Reports*, Series L (1999), 11.

[5] Asian Women's Fund, *Report of an Expert Meeting: Zero Tolerance for Domestic Violence* (Tokyo: Asian Women's Fund, 2001).

[6] WHO, *Women's Mental Health: An Evidence Based Review* (Geneva: WHO, 2000), part 4: Violence Against Women, WHO/MSD/MHP/00.1.

the female body. Domestic violence is a chronic and recurrent type of violence in the family. It has been rightly stated that wounds of the body heal sooner or later, leaving only scars, while wounds of the soul take much longer to heal and can bleed again at any time.

3. Ethical Aspects

It is evident that violence deliberately directed against anyone, other than in proportional self-defence, is always unethical, not just when directed against a person in her own home by a partner whose legal and moral duty is to defend her. The enormity of the outrage is even greater when she carries a child. The ethical violation offends against both aspects of the principle of respect for persons, in denying the person's autonomy and denying protection to both the vulnerable victim and an unborn child.

The ethical challenge in this case arises only from the victim's request that action not be taken against the suspected perpetrator, because of disadvantage the victim fears for herself and her dependent children. At the microethical level, between doctor and patient, the doctor may ethically defer to the patient's choice, even recognizing that it is not freely made. However, legislation or other compelling obligation may require the doctor to address the issue at a macroethical level, concerned with the prevention and abatement of domestic violence in the community in general. This level of approach may be appropriate if societies provide for victims' protection against consequent disadvantage to them of action taken against perpetrators of violence, for instance by provision of shelters and financial support, to make victims, including family members, domestically, economically, and otherwise independent of their abusers.

The FIGO Committee for the Ethical Aspects of Human Reproduction and Women's Health in their statement on violence against women, affirmed that

> [v]iolence against women is not acceptable whatever the setting and therefore physicians treating women are ethically obligated to:
> i.   Inform themselves about the manifestations of violence and recognize cases. Documentation must take into account the need for confidentiality to avoid potential harmful consequences for the woman, and this may need separate, non-identifiable compilation of data.
> ii.   Treat the physical and psychological results of the violence.
> iii. Affirm to their patients that violent acts towards them are not acceptable.
> iv.   Advocate for social infrastructures to provide women with the choice of seeking secure refuge and ongoing counselling.[7]

---

[7] FIGO, 'Violence against Women', in FIGO, *Recommendations on Ethical Issues in Obstetrics and Gynecology* (London: FIGO, 2000), 7–8, para. 2 at 7. Available at http://www.figo.org/default.asp?id=6115, last accessed 2 May 2002.

Research into the incidence, nature, gravity, and prevention of domestic violence may go beyond conventional medical research involving human subjects, raising ethical issues of social science and epidemiological research.[8] Pitched at the macroethical level, these studies may require compromises of confidentiality and, for instance, the consent of those whose behaviour and victimization is examined.[9]

4. *Legal Aspects*

Some countries impose legal duties on physicians to report suspected deliberate infliction of injuries, such as child abuse and, in a number of countries, abuse of elderly and mentally impaired persons. Where there is no mandatory reporting duty, however, physicians and other health care personnel have a legal discretion to report. Exercise of this discretion will be considered in law not to violate duties of confidentiality, provided that reports are made in good faith and with due care. For instance, reports should be made only to police or family welfare authorities that are equipped to respond to incidents or conditions of violence, and suspected perpetrators should be narrowly specified in order to leave innocent persons outside the net of reasonable suspicion. Police, child welfare, and comparable recipients of reports of abuse have a practice, upheld as lawful by the highest courts in several countries, of refusing to disclose informants' identities.[10] This protects informants from being disclosed as such, but at a cost of leaving both informants and non-informants liable to accusation by patients and their family members of violating information believed to be confidential.

Physicians' exercise of their lawful reporting discretion is subject to review by their licensing authorities and professional associations on grounds of professional ethics. The fact that patients have no remedies in courts of law against physicians who report confidential information does not preclude licensing authorities or professional associations, perhaps on patients' complaints, from considering whether the legal power to report has been properly exercised. For instance, negligently inappropriate reporting that exposes women to further danger, such as by informing a police station of domestic violence committed by a husband who is an officer serving at that station, may

---

[8] M. Ellsberg, L. Heise, R. Pena, S. Agurto, and A. Winkvist, 'Researching Domestic Violence against Women: Methodological and Ethical Considerations', *Studies in Family Planning*, 32 (2001), 11–16.

[9] Z. Bankowski, J. H. Bryant, and J. M. Last (eds.), *Ethics and Epidemiology: International Guidelines. Proceedings of the XXVth CIOMS Conference, Geneva, Switzerland, 7–9 November 1990* (Geneva: Council for International Organizations of Medical Sciences, 1991).

[10] *D. v. National Society for the Prevention of Cruelty to Children*, [1977] 1 All ER 589 (House of Lords, England).

attract a disciplinary sanction the licensing authority or professional association is legally empowered to impose.

Legal systems do not evolve at the same pace, and contrasts are apparent between the more progressive and the more reactionary. The imposition of non-consensual sexual intercourse is a criminal offence in every country. However, the more progressive recognize that women's consent to marry does not provide consent to any and every act of forced intercourse by a husband, and that husbands, no less than strangers, can be convicted of raping their wives. Some systems fall short of willingness to stigmatize husbands' coercion of intercourse as rape, but are willing to convict husbands of lesser offences such as assault. However, some courts, such as the Supreme Court of Mexico in June, 1997, have held that violently imposed sexual relations within marriage are not criminal at all, because they are the exercise of a legal 'right'.[11] Such callous judicial reasoning can be contrasted with court decisions[12] and statutes[13] in other countries that allow conviction of husbands for raping their wives through forceful overcoming of wives' resistance to intercourse.

5. *Human Rights Aspects*

The minimum standard of human rights protection to which actual and potential victims of violence are entitled is security of the person. The gravity, nature, and frequency of the abuse they suffer may elevate their entitlements to protection against inhuman and degrading treatment, and to protection of life itself. Different forums for exploring the protection and promotion of women's rights to freedom from domestic violence include the more obvious, such as police services and courts of law, but sometimes sources of protection obvious in theory are inaccessible in practice. Human rights ombudsmen or national human rights commissions might be more accessible, and might be encouraged to investigate domestic violence and how different police and governmental resources might be used more effectively in addressing the problem.

Domestic violence presents a paradox concerning women's protection against violence, because of ways in which the human rights protection of private and family life is occasionally applied. Some states try to be solicitous of family life by classifying activity within the home as falling within the private sphere, and therefore beyond public scrutiny and governmental intervention. This principle has served families well, concerning, for instance, consensual

[11] Cited in Center for Reproductive Law and Policy, *Reproductive Rights 2000: Moving Forward* (New York: CRLP, 2000), 47.
[12] *SW v. United Kingdom* and *CR v. United Kingdom* (1995) 21 EHRR 363 (European Court of Human Rights).
[13] See, for instance, the Criminal Code of Canada, Sec. 278.

contraceptive practice, but is dysfunctional when the principle is invoked to deny or obstruct police and other governmental intervention in non-consensual incidents of domestic violence, including marital rape. Studies have shown that criminal justice systems have yet to be adequately and equally applied to satisfy women's needs for protection against assaults inside and outside the home.[14] A challenge to criminal law enforcement is that the only adult witness to domestic violence may be the victim, and her protective refusal to testify may be difficult to overcome without threatening her with police or judicial punishment, such as for contempt of court in refusing to testify or to identify her assailant.

Governmental restraint from intervention in violent and otherwise abusive conduct within families may perpetuate a culture of violence against women, both sexual and non-sexual, and violate provisions, for instance, of the Women's Convention, by which states undertake to implement appropriate measures 'to modify the social and cultural patterns of conduct . . . which are based on the idea of the inferiority or the superiority of either of the sexes or on stereotyped roles for men and women' (Article 5(*a*)). The human right to private and family life is of special importance, but cannot be tolerated to condone private conduct within families in which one partner enforces dominance by violence over the other. The key human rights principle is that violence deliberately directed against any other person is never a purely private matter.

6. *Approaches*

6.1. *Clinical duty*

Dr O must treat Mrs N's presenting physical condition, and act in consultation with her regarding the effect of treatment options on her, her foetus, and her means to care for her children and others. Dr O must similarly treat Mrs N's psychological condition, addressing whether she recognizes or is in denial of her vulnerability to domestic violence, and the potential for her to react to violence with violence, directed perhaps against her children. Dr O should also consider Mrs N's protection against future violence, possibly through counselling her on means to avoid, diffuse, or escape from volatile or emotionally explosive situations. Attention should be directed both to Mrs N's welfare during pregnancy and childbirth, and to her and her family's well-being thereafter.

If Mrs N is protective of her husband for economic reasons, Dr O may defer to her judgement, and accept the compromise of any capacity the doctor

---

[14] Human Rights Watch, *Criminal Injustice: Violence against Women in Brazil* (New York: Human Rights Watch, 1991).

possesses to involve police authorities in Mr N's possible abuse of her. However, Dr O may guide Mrs N to any accessible less invasive means of protection.

This discharge of Dr O's ethical duty of beneficence requires care not to risk violation of the reciprocal duty of non-maleficence, in provoking the husband's anger directed at his wife and family. If appropriate, Dr O may advise Mr N of the potential for punitive justice if his conduct causes injury, and of any reporting responsibilities the law imposes on Dr O to inform police authorities of evidence of incidents of non-accidental injury. Attention must also be given to Mrs N's possible exposure to violence from other family members, such as in-laws with whom she may live. If Dr O practises within a health care environment where administrative or other staff can collaborate in Mr N's counselling, general reporting duties may be addressed by others, such as a health centre's administrative officer, or a religious official.

6.2. *Health care systems obligations*

Dr O has the power and responsibility to educate colleagues in their understanding of the reality, scope, and forms of domestic violence. Dr O might help initiate development, through hospitals and health centres of practice guidelines or protocols to be followed on identification of patients' injuries that may be due to violence.[15] In addition, Dr O might initiate the introduction of curricular and specialist training of health care providers including obstetricians/gynaecologists, pursuant to the call of the International Federation of Gynecology and Obstetrics (FIGO) General Assembly inviting member societies to 'ensure that violence against women is included in the curricula of all reproductive health care providers, in the specialist training of obstetricians/gynecologists and in programmes for continuing education'.[16]

6.3. *Social action for underlying conditions*

The FIGO Committee for the Ethical Aspects of Human Reproduction and Women's Health has explained that 'violence against women is one reflection of the unequal power relationship of men and women in societies', and that '[t]he physical, financial and social vulnerabilities of women are fundamentally harmful to the future of a society. Not redressing them fails to prevent harm to

---

[15] S. MacDonald, J. Wyman, and M. Addision, *Guidelines and Protocols for the Sexual Assault Nurse Examiner* (Toronto: Sexual Assault Care Centre, Women's College Hospital, 1995).
[16] FIGO, *General Assembly Resolution on Violence against Women, FIGO/WHO, Pre-congress Workshop on Violence against Women: In Search of Solutions* (Geneva: WHO, 1998), 33–4. WHO/FRH/WHD/97.38. Also available at http://www.figo.org/default.asp?id=/00000087.htm, last accessed 6 May 2002.

subsequent generations and contributes to the cycle of violence.' The Committee also noted that 'there is a need for wider awareness of the magnitude of the problem of violence against women', and that 'physicians are uniquely placed to assist in this. Only if a problem is recognized can it be addressed.' The Committee concluded that '[t]here is therefore a duty for professional societies and physicians to publicize information about the frequency of types of violence against women'.[17]

Dr O's awareness of the high prevalence of domestic violence in the community provides a basis to inspire and work with community leaders, health care facilities, and professional and women's health organizations to address this destructive feature of domestic life.[18] These leaders and organizations will need to publicize the extent and harms of domestic violence, and to take initiatives for its relief, reduction, and eventual removal. Given the high prevalence of domestic violence in the community, Dr O might want to explore with women's organizations the feasibility of establishing counselling hotlines and, for example, shelters for victims of domestic violence. Where laws against domestic violence are inadequate or inadequately enforced, Dr O might explore with legislators or prosecutors how appropriate legal steps might be taken to improve preventive strategies and effective law enforcement.

[17] FIGO, 'Violence against Women'.
[18] R. F. Jones and D. L. Horan, 'The American College of Obstetricians and Gynecologists: A Decade of Responding to Violence against Women', *Int. J. Gynecol. Obstet.* 58 (1997), 43–50.

16

A Maternal Death

Case Study

Dr AB works in the department of obstetrics and gynaecology of a regional hospital. Mrs X was admitted to the hospital's emergency room suffering from severe bleeding from the vagina. She was in her last month of pregnancy, and had six living children (two boys and four girls). Mrs X was in a state of shock because of blood loss, and Dr AB was called in to perform abdominal delivery, but Mrs X and the child died during the operation. Dr AB and a hospital colleague reviewed all of the procedures undertaken at the hospital and other circumstances of the case. What more should Dr AB do to discharge medical, ethical, legal, and human rights responsibilities?

1. Background

Although maternal deaths are now very rare events in developed countries, they unfortunately remain common events in developing countries. Estimates of maternal mortality revised to 1995 indicate that every year about 515,000 women die from causes related to pregnancy and childbirth,[1] a rate of over 1,400 maternal deaths each day, and little short of one death every minute. A 1993 World Bank report ranked maternity as the primary health problem in young adult women (ages 15–44) in developing countries, accounting for 18 per cent of the total disease burden.[2] Women who die are in the prime period of their lives. As mothers, their deaths have major health and social impacts on their families. Moreover, maternal mortality should be viewed as only the tip of an iceberg of maternal morbidity and acute or chronic suffering. For every maternal death, there are many women who survive serious illness with

---

[1] WHO, *Maternal Mortality in 1995: Estimates Developed by WHO, UNICEF, UNFPA* (Geneva: WHO, 2001), 2, 42–7, WHO/RHR/01.9.

[2] World Bank, *World Development Report: Investing in Health* (New York: Oxford University Press, 1993).

continued suffering and incapacity,[3] for example through problems associated with obstructed labour, such as obstetric fistulae (holes in the vaginal wall communicating to the bladder or the rectum).[4]

Maternal mortality in developing countries is also a tragedy in terms of equity and social justice. The 1995 revised estimates indicate that the global figure for the maternal mortality ratio (MMR) is 400 maternal deaths per 100,000 live births.[5] The maternal mortality ratio indicates the risk of maternal death among pregnant or recently pregnant women. It reflects a woman's basic health status, her access to care, and the quality of care she receives.[6]

The differences by region are great, in terms of number of deaths and maternal mortality ratios.[7] The inequity is even more dramatic by reference to the lifetime risk, which is the probability of maternal death faced by an average woman over her entire reproductive life-span.[8] More detail on the magnitude of inequity has been presented in Part I, Chapter 2, on Reproductive and Sexual Health. Table III.1.1 includes country data on maternal mortality ratio.

2. *Medical Aspects*

All pregnant women face some unpredictable, and often unpreventable, risks during pregnancy and childbirth.[9] From a global standpoint, the majority of maternal deaths are caused by severe bleeding (25 per cent), infection (15 per cent), eclampsia (convulsions) (12 per cent), obstructed labour (8 per cent), and unsafe abortion (13 per cent).[10]

The tragedy of maternal death is not just that it is a death that occurs at a time of expectation and joy; it is one of the most terrible ways to die. A woman can see herself bleeding to death with no help able to stop the bleeding. Severe sepsis after delivery exhausts a woman already weakened by the trauma of childbirth. Seeing a woman in the agony of convulsive fits in eclampsia is a scene that cannot be forgotten. In obstructed labour, the uncontrollable

---

[3] J. A. Fortney and J. B. Smith, 'Measuring Maternal Morbidity', *Reproductive Health Matters*, special edition (1999), 43–50.

[4] WHO, *Obstetric Fistulae: A Review of Available Information* (Geneva: WHO, 1991), WHO/MCH/MSM/91.5.

[5] WHO, *Maternal Mortality*.

[6] A. Starrs, *The Safe Motherhood Action Agenda: Priorities for the Next Decade. Report of the Safe Motherhood Technical Consultation, Colombo, Sri Lanka, 1997* (New York: Family Care International, 1998), 62.

[7] WHO, *Maternal Mortality*.   [8] Ibid.

[9] M. F. Fathalla, 'Chapter 9: Pregnancy and Childbirth: A Risky Business', in *Obstetrics and Gynecology to Women's Health: The Road Ahead* (New York and London: Parthenon, 1997), 103–22.

[10] WHO, *Mother–Baby Package: Implementing Safe Motherhood in Countries* (Geneva: WHO, 1994), 2. WHO/FHE/MSM/94.11.

involuntary severe uterine contractions continue until the uterus gives way and is ruptured, with internal haemorrhage taking place. Unsafe abortion can cause death from uncontrollable bleeding, from trauma to the uterus and to the pelvic organs and from severe sepsis.

It is estimated that about 15 per cent of pregnant women will require medical care to avoid death or disability from life-threatening complications. Trained midwives have an important role in community education, early detection, and referrals to health facilities. To deal with the serious complications, a facility should be able to provide essential obstetric services, including surgical procedures, anaesthesia, blood transfusions, management of pre-eclampsia and eclampsia, and special care of the newborn. Pre-eclampsia is the term given to a triad of oedema, hyptertension, and albumin in urine, of which hypertension is the most significant. It precedes the development of convulsions (eclampsia), if the blood pressure is not controlled.

The World Health Organization estimates that, on average, only 57 per cent of deliveries in the world today are attended by skilled birth attendants; the figure is 99 per cent for more developed regions; the range among less developed regions is 34 to 86 per cent.[11] The term 'skilled birth attendant' means a health professional who has the necessary training to detect, early diagnose, and, when needed, refer women with life-threatening complications to where they can get the necessary help. Only 46 per cent of all deliveries take place in health facilities; the figure for more developed regions is 98 per cent and for less developed regions is 40 per cent (with a range among regions of 26 to 78 per cent).

3. *Ethical Aspects*

At the microethical level of analysis, respect for persons requires that women be given the information and means to make a free and informed choice regarding whether or not they want to become pregnant. Every pregnancy should be a wanted pregnancy. Unwanted and unplanned pregnancies expose women to risks to their physical, mental, and social well-being that could have been avoided.

At macroethical and mesoethical levels of analysis, a rational allocation of resources in the health sector demands the ranking of diseases at different orders of priority. Ranking can be done through a rough indicator of a 'body count' or, in a more refined way, by using a criterion such as disability-adjusted life years (DALYs) lost. Although this approach is generally valid for setting

---

[11] WHO, *Coverage of Maternity Care: A Listing of Available Information* (Geneva: WHO, 1997). WHO/RHT/MSM/96.28.

priorities among diseases, the question should be raised whether society would be justified in ranking maternal health problems with other diseases.

Maternity is not a disease. It is an essential function that women fulfil for the survival of our species. Society has at least the same obligation to prevent maternal deaths as to prevent deaths from other conditions and diseases, but it might have additional obligations to ensure safe maternity. Some national constitutions require that special protection be given to mothers during maternity, because of the social function of motherhood. Moreover, ethical principles of protection of the vulnerable and beneficence, or doing good, reinforce the justice principle of non-discrimination on grounds of sex, to support health resource allocations to address women's avoidable deaths from pregnancy-related causes.

Resources allocated for maternal health are generally lumped together with resources for child health, in a maternal and child health (MCH) package. The role of maternal health in MCH has often been seen as an instrumental means to serve child health and not an end in itself. Health investments are often directed to low-cost interventions that benefit children, and much less to essential obstetric functions and referral services that can save the lives of pregnant women and women about to give birth in high-risk situations.

The value system underlying judgements about the monetary value of human life does not address questions of economics alone. It also addresses questions of social ethics and social justice, particularly where women are concerned.[12] Many societies in developing countries tend to invest less in girls than in boys, and to ignore or underestimate the economic contributions of women. Investment in girls' education is lagging behind investment in that of boys. Globally, two-thirds of children not attending school are girls.[13] A common belief is that women contribute a minor share of the world's economic product. Conventional measures of economic activity undercount women's paid labour and do not include the value of their unpaid labour. A hard-working housewife and mother is often described in economic measurements as 'not working'.

When resources are limited, decisions have to be made, which are often tough decisions, on who shall live and who shall die. Women are a minority among decision-makers. Although they comprise 50 per cent of the world's enfranchised population, women hold very few seats in national legislatures; in many governments there are no women in the highest decision-making body of the country, and in those cabinets where women are included, there are usually only one or two women. Institutions that exercise power within countries, such

---

[12]   M. F. Fathalla, 'Imagine a World where Motherhood is Safe for All Women', *Int. J. Gynecol. Obstet.* 72 (2001), 207–13.

[13]   United Nations Children's Fund (UNICEF), *Girls' Education: A Framework for Action* (New York: UNICEF, 2000), http://www.unicef.org/pdeduc/education/pdf/framework.pdf, last accessed 2 May 2002.

as religious, military, commercial, industrial, professional, and educational institutions, often lack women leaders, and may even exclude women from influential participation, which reduces the credibility and influence of such institutions as sources of ethical authority.

4. *Legal Aspects*

The law sets minimum standards beneath which medical practitioners must not perform in care of their patients. Medical practice falling below that standard puts medical practitioners, and possibly health care facilities, in breach of their legal duties to members of the communities they claim to serve. Residents of a hospital's or other facility's catchment area have stronger legal entitlements to admission for care than other people, but all people admitted, including to an emergency department, are legally entitled to adequate diagnosis and treatment. Further, admission and care of persons needing emergency care, because their lives or continuing health are at serious risk, should not be delayed to determine whether they have the means to pay for the indicated care. Accordingly, an unsuccessful outcome of a patient's care raises the issues of adequacy of care-givers' skills, and of the resources available to them.

Courts are often reluctant to review whether governmental officers such as treasurers, finance ministers, or health ministers have allocated resources appropriately, since judges regard these decisions as falling within the exclusive domain of governments. However, in exceptional cases, such as when the allocation of available resources fails to achieve due respect for at least minimal standards of human dignity and human rights, courts may make decisions that require governments to review their refusals or failures to fund an appropriate level of services.

Courts may be more interventionist when health care providers decide, on grounds of economy, to withhold available resources from their patients' care when application of those resources could benefit patients. Providers who act as double agents, balancing clinical duties to their patients against public or institutional duties they perceive to use resources economically in the interests of other patients, including other providers' patients, are in a conflict of interest. This is both unethical and unlawful. Patients are entitled to their health care providers' undivided allegiance, particularly when their lives or continuing health are at stake. Health care providers who compromise care of their patients in order to serve interests of governmental administrations, health facility budgetary officers, or public or private health care insurance providers, face legal liability for negligence, breach of contract, or, for instance, breach of fiduciary duties owed to their patients. They may also face professional disciplinary proceedings, for instance by licensing authorities, for unethical conduct.

5. *Human Rights Aspects*

Those drafting the Constitution of the World Health Organization in 1946 were vigilant to condemn all types of discrimination in health, exercised on the basis 'of race, religion, political belief, economic or social condition'.[14] However, they did not include sex as a prohibited ground of discrimination, because sex discrimination was not well understood at that time. The failure to address the avoidable causes of maternal mortality is a form of discrimination against women. That is, the neglected tragedy of maternal mortality is not just a health problem; it is a violation of women's human rights.[15] International tolerance of over half a million avoidable maternal deaths each year is explicable by reference to the deaths being of women. Military conflict that imposed such a toll on soldiers' lives would be considered a disaster that compelled international intervention. The crash of an aeroplane that costs over 350 civilian lives would be considered a major international disaster and compel investigation, but it passes almost unnoticed that, for pregnant women worldwide, the equivalent of four such crashes occurs every day of the year. National and international human rights perceptions and institutions have been slow to identify women's disadvantages as injustices amenable to remedy and prevention, even when life itself is at risk.

Avoidably high levels of maternal mortality violate women's right to life, and high levels of maternal morbidity compromise the right to the highest attainable standard of health. Breaches of both of these rights deny the rights to family life not only of women but also of their husbands and often their existing and newborn children. Neglect of medical procedures that only women need, such as those services necessary to ensure safe pregnancy and childbirth, constitutes a form of discrimination against women, thus offending the right to sexual non-discrimination found in most national constitutions and in regional and international human rights conventions.[16]

These violations may result from denials of human rights that women suffered earlier in their lives, such as devaluation and neglectful care when they were girl children, and in their reproductive lives, such as denial of their ability to space pregnancies to protect their lives and health. Women's greatest loss in maternal mortality reflects the greatest cumulative denials of their human rights.

---

[14] WHO, *Constitution* (Geneva: WHO, 1985).   [15] Fathalla, 'Imagine a World'.
[16] R. J. Cook, B. M. Dickens, O. A. Wilson, and S. E. Scarrow, *Advancing Safe Motherhood through Human Rights* (Geneva: WHO, 2001).

6. *Approaches*

6.1. *Clinical duty*

Dr AB should not feel that reviewing the case of Mrs X alone is enough. She was not the only unfortunate woman who had to sacrifice her life in the process of pregnancy and childbirth. Dr AB, in collaboration with key health care personnel involved in maternity care, should review the hospital records of the maternal deaths and near misses that had occurred in the hospital in at least the previous three years. The review of these adverse events should be undertaken in a non-judgemental way, with a view towards identifying what might be done to avoid the tragedy of maternal deaths in the future.[17] The review may well confirm that many maternal deaths could have been avoided if there was no *delay* in women deciding to seek treatment, no *delay* in reaching the health care facility, and no *delay* in the health facility in instituting the proper treatment.[18]

In the case of Mrs X, for example, her history may reveal, for instance, that she had two minor episodes of bleeding before this major haemorrhage. However, she, her family and the traditional birth attendant in the village may not have understood the significance of the bleeding episodes as indicating the threat of a serious bleeding because of a low-lying placenta. It took Mrs X several hours to reach hospital because of the lack of emergency transport, with the result that she lost a large amount of blood and arrived at the hospital in severe shock. In the hospital, blood transfusion was not readily available, and the operation was performed after a wait of two hours. The anaesthetist had to be summoned from home. The 'three delays' operated in one way or another in other cases.

Based on these findings Dr AB and his colleagues may agree to take the necessary steps to avoid delays in the management of obstetric emergencies in the hospital. They may also decide to keep an ongoing system of confidential inquiry into all maternal deaths in the hospital, with the objective of identifying avoidable factors that can be remedied. However, they know that these steps are necessary but not sufficient to significantly reduce maternal mortality, and that they have a professional responsibility to advocate for action by the health care system and by the society at large.

6.2. *Health care systems obligations*

The death of Mrs X is only one of several maternal deaths in the hospital. Maternal deaths in the hospital are only a fraction of the maternal deaths in the

[17] L. B. Andrews, C. Stocking, T. Krizek, *et al.*, 'An Alternative Strategy for Studying Adverse Events in Medical Care', *Lancet*, 349 (1997), 309–12.
[18] D. Maine, M. Z. Akalin, V. M. Ward, and A. Kamara, *The Design and Evaluation of Maternal Mortality Programs* (New York: Center for Population and Family Health, Columbia University School of Public Health, 1997), 11–13.

community. Moreover, these maternal deaths are only the very unfortunate among many more near fatal misses of women who survived but may suffer from serious morbidities. Dr AB, in joint discussion with colleagues, may decide to urge medical and other health professional associations to advocate for women's right to safe motherhood. They have to make the case for a more rational allocation of resources in the health care system, so that every woman is attended by a skilled birth attendant, and emergency obstetric care is made available, accessible, and efficient for those women who need such care. Stories of maternal deaths, like that of Mrs X, need to be publicized not only as medical cases, but also as cases of violations of women's right to life. To achieve universal coverage of maternity services, obstetricians should play the role of team leaders, and delegate certain responsibilities as appropriate to other categories of health care providers.

The professional society of obstetricians and gynaecologists should develop training curricula for obstetricians, general practitioners, midwives, and other categories of health workers, as appropriate, on how to deal with obstetric emergencies.

6.3. *Social action for underlying conditions*

Mrs X already had six children, including two boys. The fatal pregnancy in all likelihood was not wanted or planned. But her need for family planning services was not met. She had neither the information nor the means to control her fertility.

She was probably married early, and did not get a chance to continue her education. She lacked the opportunity to support her family by being gainfully employed. Her status in her community as a woman was probably low. Children were the only goods she was expected to produce. She could not seek treatment without the permission of her husband or in-laws.

Dr AB wonders whether Mrs X really died of haemorrhage, or of social injustice to women. Realizing that powerlessness of women is a serious health hazard, Dr AB feels the social responsibility to urge the local medical professional society to join with others in the community who are working to raise the status of women, and to eliminate all forms of discrimination against them.

Societies have an obligation to protect women's right to life when they go through the risky business of a social function that ensures the survival of our species. The Committee on the Elimination of Discrimination against Women, in its General Recommendation 24, requested that:

Reports [of states parties] should also include what measures states parties have taken to ensure women appropriate services in connection with pregnancy, confinement and the postnatal period. Information on the rates at which these measures have reduced maternal mortality and morbidity in their countries, in general, and in vulnerable groups, regions and communities, in particular, should also be included.

States parties should include in their reports how they supply free services where necessary to ensure safe pregnancies, childbirth and post-partum periods for women. Many women are at risk of death or disability from pregnancy-related causes because they lack the funds to obtain or access the necessary services, which include ante-natal, maternity and post-natal services. The Committee notes that it is the duty of states parties to ensure women's right to safe motherhood and emergency obstetric services and they should allocate to these services the maximum extent of available resources. (see Pt. III, Ch. 6, Sect. 2, paras. 26, 27)

PART III

Data and Sources

1

Reproductive Health Data

The purpose of this chapter is to present data on reproductive and sexual health. The data presented in each table come from sources referenced below each table. Updates of the data are usually available on the referenced websites. It needs to be stressed that, although the tables give only estimates, they present pictures, however incomplete, of the magnitude of the problems surrounding reproductive and sexual health. There is wisdom in the saying that what is only incompletely known should not be completely ignored.

The first table below provides national data on fertility rates, contraceptive use, maternal health status and services, and HIV/AIDS prevalence. The explanation of the indicators comes from *Reproductive Health Indicators for Global Monitoring: Report of the Second Interagency Meeting* (Geneva: WHO, 2001). Every effort has been made to provide the most recent data available for each indicator, as of 8 May 2002. Readers are encouraged, however, to check the referenced websites for more recent data. In the event that readers do not have access to the references used for each indicator, alternative sources of data are provided. An alphabetical listing of sources of more general use is provided, with website addresses where available. These sources were last accessed on 8 May 2002.

The second set of tables provides the estimated prevalence of female genital cutting by country where it is practised. Three sets of data are given according to the reliability of the estimates. The tables are intended to provide the most recent data available, as of 4 December 2001. Readers are again encouraged, however, to check the referenced websites for more recent data.

The third set of tables provides data on abortion mortality and complications. The first of these tables gives global and regional estimates of the incidence of unsafe abortion and of resulting mortality. The second table provides estimates of induced abortions and hospitalizations for abortion complications for selected Latin American countries. The third table presents the percentage of young women hospitalized for abortion complications in selected countries in Latin America and Africa.

Table III.1.1. Data on selected reproductive health indicators, by country

Country	Fertility and contraceptive use			Maternal health status
	Total fertility rate[a] (births per woman)	Adolescent fertility rate[b] (births per woman aged 15–19)	Contraceptive prevalence[c] (% of married women using contraception)	Maternal mortality ratio[d] (maternal deaths per 100,000 live births)
Afghanistan	6.80	—	1.6	0,820
Albania	2.27	12	—	31
Algeria	2.79	20	56.9	150
Angola	7.20	215	—	1,300
Argentina	2.44	63	—	85
Armenia	1.10	40	60.5	29
Australia	1.75	29	76.1	6
Austria	1.24	20	50.8	11
Azerbaijan	1.51	22	—	37
Bahamas	2.31	—	61.7	10
Bahrain	2.28	—	61.8	38
Bangladesh	3.56	140	53.8	600
Barbados	1.50	—	55.0	33
Belarus	1.20	22	50.4	33
Belgium	1.48	11	78.4	8
Belize	2.89	—	46.7	140
Benin	5.68	109	16.4	880
Bhutan	5.10	—	18.8	500
Bolivia	3.92	80	48.3	550
Bosnia and Herzegovina	1.30	33	—	15
Botswana	3.94	74	33.0	480
Brazil	2.15	71	76.7	260
Brunei Darussalam	2.53	—	—	22
Bulgaria	1.10	45	85.9	23
Burkina Faso	6.80	139	11.9	1,400
Burundi	6.80	53	8.7	1,900
Cambodia	4.77	13	23.8	590
Cameroon	4.70	134	19.3	720
Canada	1.58	20	74.7	6
Cape Verde	3.24	—	52.9	190

					HIV/AIDS prevalence	
and services						
Antenatal care coverage[e] (% of pregnant women covered)	% of births attended by skilled health personnel[f]	Perinatal mortality rate[g] (no. of perinatal deaths per 1,000 births)	% of live births with low birthweight[h]	% of pregnant women with anaemia[i]	% of pregnant women with HIV/AIDS in antenatal care clinics	
					major urban areas[j]	outside major urban areas[k]
8	8	—	—	—	—	—
—	—	15	5	—	—	—
58	77	55	7	42	—	—
25	17	105**	—	29	1.2	8.5
—	96	15	7	26	1.8	0.24
95*	95*	15	9	—	0.13	0
—	—	5	7	—	—	—
—	—	5	7	—	—	—
95*	95*	15	10	—	—	—
100	100	25	—	—	3.6	—
96	94	20	10	—	0.1	—
23	14	80	30	53	—	0
98	98	20	10	—	1.1	—
—	—	10	5	—	—	0.04[n]
—	—	10	8	—	—	—
96	77	30	4	—	—	—
60	38	60	15	41	3.7	1.5
51	12	75	15	—	—	0
52	46	45	8	54	0.5	0
—	—	10**	4	—	—	—
92	77	70	11	—	43.0	30.0
74	73	40	9	33	0.7	0.4
100	98	10	—	—	—	—
—	—	10	9	—	—	0.01[n]
59	43	60	18	24	7.4	4.3
88	24	85	16***	68	18.6	19.7
52	21	75	9	—	3.8	2.3
73	58	70	10	44	5.5	9.2
—	—	5	6	—	—	—
99	—	25**	13	—	—	—

Table III.1.1. (*cont.*)

Country	Fertility and contraceptive use			Maternal health status
	Total fertility rate[a] (births per woman)	Adolescent fertility rate[b] (births per woman aged 15–19)	Contraceptive prevalence[c] (% of married women using contraception)	Maternal mortality ratio[d] (maternal deaths per 100,000 live births)
Central African Republic	4.92	128	14.8	1,200
Chad	6.65	185	4.1	1,500
Chile	2.35	44	—	33
China	1.80	15	83.8	60
Colombia	2.62	84	76.9	120
Comoros	4.96	—	21.0	570
Congo, Democratic Republic of	6.70	211	7.7	940
Costa Rica	2.67	76	75.0	35
Côte d'Ivoire	4.64	128	15.0	1,200
Croatia	1.70	18	—	18
Cuba	1.55	67	70.0	24
Cyprus	1.92	—	—	0
Czech Republic	1.16	23	68.9	14
Democratic People's Republic of Korea	2.07	2	61.8	35
Denmark	1.65	9	78.0	15
Djibouti	5.77	—	—	520
Dominican Republic	2.71	12	63.7	110
East Timor	3.85	—	—	850
Ecuador	2.76	73	65.8	210
Egypt	2.88	61	56.1	170
El Salvador	2.88	104	59.7	180
Equatorial Guinea	5.89	—	—	1,400
Eritrea	5.28	116	5.0	1,100
Estonia	1.20	25	70.3	80
Ethiopia	6.75	151	8.1	1,800
Fiji	2.98	—	41.0	20
Finland	1.55	11	77.4	6
France	1.80	9	74.6	20
French Polynesia	2.47	—	—	20

| and services | | | | | HIV/AIDS prevalence | |
| Antenatal care coverage[e] (% of pregnant women covered) | % of births attended by skilled health personnel[f] | Perinatal mortality rate[g] (no. of perinatal deaths per 1,000 births) | % of live births with low birthweight[h] | % of pregnant women with anaemia[i] | % of pregnant women with HIV/AIDS in antenatal care clinics | |
					major urban areas[j]	outside major urban areas[k]
67	46	70	13***	67	12.8	12.2
30	15	70	24	37	6.2	4.7
91	98	10	5	13	0.1	0
79	85	35	6	52	—	0.4
83	85	35	7	24	0.5	0.1
69	24	50	18	—	0	—
—	—	65**	15	—	4.1	8.5
95	97	15	6	27	0.3	0.1
83	45	95	17	34	10.6	10
—	—	10	6	—	—	—
100	99	10	6	47	0	—
100	98	5**	—	—	—	0
—	—	5	6	23	—	0.005[n]
100	100	60**	—	71	—	—
—	—	5	6	—	—	—
76	79	75**	—	—	2.9	—
97	90	40	13	—	1.4	2.1
—	—	125**	—	—	—	—
75	64	30	16	17	—	0.3
53	46	55	10	24	0	0
69	87	25	13	14	0	—
37	5	60**	—	—	0.7	0.3
19	6	50	14	—	—	3
—	—	5	5	—	—	—
20	8	100	12	42	17.6	9.2
100	100	15	12***	—	—	—
—	—	5	6	—	0	0.01[n]
—	—	5	6	—	0.4	—
95	98	10**	—	—	—	—

Table III.1.1. (*cont.*)

Country	Fertility and contraceptive use			Maternal health status
	Total fertility rate[a] (births per woman)	Adolescent fertility rate[b] (births per woman aged 15–19)	Contraceptive prevalence[c] (% of married women using contraception)	Maternal mortality ratio[d] (maternal deaths per 100,000 live births)
Gabon	5.40	162	32.7	620
Gambia	4.79	167	11.8	1,100
Georgia	1.39	31	40.5	22
Germany	1.29	14	74.7	12
Ghana	4.22	84	22.0	590
Greece	1.24	17	—	2
Guadeloupe	2.02	—	43.6	5
Guam	3.95	—	—	12
Guatemala	4.41	109	38.2	270
Guinea	5.83	162	6.2	1,200
Guinea-Bissau	5.99	183	—	910
Guyana	2.31	—	31.4	150
Haiti	3.98	66	28.1	1,100
Honduras	3.72	108	50.0	220
Hong Kong, China	1.17	5	86.2	—
Hungary	1.20	27	77.4	23
Iceland	1.90	—	—	16
India	2.97	107	48.2	440
Indonesia	2.27	57	57.4	470
Iran	2.76	48	72.9	130
Iraq	4.77	38	13.7	370
Ireland	2.02	14	—	9
Israel	2.70	20	—	8
Italy	1.20	8	60.2	11
Jamaica	2.37	92	65.9	120
Japan	1.33	3	58.6	12
Jordan	4.31	32	52.6	41
Kazakhstan	1.95	39	66.1	80
Kenya	4.15	106	39.0	1,300
Kuwait	2.66	32	50.2	25
Kyrgyszstan	2.34	34	59.5	80

and services					HIV/AIDS prevalence	
Antenatal care coverage[e] (% of pregnant women covered)	% of births attended by skilled health personnel[f]	Perinatal mortality rate[g] (no. of perinatal deaths per 1,000 births)	% of live births with low birthweight[h]	% of pregnant women with anaemia[i]	% of pregnant women with HIV/AIDS in antenatal care clinics	
					major urban areas[j]	outside major urban areas[k]
86	80	40**	—	—	4.0	1.2
91	44	75	14	80	1.0	2.4
95*	95*	20	6	—	0	—
—	—	5	7	—	0.06	0.01
86	44	80	9	64	3.4	3.4
—	—	10	7	—	—	—
—	—	10	—	—	—	—
97	100	10**	—	—	—	—
53	35	30	12	45	2.9	1.9
59	31	115	10	—	1.5	1.4
50	—	100**	20	74	2.7	—
95	93	55	14	—	3.8	—
68	20	40	28***	64	10	4.8
73	47	25	6	14	2.9	3
100	100	5	—	—	—	—
—	—	5	9	—	—	0_n
—	—	5	4	—	—	—
62	35	70	26	88	2	0.3
82	36	40	9	64	—	0
62	74	55	7	17	0	0
59	54	30	23	18	—	0
—	—	10	4***	—	—	—
90	99	5	8	—	—	—
—	—	5	6	—	0.15	0.1_n
98	92	30	11	40	1	—
—	—	5	7***	—	0	0
80	87	20	10	50	0_n	0
92	99	35	6	27	—	—
95	45	40	9	35	15.2	12.7
99	99	20	7	40	0	0
90*	95*	30	6	—	—	—

Table III.1.1. (*cont.*)

Country	Fertility and contraceptive use			Maternal health status
	Total fertility rate[a] (births per woman)	Adolescent fertility rate[b] (births per woman aged 15–19)	Contraceptive prevalence[c] (% of married women using contraception)	Maternal mortality ratio[d] (maternal deaths per 100,000 live births)
Lao People's Democratic Republic	4.80	41	18.6	650
Latvia	1.10	31	48.0	70
Lebanon	2.18	25	61.0	130
Lesotho	4.45	81	23.2	530
Liberia	6.80	—	6.4	1,000
Libyan Arab Jamahiriya	3.31	53	39.7	120
Lithuania	1.20	35	58.5	27
Luxembourg	1.76	—	—	0
Macedonia (The Former Yugoslav Republic of)	1.48	36	—	17
Madagascar	5.68	167	19.4	580
Malawi	6.34	151	30.6	580
Malaysia	2.90	24	54.5	39
Maldives	5.37	—	—	390
Mali	7.00	174	6.7	630
Malta	1.77	—	—	0
Martinique	1.70	—	51.3	4
Mauritania	6.00	129	3.3	870
Mauritius	1.90	40	74.7	45
Mexico	2.49	70	66.5	65
Mongolia	2.32	50	59.9	65
Morocco	3.03	47	50.3	390
Mozambique	5.86	159	5.6	980
Myanmar	2.80	24	32.7	170
Namibia	4.87	101	28.9	370
Nepal	4.48	117	28.5	830
Netherlands	1.50	5	78.5	10
Netherlands Antilles	2.09	—	—	20

nd services					HIV/AIDS prevalence	
Antenatal care coverage[e] (% of pregnant women covered)	% of births attended by skilled health personnel[f]	Perinatal mortality rate[g] (no. of perinatal deaths per 1,000 births)	% of live births with low birthweight[h]	% of pregnant women with anaemia[i]	% of pregnant women with HIV/AIDS in antenatal care clinics	
					major urban areas[j]	outside major urban areas[k]
25	30*	110**	—	62	0.4	—
—	—	15	5	—	—	0.06[n]
85	45	25	6	49	—	0
91	50	60**	—	7	31.3	27.1
83	58	80**	—	—	4.0	10.1
00	76	30	7***	—	—	0
	—	10	4	—	0	0[u]
—	—	10	4	—	—	—
—	—	30	6	—	—	—
78	57	55	15	—	0	0
90	55	70	13***	55	26.0	18.2
90	98	10	9	56	0.03	0.05
95	90	75	12	—	—	—
25	24	115	16	58	2.7	2.9
—	—	10	7	—	—	—
—	—	10	—	—	—	—
49	40	130	—	24	0.5	0
99	97	35	13	29	0	—
71	69	20	9	41	0	0.36
90	97	55	6	45	—	—
45	40	40	9***	45	0.02[n]	0
54	30	90	13	58	11.2	17.0
80	52	85**	16	58	0.65	1.5
88	68	60	15***	16	25.9	15.0
15	8	70	21	65	0	0
—	—	10	—	—	0.33	—
95*	95*	15**	—	—	—	—

Table III.1.1. (*cont.*)

Country	Fertility and contraceptive use			Maternal health status
	Total fertility rate[a] (births per woman)	Adolescent fertility rate[b] (births per woman aged 15–19)	Contraceptive prevalence[c] (% of married women using contraception)	Maternal mortality ratio[d] (maternal deaths per 100,000 live births)
New Caledonia	2.47	—	—	10
New Zealand	1.97	30	74.9	15
Nicaragua	3.82	130	60.3	250
Niger	8.00	211	8.2	920
Nigeria	5.42	114	15.3	1,100
Norway	1.70	12	73.8	9
Oman	5.46	61	23.7	120
Pakistan	5.08	100	23.9	200
Panama	2.42	77	58.2	100
Papua New Guinea	4.32	66	25.9	390
Paraguay	3.84	81	57.4	170
Peru	2.64	65	64.2	240
Philippines	3.24	43	46.0	240
Poland	1.26	21	49.4	12
Portugal	1.45	22	66.3	12
Puerto Rico	1.90	64	77.7	30
Qatar	3.34	—	43.2	41
Republic of Korea	1.51	4	80.5	20
Republic of Moldova	1.40	53	73.7	65
Romania	1.32	41	63.8	60
Russian Federation	1.14	42	—	75
Rwanda	5.77	54	13.2	2,300
Samoa	4.24	—	—	15
Saudi Arabia	5.54	107	31.8	23
Senegal	5.11	99	12.9	1,200
Sierra Leone	6.50	196	—	2,100
Singapore	1.45	9	74.2	9
Slovakia	1.28	62	74.0	14
Slovenia	1.14	65	—	17
Solomon Islands	5.26	—	—	60
Somalia	7.25	—	—	1,600
South Africa	2.85	45	56.3	340
Spain	1.13	8	80.9	8

Antenatal care coverage[e] (% of pregnant women covered)	% of births attended by skilled health personnel[f]	Perinatal mortality rate[g] (no. of perinatal deaths per 1,000 births)	% of live births with low birthweight[h]	% of pregnant women with anaemia[i]	HIV/AIDS prevalence % of pregnant women with HIV/AIDS in antenatal care clinics	
					major urban areas[j]	outside major urban areas[k]
98	98	15	—	—	—	—
—	—	10	6	—	—	—
71	61	20	13	36	—	—
30	15	150	12	41	1.3	4.7
60	31	100	9	55	4.5	4.9
—	—	10	5	—	—	0.01[n]
98	92	15	8	54	—	—
27	18	65	21***	37	0	0
72	84	30	10	—	0.3	0.9
70	33	80	—	16	0.2	0
83	66	25	9	44	0	—
64	53	30	10	53	0.3[n]	0.04[n]
83	53	25	18	48	—	—
—	—	15	6	—	—	—
—	—	5	7	—	0.2	—
99	99	15	—	—	—	—
00	97	15*	10	—	—	—
96	95	5	—	—	—	—
—	—	15	7	20	—	0[n]
—	—	15	9	31	—	—
—	—	15	7	30	—	0.005[n]
94	26	70	12***	—	19	7.5
52	52	15**	—	—	—	—
87	90	20	3	—	—	—
74	47	85	12	26	0.5	0.5
30*	25*	160**	22	31	2	—
00	100	5	8	—	—	—
—	—	10	7	—	—	0[n]
—	—	10	6	—	—	0[n]
71	85	35**	—	—	—	—
40*	2	85**	—	—	0	2.0
89	82	25	—	37	19.2	21.3
—	—	5	6	—	0.13	0.15[n]

Table III.1.1. (*cont.*)

Country	Fertility and contraceptive use			Maternal health statu
	Total fertility rate[a] (births per woman)	Adolescent fertility rate[b] (births per woman aged 15–19)	Contraceptive prevalence[c] (% of married women using contraception)	Maternal mortality ratio[d] (maternal deaths per 100,000 live births)
Sri Lanka	2.09	21	66.1	60
Sudan	4.47	53	8.3	1,500
Suriname	2.05	—	—	230
Swaziland	4.44	—	19.9	370
Sweden	1.29	9	78.0	8
Switzerland	1.38	4	82.0	8
Syrian Arab Republic	3.65	41	36.1	200
Tajikistan	2.87	28	—	120
Thailand	2.00	76	72.2	44
Togo	5.36	84	23.5	980
Trinidad and Tobago	1.53	42	52.7	65
Tunisia	2.10	11	60.0	70
Turkey	2.30	56	63.9	55
Turkmenistan	3.17	16	61.8	65
Uganda	7.10	189	14.8	1,100
Ukraine	1.10	34	67.5	45
United Arab Emirates	2.86	71	27.5	30
United Kingdom	1.61	28	82.0	10
United Rep. of Tanzania	5.03	130	24.2	1,100
United States of America	1.93	50	76.4	12
Uruguay	2.30	66	—	50
Uzbekistan	2.29	42	55.6	60
Vanuatu	4.26	—	—	32
Venezuela	2.72	95	49.3	43
Vietnam	2.25	34	75.3	95
Yemen	7.60	100	20.8	850
Yugoslavia	1.55	32	55.0	15
Zaire	—	—	—	—
Zambia	5.66	138	25.0	870
Zimbabwe	4.50	85	53.5	610

nd services					HIV/AIDS prevalence	
Antenatal care coverage^e (% of pregnant women covered)	% of births attended by skilled health personnel^f	Perinatal mortality rate^g (no. of perinatal deaths per 1,000 births)	% of live births with low birthweight^h	% of pregnant women with anaemia^i	% of pregnant women with HIV/AIDS in antenatal care clinics	
					major urban areas^j	outside major urban areas^k
00	94	30	17	39	0	0
54	86^0	65	—	36	0.5	3.8
00	91	25**	11	—	0.8	—
70	56	35	—	—	30.3	31.5
—	—	5	4	—	—	0.01^n
—	—	5	6	—	—	—
33	67	45	6	—	0	—
90*	92	35	13	50	—	—
77	71	20	7	57	1.28	1.71
43	32	80	13	48	6.8	4.6
98	98	10	—	53	1	—
71	90	35	5	38	0	0
62	76	30	15	74	—	—
90*	90*	25	5	—	—	—
87	38	50	13	30	13.8	7.7
—	—	10	6	—	0.15	0.05^n
95	96	20	—	—	—	—
—	—	10	8	—	0.19	0.02
92	44	65	11	59	13.7	18.6
—	—	5	8	—	—	—
80	96	15	—	20	0	0
90*	90*	15	6	—	—	—
90	79	45**	7***	—	—	—
74	97	15	6	29	0	0
78	79	30	19	—	0.17	0
26	16	60	26	—	—	—
—	—	15	5	—	—	—
66	—	—	—	—	—	—
92	51	65	11	34	27.0	13.9
93	69	75	10	—	29.7	30.0

Notes to Table III.1.1.

n = nationwide number that does not allow for an urban/rural breakdown
o = data that are locally defined;
* indicates that the number is rounded;
** estimates for countries for which no data were available;
*** data for periods outside 1995–2000 that differ from standard of definition or refer to part of a country.

ᵃ The total fertility rate measures the total number of children a woman would have by the end of her reproductive period if she experienced the currently prevailing age-specific fertility rates throughout her childbearing life. Total fertility rate is useful as a measure of poor physical reproductive health, since high parity births (>5) are one of the risk factors for maternal morbidity and mortality. The indicator also complements measures of contraceptive prevalence. Low, medium, and high estimates are made. The medium variant estimates are used for 2000–5. *Sources*: UN Population Division, *World Population Prospects: The 2000 Revision*, i. *Comprehensive Tables* (New York: United Nations, 2000), 584–91. Also: World Bank, *World Indicators 2001*, table 2.17, pp. 106–9; UNFPA, *State of World Population 2001*, 70–3; Population Reference Bureau, *2001 World Population Data Sheet*.

ᵇ The adolescent fertility rate estimates the births per 1,000 women aged 15–19. Figures are for 1999. *Sources*: World Bank, *World Indicators 2001*, table 2.17, pp. 106–9. Also: UNFPA, *State of World's Population 2001*, 67–9, gives country data on births per 1,000 women aged 15–19; Population Reference Bureau, *World's Youth 2000*, 18–24, estimates the percentage of the total fertility rate attributed to births by women aged 15–19.

ᶜ The contraceptive prevalence measures the percentage of married or cohabiting women of reproductive age who are using (or whose partner is using) any method of contraception. The methods include female and male sterilization, injectables and oral hormones, intrauterine devices, diaphragms, spermicides and condoms, natural family planning, and lactational amenorrhoea. While efforts are being made to cover all women aged 15–49, irrespective of their marital status, who are at risk of pregnancy, i.e. sexually active women who are not infecund, pregnant, or amenorrhoeic, these data refer only to married women including women in consensual and other forms of informal unions. Figures are for 2001. *Sources*: United Nations, Wall Chart on World Contraceptive Use 2001 (New York: United Nations, 2002), also available on www.unpopulation.org. Also: UN Population Division, *Levels and Trends of Contraceptive Use as Assessed in 1998* (New York: UN, 2000); World Bank, *World Indicators 2001*, table 2.17, pp. 106–9; UNFPA, *State of World Population 2001*, 67–9; and UNDP, *Human Development Report 2000*, 158–62; Population Reference Bureau, *2001 World Population Data Sheet*.

ᵈ The maternal mortality ratio measures the annual number of maternal deaths per 100,000 live births. These estimated numbers are for 1995. They are indicative of orders of magnitude and are not intended to serve as precise estimates. *Sources*: World Health Organization, *Maternal Mortality in 1995: Estimates developed by WHO, UNICEF and UNFPA* (Geneva: WHO, 2001), 42–7. Also: WHO and World Bank, 'Maternal Health Around the World' poster, 1997; UNFPA, *State of World Population 2001*, 67–9; UNDP, *Human Development Report 2001*, 166–70; World Bank, *World Indicators 2001*, table 2.17, pp. 106–9; UNICEF, *State of the World's Children 2002*, 36–9.

ᵉ Antenatal care coverage estimates the percentage of women attended at least once during pregnancy by skilled health personnel for reasons related to pregnancy. Skilled health personnel includes doctors (specialist or non-specialist), and persons with midwifery skills who can diagnose and manage obstetrical complications as well as normal deliveries. The estimates should be understood as indicating the orders of magnitude rather than precise figures. They are based on analysis of data from developing countries up to mid-1996. Antenatal care provides an important opportunity for discussion between a pregnant woman and a health care provider, and is important as well for preventive care and for early diagnosis and treatment of complications. *Sources*: WHO, *Coverage of Maternity Care: A Listing of Available Information*, 1997, 15–19. This source is limited to developing countries. Also: UNICEF, *State of the World's Children 2002*, 36–9; UN, *The World's Women 2000*, table 3B.

[f] This indicator estimates the percentage of total births attended by skilled health personnel irrespective of outcome (live birth or foetal death). Skilled health personnel include doctors (specialist or non-specialist), and persons with midwifery skills who can diagnose and manage obstetrical complications as well as normal deliveries. The estimates should be understood as indicating the orders of magnitude rather than precise figures. They are based on analysis of data from developing countries up to mid-1996. The share of births attended by skilled health staff is an indicator of a health system's ability to provide adequate care for pregnant women. Good antenatal and postnatal care improves maternal health and reduces maternal and infant mortality, and other indicators may not reflect such improvements because health information systems are often weak, maternal deaths are underreported, and rates of maternal mortality are difficult to measure. *Sources*: WHO, *Coverage of Maternity Care*, 15–19. This source is limited to developing countries. Also: World Bank, *World Development Indicators 2001*, Table 2.17: Reproductive Health, pp. 106–9; Population Reference Bureau, *World's Youth 2000*, pp. 18–24; UNFPA, *State of World Population 2001*, 70–3; UNICEF, *State of World's Children 2002*, 36–9; UN, *The World's Women 2000*, table 3B.

[g] The perinatal mortality rate estimates the number of perinatal deaths per 1,000 births. Perinatal deaths are those that occur during late pregnancy (at 22 completed weeks gestation and over), during childbirth and up to seven completed days of life. Figures are for 1999. *Source*: WHO/Reproductive Health and Research (RHR), provided by Jelka Zupan of RHR, 10 Apr. 2002.

[h] The low-birthweight indicator estimates the percentage of live births with a birthweight of less than 2,500 grams, with the measurement taken within the first hours of life, before significant postnatal weight loss has occurred. This indicator is a direct measure of newborn health and chance of survival. It is also an efficient marker of the health status of the mother. Data are for the most recent year during 1995–2000. *Source*: UNICEF, *State of the World's Children 2002*, 16–19. Also: UNDP, *Human Development Report 2001*, 162–6; World Bank, *World Indicators 2001*, table 2.18, pp. 110–13.

[i] The percentage of pregnant women who are anaemic, measured by haemoglobin levels less than 11 grams per deciliter. This indicator is useful as a direct measure of health status because anaemia is directly injurious to health. It can also be used as a proxy measure of general nutritional status. Data are for the most recent year available in 1985–99. *Source*: World Bank, *World Development Indicators 2001*, 110–13.

[j] The percentage of pregnant women tested in antenatal care clinics in major urban areas who were found to be infected with HIV. The medium variant is reported. Data are for the most recent year available in 1992–5. *Sources*: Joint United Nations Programme on HIV/AIDS, *Report*, 123–35. Country data on the percentage of adults (men and women) in 1999 who were found to be HIV positive are available in World Bank, *World Indicators 2001*, table 2.18, pp. 110–13; country data on the estimated number of people with HIV/AIDS at the end of 1997 and the percentage of those estimates that are women is reported in *The*

World's Women 2000, table 3B, pp. 79–80; country data on the percentage of men and women aged 15–24 who have HIV in UNFPA, *State of World Population 2001*, 67–9.

ᵏ The percentage of pregnant women tested in antenatal care clinics outside major urban areas who were found to be infected with HIV. The medium variant is reported. Data are for the most recent year available in 1992–9. *Sources*: Joint United Nations Programme on HIV/AIDS, *Report*, 123–35. See also n. j.

Acknowledgements

Iqbal Shah, Jelka Zupan, Wilma Doedens, Vasantha Kandiah, Metin Gulvezoglu, Noah Gitterman, Jeanette Williams, Tracey Pegg.

Sources

Joint United Nations Programme on HIV/AIDS (UNAIDS), *Report on the Global Aids Epidemic, June 2000* (Geneva: UNAIDS, 2000) at http://www.unaids.org/epidemic_update/report/index.html

Population Reference Bureau, *2001 World Population Data Sheet* (Washington: Population Reference Bureau, 2002) at http://www.prb.org

—— *World's Youth 2000* (Washington.: Population Reference Bureau, 2000) at http://www.prb.org

——*World's Youth 2001* (Washington: Population Reference Bureau, 2001) at http://www.prb.org

United Nations, *The World's Women 2000, Trends and Statistics* (New York: UN, 2000) at http://www.un.org/Depts/unsd/ww2000/tables.htm

United Nations, Population Division, Department of Economic and Social Affairs, *Charting the Progress of Populations* (New York: UN, 2000) at http://www.unpopulation.org

—— *World Population Prospects: The 2000 Revision*, i. *Comprehensive Tables* (New York: UN, 2000) at http://www.unpopulation.org

United Nations Development Programme, *Human Development Report 2001* (New York: Oxford University Press, 2001) at http://www.undp.org/hdr2001/home.html

UNFPA, *State of World Population 2001* (New York: UNFPA, 2001) at http://www.unfpa.org/swp/2001/english/indicators/indicators2.html

UNICEF, *State of the World's Children* 2002 (New York: UNICEF, 2002) at http://www.unicef.org/sowc02summary/index.html

World Bank, *World Indicators 2001* (Washington: International Bank for Reconstruction and Development, 2001) at http://www.worldbank.org/data/databytopic/databytopic.html

World Health Organization (WHO), *Coverage of Maternity Care: A Listing of Available Information* (Geneva: WHO, 1997).

—— *Reproductive Health Indicators for Global Monitoring: Report of the Second Interagency Meeting* (Geneva: WHO, 2001) at http://www.who.int/reproductive-health/index.htm

—— and World Bank, 'Maternal Health Around the World 1997' poster at www.safemotherhood.org

Searchable databases include: World Population Prospects Population Database at http://esa.un.org/unpp; Demographic and Health Surveys by Macro International, Inc. at http://www.measuredhs.com

Table III.1.2.   Female genital cutting (FGC), estimated prevalence

III.1.2.1.   Most reliable estimates: national surveys

Country	Prevalence (%)[a]	Year[b]
Burkina Faso	72	1998/9
Central African Republic	43	1994/5
Côte d'Ivoire	43	1994
Egypt	97	1995
Eritrea	95	1995
Guinea	99	1999
Kenya	38	1998
Mali	94	1995/6
Niger	5	1998
Nigeria	25	1999
Somalia	96–100	1982–93
Sudan	89	1989/90
Tanzania	18	1996
Togo	12	1996
Yemen	23	1997

[a] Prevalence measures the percentage of women aged 15–49 who have undergone genital cutting by the year specified. It is important to emphasize that these percentages are estimates. Moreover, these estimates are for all forms of genital cutting.

[b] Year refers to the year of the survey, except for Somalia, where year refers to the publication date of the MOH report. Note that some DHS reports are dated a year after the survey itself.

Sources

The source for the above estimates (with the exception of Somalia and Togo) is D. Carr, *Female Genital Cutting: Findings from the Demographic and Health Surveys* (DHS) (Calverton, Md.: Macro International Inc., 1997), available from http://www.measuredhs. int. The data are available on the WHO website: http:///.who.int/frh-whd/fgm, most recently updated May 2001, last accessed 4 Dec. 2001.

For Somalia, the estimate comes from a 1983 national survey by the Ministry of Health, *Fertility and Family Planning in Urban Somalia, 1983*, Ministry of Health, Mogadishu and Westinghouse. The survey found a prevalence of 96%. Five other surveys, carried out between 1982 and 1993 on diverse populations, found prevalences of 99–100%. Details about these sources can be found in C. Makhlouf Obermeyer, 'Female Genital Surgeries: The Known, the Unknown, and the Unknowable', *Medical Anthropology Quarterly*, 13/1 (1999), 79–106.

For Togo, the source is a national survey carried out by the Unité de Recherche Démographique (URD) in 1996 (The reference of the unpublished report is E. Agounke, M. Janssens, and K. Vignikin K, 'Prévalence et facteurs socio-économiques de l'excision au Togo, rapport provisoire', Lomé, June 1996. Results are given in T. Locoh, 'Pratiques, opinions et attitudes en matière d'excision en Afrique', *Population* 6 (1998), 1227–40.

III.1.2.2. Other estimates

Country	Prevalence (%)	Year[a]	Source
Benin	50	1993	National Committee study, unpub., cit. in Toubia (1995); Toubia and Izett (1998)
Chad	60	1991	UNICEF sponsored study, unpub., cit. in Toubia (1995); Toubia and Izett (1998)
Ethiopia	85	1985; 1990	Ministry of Health study sponsored by UNICEF; Inter-African Committee study; cit. in Toubia and Izett (1998)
Gambia	80	1985	Study, cited in Toubia (1995); Toubia and Izett (1998)
Ghana	30[b]	1986; 1987	Two studies cit. in Toubia (1995); Toubia and Izett (1998); on different regions, divergent findings
Liberia	60[c]	1984	Unpub. study, cit. in Toubia (1995); Toubia and Izett (1998)
Senegal	20	1990	National study cit. in Toubia (1995); Toubia and Izett (1998)
Sierra Leone	90	1987	Koso-Thomas (1987)

[a] For published studies year refers to year of publication. For unpublished studies, it is not always clear whether year refers to year of the report or year of the survey. Where no year is indicated, the information is not available.

[b] One study found prevalences ranging from 75 to 100% among ethnic groups in the north; another study in the south found FGC only among migrants; the 30% comes from Toubia (1995).

[c] A limited survey found that all but three groups practise FGC, and estimated prevalence at 50–70%; the 60% comes from Toubia (1995).

Sources

The data are available on the WHO website: http:///.who.int/frh-whd/fgm, most recently updated May 2001, last accessed 4 Dec. 2001.

Koso-Thomas, O., *The Circumcision of Women: A Strategy for Eradication* (London: Zed Press, 1987).

Makhlouf Obermeyer, C., 'Female Genital Surgeries: The Known, the Unknown, and the Unknowable', *Medical Anthropology Quarterly*, 13/1 (1999), 79–106.

Toubia, N., *Female Genital Mutilation: A Call for Global Action* (2nd edn.; New York: Rainbo, 1995) (http://www.rainbo.org) (some figures are updated in the 1996 Arabic version of the document).

—— and Izett, S., *Female Genital Mutilation: An Overview* (Geneva: WHO, 1998).

III.1.2.3. Questionable estimates

Country	Prevalence (%)
Cameroon	20
Democratic Republic of the Congo	5
Djibouti	98
Guinea-Bissau	50
Mauritania[a]	25
Uganda	5

[a] A national survey carried out by the DHS.

Source

These estimates are available on the WHO website: http:///.who.int/frh-whd/fgm, most recently updated May 2001, last accessed 4 Dec 2001. They are based on anecdotal evidence, and are cited in Toubia (1995) and Toubia and Izett (1998).

Table III.1.3. Abortion mortality and complications

III.1.3.1. Incidence of and mortality due to unsafe abortion, global and regional annual
estimates, 1995–2000

Region	Estimated no. of unsafe abortions (000s)[a]	Incidence rate[b]	Incidence ratio[c]	Estimated no. of deaths due to unsafe abortion[d]	Mortality ratio[e]	Proportion of maternal deaths[f]
World Total	**20,000**	**13**	**15**	**78,000**	**57**	**13**
More Developed Regions	900	3	7	500	4	13
Less Developed Regions	19,000	16	16	77,500	63	13
Africa	**5,000**	**27**	**16**	**34,000**	**110**	**13**
Eastern Africa	1,900	36	19	16,000	153	14
Middle Africa	600	28	14	4,000	98	10
Northern Africa	600	15	13	1,200	24	7
Southern Africa	200	16	13	800	49	19
Western Africa	1,600	31	16	12,000	121	12
Asia	**9,900**	**11**	**13**	**38,500**	**48**	**12**
Eastern Asia	—	—	—	—	—	—
South-Central Asia	6,500	19	17	29,000	72	13
South-Eastern Asia	2,800	21	23	8,100	66	15
Western Asia	500	12	11	1,100	20	6
Europe	**900**	**5**	**12**	**500**	**6**	**17**
Eastern Europe	800	10	25	500	15	24
Northern Europe	<30	1	2	<20	0.2	2
Southern Europe	<90	2	6	<20	1	10
Western Europe	—	—	—	—	—	—
Latin America and Caribbean	**4,000**	**30**	**36**	**5,000**	**41**	**21**
Caribbean	200	17	21	600	71	18
Central America	900	26	26	700	20	14
South America	3,000	34	42	3,500	47	24
North America	—	—	—	—	—	—
Oceania	**30**	**15**	**12**	**150**	**51**	**8**

Note: Figures may not add to totals due to rounding. For regions where the incidence is negligible no estimates
are shown. Australia, Japan, and New Zealand have been excluded from the regional estimates, but are
included in the total for developed countries.

ᵃ 19 million of the estimated 20 million unsafe abortions take place each year in the less developed countries where abortion laws are the most restrictive.

ᵇ Incidence rate: 'The unsafe abortion *rate* is the number of unsafe abortions per 1,000 women of reproductive age (15–49) per year.'

ᶜ Incidence ratio: 'The unsafe abortion *ratio* is the number of unsafe abortions relative to 100 live births (as a proxy for all pregnancies), expressed as a percentage. The abortion ratio indicates the probability that a pregnant woman will resort to unsafe abortion [in a given year].'

ᵈ It is likely that about 77,500 women in less developed regions die each year from complications following unsafe abortion. Country estimates are available, WHO, *Unsafe Abortion*, 27–109. They vary according to available data, and therefore are not necessarily comparable across countries. However for a particular country, the data estimate the frequency of unsafe abortion, often measured by hospital admissions to treat unsafe abortion, and the mortality due to unsafe abortion. Even though these figures are estimates, they suggest that more needs to be done to reduce unsafe abortion. Measures include improving the quality of abortion services and the conditions that enable safe abortions, such as liberalizing and implementing abortion laws, and decreasing the need to resort to unsafe procedures such as by improving access to effective contraception and its use by both men and women and reducing rape and sexual abuse.

ᵉ Mortality ratio: 'The unsafe abortion mortality ratio is the number of deaths due to unsafe abortion per 100,000 live births during the same period. This is a subset of the maternal mortality ratio and represents the risk of death due to unsafe abortion.'

ᶠ Deaths due to unsafe abortion [are estimated] as a percentage of all maternal deaths. The total number of maternal deaths has been calculated using the revised 1990 ratios: WHO and UNICEF, *Revised 1990 Estimates of Maternal Mortality: A New Approach by WHO and UNICEF* (Geneva: WHO, 1996). Another estimate that is used is the case fatality rate. While not provided in this table, case fatality rates are given for some countries, WHO, *Unsafe Abortion*, 27–109. 'The unsafe abortion fatality rate expresses the estimated number of deaths per 100 estimated number of unsafe abortion procedures.'

Source

WHO *Unsafe Abortion: Global and Regional Estimates of Incidence of and Mortality Due to Unsafe Abortion with a Listing of Available Country Data* (3rd edn.; Geneva: WHO, 1997), 8–9. This WHO study explains (p. 3) that unsafe abortion is an 'abortion not provided through approved facilities and/or persons'.

III.1.3.2. Measures of induced abortion and hospitalization for abortion complications
for selected Latin American countries

Country and year	Abortions				Hospitalizations for abortion complications	
	Best estimate of annual no. of abortions	Range	Rate (abortions per 1,000 women aged 15–44)	Ratio (abortions per 100 pregnancies)	No.	Rate (% of women hospitalized for abortion complications
Brazil, 1991	1,444,000	1,021,000–2,021,000	40.8	29.8	288,700	8.1
Chile, 1990	160,000	128,000–224,000	50.0	35.3	31,000	10.0
Colombia, 1989	288,000	288,000–404,000	36.3	26.0	57,000	7.2
Dominican Republic, 1990	82,000	58,000–115,000	47.0	27.9	16,500	9.8
Mexico, 1990	533,000	297,000–746,000	25.1	17.1	106,500	5.4
Peru, 1989	271,000	271,000–380,000	56.1	30.0	54,200	10.9
Total (above 6 countries)	2,768,150		33.9		555,630	
Estimated total for Latin America*	4,000,000		33.9		800,000	

Note: Numbers are estimated on the assumption that these six countries account for 70% of the population of Latin Americ
and that all countries in the region have similar hospitalization levels; rounded to the nearest 100,000. AGI, *Overview*, at
and 5.

Sources

S. K. Henshaw, S. Singh, and T. Haas, 'The Incidence of Abortion Worldwide', *International Family Planning Perspectives*
25 (suppl.) (1999), S30–S38; S. Singh and D. Wulf, 'Estimated Level of Induced Abortion in Six Latin American Countries
International Family Planning Perspectives, 20/1 (1994), 4–13; Alan Guttmacher Institute (AGI), *An Overview of Clandestin
Abortion in Latin America: Issues Brief* (New York: AGI, 1996). These studies explain that one way of obtaining informatio
about women having abortions in countries where abortion is legally very restricted is to examine data on women hospita
ized for abortion complications. The studies point out, however, that hospitalized women are not necessarily representativ
of all women having induced abortions in that country. Moreover, Henshaw *et al.* point out (S35) that 'the proportion c
women hospitalized for complications of abortion is based on several variables for which accurate measurement is not pos
sible. The extent to which safe abortion is practiced, the probability of complications arising from procedures provided b
nonphysicians and the ease of access to a hospital are all reflected in this factor.'

   Other sources for abortion data for Latin American countries include AGI, *Clandestine Abortion: A Latin America
Reality* (New York: AGI, 1994); J. M. Paxman, A. Rizo, L. Brown, and J. Benson, 'The Clandestine Epidemic: The Practic
of Unsafe Abortion in Latin America', *Studies in Family Planning*, 24/4 (1993), 205–26.

III.1.3.3. Young women hospitalized for abortion complications in selected Latin American and African countries

Country	% of women hospitalized for abortion complications		Sample size
	<20 years old	<24 years old	
Brazil[a]	23	59	2,083
Dominican Republic[b]	16	49	352
Mexico[c]	28	57	134
Kenya[d]	18(<19)	38	1,404
Mauritius[e]	10	36	475
Tanzania[f]	33	62	455

[a] C. Misago and W. Fonseca, 'Determinants and Medical Characteristics of Induced Abortion Among Poor Women in North-East Brazil', in A. I. Mundigo and C. Indriso (eds.), *Abortion in the Developing World* (Geneva and New Delhi: WHO and Vistaar, 1999), 217–27.

[b] D. Paiewonsky, 'Social Determinants of Induced Abortion in the Dominican Republic', in Mundigo and Indriso (eds.), *Abortion*, 131–50.

[c] M. C. Elu, 'Between Political Debate and Woman's Suffering in Mexico', in Mundigo and Indriso (eds.), *Abortion*, 245–58.

[d] J. Solo, D. L. Billings, C. Aloo-Opbunga, A. Ominde, and M. Makumi, 'Creating Linkages between Incomplete Abortion Treatment and Family Planning Services in Kenya', in D. Huntington and N. J. Piet-Pelon (eds.), *Postabortion Care: Lessons from Operations Research* (New York: Population Council, 1999), 38–60.

[e] G. Oodit and U. Bhowon, 'The Use of Induced Abortion in Mauritius: An Alternative to Fertility Regulation or an Emergency Procedure', in Mundigo and Indriso (eds.), *Abortion*, 151–66.

[f] G. S. Mpangile, M. T. Leshabari, and D. J. Kihwele, 'Induced Abortion in Dar es Salaam, Tanzania: The Plight of Adolescents', in Mundigo and Indriso (eds.), *Abortion*, 387–403.

Sources

With the exception of Kenya, the data are presented in S. Bott, 'Unwanted Pregnancy and Induced Abortion among Adolescents in Developing Countries: Findings from WHO Case Studies', in C. Chandraburi and P. Van Look, *Proceedings from the International Conference on Reproductive Health, 15–19 Nov 1998, Mumbai, India* (Geneva: WHO, 1999). The source of each country case study is given in the notes.

2

World Medical Association Declaration of Helsinki: Ethical Principles for Medical Research Involving Human Subjects

Adopted by the 18th WMA General Assembly, Helsinki, Finland, June 1964, and amended by the 29th WMA General Assembly, Tokyo, Japan, October 1975, 35th WMA General Assembly, Venice, Italy, October 1983, 41st WMA General Assembly, Hong Kong, September 1989, 48th WMA General Assembly, Somerset West, Republic of South Africa, October 1996, and the 52nd WMA General Assembly, Edinburgh, Scotland, October 2000

A. Introduction

1. The World Medical Association has developed the Declaration of Helsinki as a statement of ethical principles to provide guidance to physicians and other participants in medical research involving human subjects. Medical research involving human subjects includes research on identifiable human material or identifiable data.

2. It is the duty of the physician to promote and safeguard the health of the people. The physician's knowledge and conscience are dedicated to the fulfillment of this duty.

3. The Declaration of Geneva of the World Medical Association binds the physician with the words, 'The health of my patient will be my first consideration', and the International Code of Medical Ethics declares that, 'A physician shall act only in the patient's interest when providing medical care which might have the effect of weakening the physical and mental condition of the patient.'

4. Medical progress is based on research which ultimately must rest in part on experimentation involving human subjects.

5. In medical research on human subjects, considerations related to the well-being of the human subject should take precedence over the interests of science and society.

6. The primary purpose of medical research involving human subjects is to improve prophylactic, diagnostic and therapeutic procedures and the understanding of the aetiology and pathogenesis of disease. Even the best proven

prophylactic, diagnostic, and therapeutic methods must continuously be challenged through research for their effectiveness, efficiency, accessibility and quality.

7. In current medical practice and in medical research, most prophylactic, diagnostic and therapeutic procedures involve risks and burdens.

8. Medical research is subject to ethical standards that promote respect for all human beings and protect their health and rights. Some research populations are vulnerable and need special protection. The particular needs of the economically and medically disadvantaged must be recognized. Special attention is also required for those who cannot give or refuse consent for themselves, for those who may be subject to giving consent under duress, for those who will not benefit personally from the research and for those for whom the research is combined with care.

9. Research Investigators should be aware of the ethical, legal and regulatory requirements for research on human subjects in their own countries as well as applicable international requirements. No national ethical, legal or regulatory requirement should be allowed to reduce or eliminate any of the protections for human subjects set forth in this Declaration.

B. Basic Principles for All Medical Research

10. It is the duty of the physician in medical research to protect the life, health, privacy, and dignity of the human subject.

11. Medical research involving human subjects must conform to generally accepted scientific principles, be based on a thorough knowledge of the scientific literature, other relevant sources of information, and on adequate laboratory and, where appropriate, animal experimentation.

12. Appropriate caution must be exercised in the conduct of research which may affect the environment, and the welfare of animals used for research must be respected.

13. The design and performance of each experimental procedure involving human subjects should be clearly formulated in an experimental protocol. This protocol should be submitted for consideration, comment, guidance, and where appropriate, approval to a specially appointed ethical review committee, which must be independent of the investigator, the sponsor or any other kind of undue influence. This independent committee should be in conformity with the laws and regulations of the country in which the research experiment is performed. The committee has the right to monitor ongoing trials. The researcher has the obligation to provide monitoring information to the committee, especially any serious adverse events. The researcher should also submit to the committee, for review, information regarding funding, sponsors, institutional affiliations, other potential conflicts of interest and incentives for subjects.

14. The research protocol should always contain a statement of the ethical considerations involved and should indicate that there is compliance with the principles enunciated in this Declaration.

15. Medical research involving human subjects should be conducted only by scientifically qualified persons and under the supervision of a clinically competent medical person. The responsibility for the human subject must always rest with a medically qualified person and never rest on the subject of the research, even though the subject has given consent.

16. Every medical research project involving human subjects should be preceded by careful assessment of predictable risks and burdens in comparison with foreseeable benefits to the subject or to others. This does not preclude the participation of healthy volunteers in medical research. The design of all studies should be publicly available.

17. Physicians should abstain from engaging in research projects involving human subjects unless they are confident that the risks involved have been adequately assessed and can be satisfactorily managed. Physicians should cease any investigation if the risks are found to outweigh the potential benefits or if there is conclusive proof of positive and beneficial results.

18. Medical research involving human subjects should only be conducted if the importance of the objective outweighs the inherent risks and burdens to the subject. This is especially important when the human subjects are healthy volunteers.

19. Medical research is only justified if there is a reasonable likelihood that the populations in which the research is carried out stand to benefit from the results of the research.

20. The subjects must be volunteers and informed participants in the research project.

21. The right of research subjects to safeguard their integrity must always be respected. Every precaution should be taken to respect the privacy of the subject, the confidentiality of the patient's information and to minimize the impact of the study on the subject's physical and mental integrity and on the personality of the subject.

22. In any research on human beings, each potential subject must be adequately informed of the aims, methods, sources of funding, any possible conflicts of interest, institutional affiliations of the researcher, the anticipated benefits and potential risks of the study and the discomfort it may entail. The subject should be informed of the right to abstain from participation in the study or to withdraw consent to participate at any time without reprisal. After ensuring that the subject has understood the information, the physician should then obtain the subject's freely-given informed consent, preferably in writing. If the consent cannot be obtained in writing, the non-written consent must be formally documented and witnessed.

23. When obtaining informed consent for the research project the physician should be particularly cautious if the subject is in a dependent relationship with the physician or may consent under duress. In that case the informed consent should be obtained by a well-informed physician who is not engaged in the investigation and who is completely independent of this relationship.

24. For a research subject who is legally incompetent, physically or mentally incapable of giving consent or is a legally incompetent minor, the investigator must obtain informed consent from the legally authorized representative in accordance with applicable law. These groups should not be included in research unless the research is necessary to promote the health of the population represented and this research cannot instead be performed on legally competent persons.

25. When a subject deemed legally incompetent, such as a minor child, is able to give assent to decisions about participation in research, the investigator must obtain that assent in addition to the consent of the legally authorized representative.

26. Research on individuals from whom it is not possible to obtain consent, including proxy or advance consent, should be done only if the physical/mental condition that prevents obtaining informed consent is a necessary characteristic of the research population. The specific reasons for involving research subjects with a condition that renders them unable to give informed consent should be stated in the experimental protocol for consideration and approval of the review committee. The protocol should state that consent to remain in the research should be obtained as soon as possible from the individual or a legally authorized surrogate.

27. Both authors and publishers have ethical obligations. In publication of the results of research, the investigators are obliged to preserve the accuracy of the results. Negative as well as positive results should be published or otherwise publicly available. Sources of funding, institutional affiliations and any possible conflicts of interest should be declared in the publication. Reports of experimentation not in accordance with the principles laid down in this Declaration should not be accepted for publication.

C. Additional Principles for Medical Research Combined with Medical Care

28. The physician may combine medical research with medical care, only to the extent that the research is justified by its potential prophylactic, diagnostic or therapeutic value. When medical research is combined with medical care, additional standards apply to protect the patients who are research subjects.

29. The benefits, risks, burdens and effectiveness of a new method should be tested against those of the best current prophylactic, diagnostic and therapeutic

methods. This does not exclude the use of placebo, or no treatment, in studies where no proven prophylactic, diagnostic or therapeutic method exists.

30. At the conclusion of the study, every patient entered into the study should be assured of access to the best proven prophylactic, diagnostic and therapeutic methods identified by the study.

31. The physician should fully inform the patient which aspects of the care are related to the research. The refusal of a patient to participate in a study must never interfere with the patient–physician relationship.

32. In the treatment of a patient, where proven prophylactic, diagnostic and therapeutic methods do not exist or have been ineffective, the physician, with informed consent from the patient, must be free to use unproven or new prophylactic, diagnostic and therapeutic measures, if in the physician's judgement it offers hope of saving life, re-establishing health or alleviating suffering. Where possible, these measures should be made the object of research, designed to evaluate their safety and efficacy. In all cases, new information should be recorded and, where appropriate, published. The other relevant guidelines of this Declaration should be followed.

3

Human Rights Treaties and UN Conference Documents

1. International Human Rights Treaties

Universal Declaration of Human Rights, 10 Dec. 1948, GA Res. 217A (III), UN Doc. A/810, at 71.
www.un.org/Overview/rights.html

International Covenant on Civil and Political Rights, 16 Dec. 1966, 999 UNTS 171, entered into force 23 Mar. 1976.
Text: www1.umn.edu/humanrts/instree/b3ccpr.htm
Ratifications: www.unhchr.ch/tbs/doc.nsf

Optional Protocol to the International Covenant on Civil and Political Rights, 16 Dec. 1966, 999 UNTS 302, entered into force 23 Mar. 1976.
Text: www1.umn.edu/humanrts/instree/b4ccprp1.htm
Ratifications: www.unhchr.ch/tbs/doc.nsf

International Covenant on Economic, Social and Cultural Rights, 16 Dec. 1966, 993 UNTS 3, entered into force 3 Jan. 1976.
Text: www.unhchr.ch/html/menu3/b/a_cescr.htm
Ratifications: www.unhchr.ch/tbs/doc.nsf

Convention against Torture and Other Cruel and Inhuman and Degrading Treatment, 10 Dec. 1984, GA Res. 39/46, annex, 39 UN GAOR Supp. (No. 51) at 197, UN Doc. A/39/51 (1984), entered into force 26 June 1987.
Text: www.unhchr.ch/html/menu3/b/h_cat39.htm
Ratifications: www.unhchr.ch/pdf/report.pdf

Convention on the Elimination of All Forms of Discrimination against Women, 18 Dec. 1979, GA Res. 34/180, UN GAOR, 34th Sess., Supp. No. 46 at 193, UN Doc. A/34/46, entered into force 3 Sept. 1981.
Text: www1.umn.edu/humanrts/instree/e1cedaw.htm
Ratifications: www.unhchr.ch/tbs/doc.nsf

Optional Protocol to the Convention on the Elimination of All Forms of Discrimination against Women, 6 Oct. 1999, GA Res. 54/4, entered into force 22 Dec. 2000.
Text: www.un.org/womenwatch/daw/cedaw/protocol/current.htm
Ratifications: www.unhchr.ch/tbs/doc.nsf

International Convention for the Elimination of All Forms of Racial Discrimination, 21 Dec. 1965, 660 UNTS 195, entered into force 4 Jan. 1969.
Text: www1.umn.edu/humanrts/instree/d1cerd.htm
Ratifications: www.unhchr.ch/tbs/doc.nsf

Convention on the Rights of the Child, 20 Nov. 1989, GA Res. 44/25 (XLIV), UN GAOR, 44th Sess., Supp. No. 49 at 167, UN Doc. A/44/49, entered into force 2 Sept. 1990.
Text: www1.umn.edu/humanrts/instree/k2crc.htm
Ratifications: www.unhchr.ch/tbs/doc.nsf

2. *Regional Human Rights Treaties*

African [Banjul] Charter on Human and Peoples' Rights, 27 June 1981, OAU Doc. CAB/LEG/67/3 Rev. 5, 21 ILM 58 (1982), entered into force 21 Oct. 1986.
Text: www1.umn.edu/humanrts/instree/z1afchar.htm
Ratifications: www1.umn.edu/humanrts/instree/ratz1afchar.htm (as of 1 Aug. 1994)

African Charter on the Rights and Welfare of the Child, July 1990, OAU Doc. CAB/LEG/24.9/49 (1990), entered into force 29 Nov. 1999.
Text: www1.umn.edu/humanrts/africa/afchild.htm
Ratifications: www1.umn.edu/humanrts/instree/afchildratifications.html

American Declaration of the Rights and Duties of Man, (1948) OAS Res. XXX, reprinted in Basic Documents Pertaining to Human Rights in the Inter-American System, OEA/Ser.L.V./II.82 doc.6 rev.1 at 17 (1992).

American Convention on Human Rights 'Pact of San Jose, Costa Rica', 22 Nov. 1969, OAS Treaty Series No. 36, 1144 UNTS 144, entered into force 18 July 1978.
For texts and ratification of this and the following Additional Protocol, see: www.cidh.oas.org/basic.htm

Additional Protocol to the American Convention on Human Rights in the Area of Economic, Social and Cultural Rights 'Protocol of San Salvador', 17 Nov. 1988, OAS Treaty Series No. 69, entered into force 16 Nov. 1999.

Arab Charter on Human Rights, 15 Sept. 1994, Council of the League of Arab States, 102d Sess, Res. 5437, reprinted in 56 Review of the International Commission of Jurists 57 (1997) and 4 Int. Human Rights Reporter 850 (1997)
Text: www.al-bab.com/arab/docs/league.htm

Inter-American Convention on the Prevention, Punishment and Eradication of Violence against Women 'Convention of Belem Do Para', 9 June 1994, 33 ILM 1534 (1994), entered into force 5 Mar. 1995.

Statute of the Inter-American Commission on Human Rights, OAS Res. 447 (IX-0/79), OAS Off. Rec. OEA/Ser.P/IX.0.2/80, Vol. 1 at 88, Annual Report of the Inter-American Commission on Human Rights, OEA/Ser.L/V/11.50 doc.13 rev. 1 at 10 (1980), reprinted in Basic Documents Pertaining to Human Rights in the Inter-American System, OEA/Ser.L.V/II.82 doc.6 rev.1 at 93 (1992).

Regulations of the Inter-American Commission on Human Rights Statute of the Inter-American Court on Human Rights, reprinted in Basic Documents Pertaining to Human Rights in the Inter-American System, OEA/Ser.L.V/II.82 doc.6 rev.1 at 103 (1992).

Statute of the Inter-American Court on Human Rights, OAS Res. 448 (IX-0/79), OAS Off. Rec. OEA/Ser.P/IX.0.2/80, Vol. 1 at 98, Annual Report of the Inter-American Court on Human Rights, OEA/Ser.L/V.III.3 doc. 13 corr. 1 at 16 (1980), reprinted in Basic Documents Pertaining to Human Rights in the Inter-American System, OEA/Ser.L.V/II.82 doc.6 rev.1 at 133 (1992).

European Convention for the Protection of Human Rights and Fundamental Freedoms, 4 Nov. 1940, ETS No. 5; 213 UNTS 222, entered into force 3 Sept. 1953; as amended by Protocol Nos. 3, 5, and 8 which entered into force on 21 Sept. 1970, 20 Dec. 1971, and 1 Jan. 1990, respectively.
Text and ratifications: conventions.coe.int/treaty/EN/cadreprincipal.htm

European Protocol 12 to the Convention for the Protection of Human Rights and Fundamental Freedoms, 4 Nov. 2000, ETS No. 177, not yet entered into force.
Text and ratifications: conventions.coe.int/treaty/EN/cadreprincipal.htm

European Social Charter, 13 Oct. 1961, 529 UNTS 89, entered into force 26 Feb. 1965.
Text and ratifications: conventions.coe.int/treaty/EN/cadreprincipal.htm

European Social Charter, Revised (1996) ETS No. 163, entered into force 1 July 1999.
Text and ratifications: conventions.coe.int/treaty/EN/cadreprincipal.htm

3. *UN Conference Documents*

International Conference on Population and Development, Cairo, Egypt, 13–15 Sept. 1994, UN Document A/Conf. 171/13.
See: www.iisd.ca/linkages/cairo.html

General Assembly Special Session on the International Conference on Population and Development, General Assembly A/Res/S-21/2, 8 Nov. 1999.
See: www.unfpa.org/ICPD/icpdmain.htm

The Fourth World Conference on Women, Beijing, China, 4–15 Sept. 1995, UN Document A/CONF.177/20.
See: www.un.org/womenwatch/daw/beijing/platform/

Further Actions and Initiatives to Implement the Bejing Declaration and Platform for Action, Report of the Ad Hoc Committee of the Whole of the Twenty-Third Session of the General Assembly, UN Doc. A/S-23/10/Rev.1, GAOR, 23rd spec. sess., supp. 3, at p. 6.

4

Human Rights Relating to Reproductive and Sexual Health

This chapter identifies rights (listed on the left-hand side of Table III.4) that could be applied to advance reproductive and sexual health. These rights are expressed in the human rights instruments named in the column headings of the table, and are identified by the number of the article of each particular instrument. The human rights are clustered under the following interests in reproductive and sexual health, which are shown in the horizontal subsections of the table:

- life, survival, security, and sexuality
- reproductive self-determination, and free choice of maternity
- health and the benefits of scientific progress
- non-discrimination and due respect for difference
- information, education, and decision-making.

As human rights are increasingly applied to protect reproductive and sexual health, they may be clustered differently, depending on the facts of the alleged violation of human rights.

Table III.4. Human rights relating to reproductive and sexual health

Human rights	Declarations and conventions					
	Universal Declaration of Human Rights	Int. Covenant on Civil & Political Rights	Int. Covenant on Economic, Social & Cultural Rights	Int. Convention on the Elimination of All Forms of Racial Discrimination	Convention on the Elimination of All Forms of Discrimination against Women	Convention on the Rights of the Child & its Protocol on Prostitution and Pornography
Life, survival, security, and sexuality						
Right to life and survival	3	6				6
Right to liberty and security of the person	3	9		5(b)		37(b)–(d), Protocol 1, 2, 3, 7
Right to be free from torture, cruel, inhuman, and degrading treatment or punishment	5	7				37(a), Protocol 1, 2, 3, 7
Reproductive self-determination and free choice of maternity						
Right to maternity protection	25(2)		10(2)		5(b), 12(2)	24(d)
Right to marry and found a family	16	23	10	5(d)(iv)	16	

Convention against Torture and Other Cruel and Inhuman and Degrading Treatment or Punishment	European Convention on Human Rights & Protocols 1 and 12 European Social Charter, Revised	American Convention on Human Rights & its Protocol on Economic, Social and Cultural Rights	Inter-American Convention on the Eradication of Violence against Women	African Charter on Human & Peoples' Rights African Charter on the Rights and Welfare of the Child	Arab Charter on Human Rights	Cairo Programme of Action (1994) Cairo+5 (1999)	Beijing Declaration & Platform for Action (1995) Beijing+5 (2000)
	2	4	4(a)	4, Child Charter 5	5	Principle 1, 8.21–8.27	*See generally* 89–111, 210–33, Beijing+5 72
	5	7	4(c)	6, Child Charter 16, 21, 27, 29	5	Principle 1, 7.2–7.11	*See generally* 89–130, 210–33, Beijing+5 13–14, 59, 68(2), 69, 70
1, 4, 16	3	5	3, 4(d)	5, Child Charter 16, 21, 27, 29	13	Principle 4, 4.9, 4.10, 4.22, 4.23	*See generally* 112–30
	Charter 8	26, Protocol 15, 3(a)(b)		Child Charter 14(2)(e)	38	8.19–8.24, Cairo+5 62, 64–6	94–5, 97, 110–11, Beijing+5 11–12, 72–9
	12	17	5	18, 27(1) (duty)	38	Principle 9, 4.21, *see generally* Ch. V, 7.12–7.23	92, 274(e), 275(b), *see generally* 210–33, Beijing+5 60

Table III.4. (*cont.*)

Human rights	Declarations and conventions					
	Universal Declaration of Human Rights	Int. Covenant on Civil & Political Rights	Int. Covenant on Economic, Social & Cultural Rights	Int. Convention on the Elimination of All Forms of Racial Discrimination	Convention on the Elimination of All Forms of Discrimination against Women	Convention on the Rights of the Child & its Protocol on Prostitution and Pornography
Right to private and family life	12	17	10		16	16
Health and the benefits of scientific progress						
Right to highest attainable standard of health	25		12	5(*e*)(iv)	11(1-*f*), 12, 14(2-*b*)	24, Protocol 9(3), 10(2)
Right to procedural fairness	6, 9, 10, 11	14, 15, 16		5(*a*)	15	12(2), 37(*d*), 40, Protocol 8, 9(4)
Right to benefits of scientific progress	27		15			
Non-discrimination and due respect for difference						
Sex and gender	1, 2, 7	2(1), 3, 26	2(2), 3		1, 2, 3, 4, 5	2(1)
Marital status	1, 2, 7	2(1), 26	2(2)		1	

Convention against Torture and Other Cruel and Inhuman and Degrading Treatment or Punishment	European Convention on Human Rights & Protocols 1 and 12 European Social Charter, Revised	American Convention on Human Rights & its Protocol on Economic, Social and Cultural Rights	Inter-American Convention on the Eradication of Violence against Women	African Charter on Human & Peoples' Rights African Charter on the Rights and Welfare of the Child	Arab Charter on Human Rights	Cairo Programme of Action (1994) Cairo+5 (1999)	Beijing Declaration & Platform for Action (1995) Beijing+5 (2000)
	8, Charter 16, 19, 27	11	4(e)	4, 5, 18, 29(1) (duty), Child Charter 10, 18, 19, 20	17, 38	Principle 9, *see generally* Ch. V, 7.12–7.26	*See generally* 210–33
	Charter 3, 11, 13	26, Protocol 9, 10, 11	5	16, Child Charter 14, 15, 16, 21	39	Principle 8, *see generally* Chs. VII, VIII, Cairo+5 52–72	*See generally* 89–111, Beijing+5 11–12, 44, 72, 79
	6, 7	3, 8	4(g)	7, Child Charter 4, 17	6, 7, 16	Chs. IV, VII, VIII	*See generally* 181–95
		26, Protocol 9, 10	5	22		*See generally* Ch. XII	*See generally* 89–111
	14, Charter E, Protocol 12: 1, 2	1, 24, Protocol 3	4(f), 6	2, 3, 18(3), 19, 28 (duty) Child Charter 3, 21(b)	2, 9	Principle 1, Principle 4, 4.24–4.29, Cairo+5 39–41, 49–50	97, 277(c), *see generally* 210–33, Beijing+5 26–7, 52–3, 68
	14, Charter E, Protocol 12: 1, 2	1, 24, Protocol 3	4(f), 6	2, 3, 18(3), 19, 28, Child Charter 3, 21(b)	2, 9	Principle 1, 7.3, 7.7, 7.8, 7.12, 7.14, Cairo+5 39	*See generally* 89–111, 210–33

Table III.4. (*cont.*)

Human rights	Declarations and conventions					
	Universal Declaration of Human Rights	Int. Covenant on Civil & Political Rights	Int. Covenant on Economic, Social & Cultural Rights	Int. Convention on the Elimination of All Forms of Racial Discrimination	Convention on the Elimination of All Forms of Discrimination against Women	Convention on the Rights of the Child & its Protocol on Prostitution and Pornography
Age	1, 2, 7	2(1), 26	2(2)			2(2)
Race and ethnicity	1, 2, 7	2(1), 26	2(2)	1, 2, 3, 4		2(1)
Sexual orientation	1, 2, 6	2(1)	2(2)			2(2)
Information, education, and decision-making						
Right to receive and to impart information	19	19		5(*d*-viii)	10(*h*), 14(2-*b*), 16(1-*e*)	12, 13, 17
Right to Education	26		13, 14	5(*e*-v), 7	10, 14(2-*d*)	28, 29
Right to freedom of thought, conscience, and religion	18	18		5(*d*)(vii)		14, 30

Convention against Torture and Other Cruel and Inhuman and Degrading Treatment or Punishment	European Convention on Human Rights & Protocols 1 and 12 European Social Charter, Revised	American Convention on Human Rights & its Protocol on Economic, Social and Cultural Rights	Inter-American Convention on the Eradication of Violence against Women	African Charter on Human & Peoples' Rights African Charter on the Rights and Welfare of the Child	Arab Charter on Human Rights	Cairo Programme of Action (1994) Cairo+5 (1999)	Beijing Declaration & Platform for Action (1995) Beijing+5 (2000)
	14, Charter E, Protocol 12: 1, 2	1, 24, Protocol 3	4(*f*), 6	2, 3, 18(3), 19, 28, Child Charter 3, 21(*b*)	2, 9	Principle 1, *see generally* Chs. IV, VII, 8.12–8.27, Cairo+5 42, 73, 74	*See generally* 259–85, Beijing+5 32–3
	14, Charter E, Protocol 12: 1, 2	1, 24, Protocol 3	4(*f*), 6	2, 3, 18(3), 19, 28, Child Charter 3, 21(*b*), 26	2, 9	Principle 1, 6.21–6.27, 7.3, 7.7, 7.8, 7.12, 7.14	*See generally* 89–111, 210–33, Beijing+5 66(B)
	14, Protocol 12: 1, 2	1, 24		2, 3, 18(4), 28, Child Charter 3	2, 9	7.34–7.40, 8.34	99, 108
	10	13	5	9, Child Charter 7, 8		8.26, *see generally* Ch. XI	*See generally* 69–111, 210–33
	Protocol 1: 2	26, Protocol 13	5, 6(*b*)	17, Child Charter 11, 12, 13	34	Principle 10, 4.2, *see generally* Chs. VII, VIII, XI, Cairo+5 34–6	*See generally* 69–88, 210–33, Beijing+5 9–10, 55, 67
	9	12, 13	4(i), 5	8, Child Charter 9	26, 27		

5

States Parties to Human Rights Treaties

States commit themselves to implement human rights treaties through a process of signature usually followed by ratification, or alternatively by direct accession. When states sign and then ratify, or directly accede to a treaty, they are called States Parties to the treaty. When countries are only signatories to a treaty but have not yet ratified, they nevertheless commit themselves not to act inconsistently with the treaty. If a state wants to reacquire the option to act inconsistently, it usually first withdraws its signature. When states ratify or accede to a treaty, thus becoming States Parties to that treaty, they agree to implement the treaty. This chapter identifies states that have signed, ratified, or acceded to particular treaties, and Optional Protocols if treaties have them. The chapter also provides the total number of States Parties to each treaty, indicating that there is near universal ratification of some treaties.

Table III.5.1. States Parties to Human Rights Treaties, updated as of 8 February 2002

State	Int. Covenant on Civil and Political Rights	Optional Protocol to the Int. Covenant on Civil and Political Rights	Int. Covenant on Economic, Social and Cultural Rights	Int. Convention on the Elimination of All Forms of Racial Discrimination
Afghanistan	x		x	x
Albania	x		x	x
Algeria	x	x	x	x
Andorra				
Angola	x	x	x	
Antigua & Barbuda				x
Argentina	x	x	x	x
Armenia	x	x	x	x
Australia	x	x	x	x
Austria	x	x	x	x
Azerbaijan	x	x	x	x
Bahamas				x
Bahrain				x
Bangladesh	x		x	x
Barbados	x	x	x	x
Belarus	x	x	x	x
Belgium	x	x	x	x
Belize	x		s	x
Benin	x	x	x	x
Bhutan				s
Bolivia	x	x	x	x
Bosnia & Herzegovina	x	x	x	x
Botswana	x			x
Brazil	x		x	x
Brunei Darussalam				
Bulgaria	x	x	x	x
Burkina Faso	x	x	x	x
Burundi	x		x	x
Cambodia	x		x	x
Cameroon	x	x	x	x
Canada	x	x	x	x
Cape Verde	x	x	x	x
Central African Republic	x	x	x	x
Chad	x	x	x	x
Chile	x	x	x	x
China	s		x	x

Convention on the Elimination of All Forms of Discrimination against Women	Optional Protocol to the Convention on the Elimination of All Forms of Discrimination against Women	Convention on the Rights of the Child	Optional Protocol to the Convention on the Rights of the Child on Prostitution and Pornography	Convention against Torture and Other Cruel and Inhuman or Degrading Treatment or Punishment
		X		X
		X		X
		X		X
	s	X	X	
		X		
		X	s	X
	s	X		X
		X		X
		X	s	X
X		X	s	X
X		X	s	X
		X		
		X		X
X		X	X	X
		X		
		X		X
	s	X	s	X
		X	s	X
	s	X	s	X
		X		
X		X	s	X
	s	X	s	X
		X		X
	s	X	s	X
		X		
	s	X	s	X
		X	s	X
		X		X
		X	s	X
		X	s	X
		X	s	X
		X		X
		X		
		X		X
	s	X	s	X
		X	s	X

Table III.5.1. (*cont.*)

State	Int. Covenant on Civil and Political Rights	Optional Protocol to the Int. Covenant on Civil and Political Rights	Int. Covenant on Economic, Social and Cultural Rights	Int. Convention on the Elimination of All Forms of Racial Discrimination
Colombia	x	x	x	x
Comoros				s
Congo	x	x	x	x
Cook Islands				
Costa Rica	x	x	x	x
Côte d'Ivoire	x	x	x	x
Croatia	x	x	x	x
Cuba				x
Cyprus	x	x	x	x
Czech Rep	x	x	x	x
Democratic People's Rep. of Korea	x		x	
Democratic Republic of the Congo	x	x	x	x
Denmark	x	x	x	x
Djibouti				
Dominica	x		x	
Dominican Republic	x	x	x	x
Ecuador	x	x	x	x
Egypt	x		x	x
El Salvador	x	x	x	x
Equatorial Guinea	x	x	x	
Eritrea	x		x	x
Estonia	x	x	x	x
Ethiopia	x		x	x
Fiji				x
Finland	x	x	x	x
Former Yugoslav Rep. of Macedonia	x	x	x	x
France	x	x	x	x
Gabon	x		x	x
Gambia	x	x	x	x
Georgia	x	x	x	x
Germany	x	x	x	x
Ghana	x	x	x	x
Greece	x	x	x	x

Convention on the Elimination of All Forms of Discrimination against Women	Optional Protocol to the Convention on the Elimination of All Forms of Discrimination against Women	Convention on the Rights of the Child	Optional Protocol to the Convention on the Rights of the Child on Prostitution and Pornography	Convention against Torture and Other Cruel and Inhuman or Degrading Treatment or Punishment
	s	X	s	X
		X		s
		X		
		X		
X		X	s	X
		X		X
X		X		X
s		X	X	X
s		X	s	X
X		X		X
		X		
		X	X	X
X		X	s	X
		X		
		X		
X		X		s
s		X	s	X
		X		X
s		X		X
		X		
		X		
		X		X
		X		X
		X		
X		X	s	X
s		X	s	X
X		X	s	X
		X	s	X
		X	s	s
		X		X
X		X	s	X
s		X		X
X		X	s	X

Table III.5.1. (*cont.*)

State	Int. Covenant on Civil and Political Rights	Optional Protocol to the Int. Covenant on Civil and Political Rights	Int. Covenant on Economic, Social and Cultural Rights	Int. Convention on the Elimination c All Forms of Racial Discrimination
Grenada	x		x	s
Guatemala	x	x	x	x
Guinea	x	x	x	x
Guinea Bissau	s	s	x	s
Guyana	x	x	x	x
Haiti	x			x
Holy See				x
Honduras	x	s	x	
Hungary	x	x	x	x
Iceland	x	x	x	x
India	x		x	x
Indonesia				x
Iran (Islamic Rep. of)	x		x	x
Iraq	x		x	x
Ireland	x	x	x	x
Israel	x		x	x
Italy	x	x	x	x
Jamaica	x		x	x
Japan	x		x	x
Jordan	x		x	x
Kazakhstan				x
Kenya	x		x	x
Kiribati				
Kuwait	x		x	x
Kyrgyszstan	x	x	x	x
Lao People's Dem. Rep.	s		s	x
Latvia	x	x	x	x
Lebanon	x		x	x
Lesotho	x	x	x	x
Liberia	s		s	x
Libyan Arab Jamahiriya	x	x	x	x
Liechtenstein	x	x	x	x
Lithuania	x	x	x	x
Luxembourg	x	x	x	x
Madagascar	x	x	x	x
Malawi	x	x	x	x

Convention on the Elimination of All Forms of Discrimination against Women	Optional Protocol to the Convention on the Elimination of All Forms of Discrimination against Women	Convention on the Rights of the Child	Optional Protocol to the Convention on the Rights of the Child on Prostitution and Pornography	Convention against Torture and Other Cruel and Inhuman or Degrading Treatment or Punishment
		x		
s		x	s	x
		x		x
s		x	s	s
		x		x
		x		
		x	x	
		x		x
x		x		x
x		x	x	x
		x		s
s		x	s	x
		x		
		x		
x		x	s	s
		x	s	x
x		x	s	x
		x	s	
		x		x
		x	s	x
x		x	x	x
		x	s	x
		x		
		x		x
		x		x
		x		
		x		x
		x	s	x
s		x	s	x
		x		
		x		x
x		x	s	x
s		x		x
s		x	s	x
s		x	s	s
s		x	s	x

Table III.5.1. (*cont.*)

State	Int. Covenant on Civil and Political Rights	Optional Protocol to the Int. Covenant on Civil and Political Rights	Int. Covenant on Economic, Social and Cultural Rights	Int. Convention on the Elimination of All Forms of Racial Discrimination
Malaysia				
Maldives				x
Mali	x	x	x	x
Malta	x	x	x	x
Marshall Islands				
Mauritania				x
Mauritius	x	x	x	x
Mexico	x		x	x
Micronesia (Fed. States of)				
Monaco	x		x	x
Mongolia	x	x	x	x
Morocco	x		x	x
Mozambique	x			x
Myanmar				
Namibia	x	x	x	x
Nauru	s	s		s
Nepal	x	x	x	x
Netherlands	x	x	x	x
New Zealand	x	x	x	x
Nicaragua	x	x	x	x
Niger	x	x	x	x
Nigeria	x		x	x
Niue				
Norway	x	x	x	x
Oman				
Pakistan				x
Palau				
Panama	x	x	x	x
Papua New Guinea				x
Paraguay	x	x	x	s
Peru	x	x	x	x
Philippines	x	x	x	x
Poland	x	x	x	x
Portugal	x	x	x	x
Qatar				x

Convention on the Elimination of All Forms of Discrimination against Women	Optional Protocol to the Convention on the Elimination of All Forms of Discrimination against Women	Convention on the Rights of the Child	Optional Protocol to the Convention on the Rights of the Child on Prostitution and Pornography	Convention against Torture and Other Cruel and Inhuman or Degrading Treatment or Punishment
		X		
		X		
	X	X		X
		X	s	X
		X		
		X		
	s	X	s	X
	s	X	s	X
		X		
		X	s	X
	s	X	s	X
		X	X	X
		X		X
		X		
	X	X	s	X
		X	s	s
	s	X	s	X
	s	X	s	X
	X	X	s	X
		X		s
		X		X
	s	X	s	X
		X		
	s	X	X	X
		X		
		X	s	
		X		
	X	X	X	X
		X		
	X	X	s	X
	X	X	s	X
	s	X	s	X
		X		X
	s	X	s	X
		X	X	X

Table III.5.1. (*cont.*)

State	Int. Covenant on Civil and Political Rights	Optional Protocol to the Int. Covenant on Civil and Political Rights	Int. Covenant on Economic, Social and Cultural Rights	Int. Convention on the Elimination of All Forms of Racial Discrimination
Republic of Korea	x	x	x	x
Republic of Moldova	x		x	x
Romania	x	x	x	x
Russian Federation	x	x	x	x
Rwanda	x		x	x
St Kitts & Nevis				
St Lucia				x
St Vincent & the Grenadines	x	x	x	x
Samoa				
San Marino	x	x	x	
Sao Tome & Principe	s	s	s	s
Saudi Arabia				x
Senegal	x	x	x	x
Seychelles	x	x	x	x
Sierra Leone	x	x	x	x
Singapore				
Slovakia	x	x	x	x
Slovenia	x	x	x	x
Solomon Islands			x	x
Somalia	x	x	x	x
South Africa	x		s	x
Spain	x	x	x	x
Sri Lanka	x	x	x	x
Sudan	x		x	x
Suriname	x	x	x	x
Swaziland				x
Sweden	x	x	x	x
Switzerland	x		x	x
Syrian Arab Republic	x		x	x
Tajikistan	x	x	x	x
Thailand	x		x	
Togo	x	x	x	x
Tonga				x
Trinidad & Tobago	x		x	x
Tunisia	x		x	x

Convention on the Elimination of All Forms of Discrimination against Women	Optional Protocol to the Convention on the Elimination of All Forms of Discrimination against Women	Convention on the Rights of the Child	Optional Protocol to the Convention on the Rights of the Child on Prostitution and Pornography	Convention against Torture and Other Cruel and Inhuman or Degrading Treatment or Punishment
		X	s	X
		X		X
	s	X	X	X
	s	X		X
		X		
		X		
		X		
		X		X
		X		
		X	s	
	s	X		s
		X		X
	X	X	s	X
		X	s	X
	s	X	X	X
		X		
	X	X	s	X
	s	X	s	X
		X		
				X
		X		X
	X	X	X	X
		X		X
		X		s
		X		
		X		
	s	X	s	X
		X	s	X
		X		
	s	X		X
	X	X		
		X	s	X
		X		
		X		
		X		X

Table III.5.1. (*cont.*)

State	Int. Covenant on Civil and Political Rights	Optional Protocol to the Int. Covenant on Civil and Political Rights	Int. Covenant on Economic, Social and Cultural Rights	Int. Convention on the Elimination o All Forms of Racial Discrimination
Turkey	s		s	s
Turkmenistan	x	x	x	x
Tuvalu				
Uganda	x	x	x	x
Ukraine	x	x	x	x
United Arab Emirates				x
United Kingdom	x		x	x
United Rep. of Tanzania	x		x	x
United States of America	x		s	x
Uruguay	x	x	x	x
Uzbekistan	x	x	x	x
Vanuatu				
Venezuela	x	x	x	x
Viet Nam	x		x	x
Yemen	x		x	x
Yugoslavia	x	x	x	x
Zambia	x	x	x	x
Zimbabwe	x		x	x
TOTAL NO. OF RATIFICATIONS	148	101	145	161

Notes: x = ratification, accession, acceptance, or definitive signature; s = signature not yet followed by ratification.

To check the current ratification status of international human rights, see www.unhchr.ch/pdf/report.pdf (last accesse 9 May 2002), United Nations, *Multilateral Treaties Deposited with the Secretary-General* (New York: United Nations, Offic of Legal Affairs, 1982–).

Convention on the Elimination of All Forms of Discrimination against Women	Optional Protocol to the Convention on the Elimination of All Forms of Discrimination against Women	Convention on the Rights of the Child	Optional Protocol to the Convention on the Rights of the Child on Prostitution and Pornography	Convention against Torture and Other Cruel and Inhuman or Degrading Treatment or Punishment
	s	x	s	x
		x		x
		x		
		x		x
	s	x	s	x
		x		
		x	s	x
		x		
		s	s	x
	x	x	s	x
		x		x
		x		
	s	x	s	x
		x	s	
		x		x
		x	s	x
		x		x
		x		
68	30	191	17	128

Table III.5.2.   States Parties to the European Convention and Social Charter,
updated as of 30 April 2002

State	European Convention on Human Rights	European Social Charter	European Social Charter (Revised)	Protocol 12 to the European Convention (the Protocol against discrimination)
Albania	x		s	
Andorra	x		s	
Armenia	x		s	
Austria	x	x	s	s
Azerbaijan	x		s	
Belgium	x	x	s	s
Bosnia & Herzegovina	s			
Bulgaria	x		x	
Croatia	x	s		s
Cyprus	x	x	x	s
Czech Republic	x	x	s	x
Denmark	x	x	s	
Estonia	x		x	s
Finland	x	x	s	s
France	x	x	x	
Georgia	x		s	x
Germany	x	x		s
Greece	x	x	s	s
Hungary	x	x		s
Iceland	x	x	s	s
Ireland	x	x	x	s
Italy	x	x	x	s
Latvia	x	x		s
Liechtenstein	x	s		s
Lithuania	x		x	
Luxembourg	x	x	s	s
Malta	x	x		
Moldova	x		x	s
Netherlands	x	x		s
Norway	x	x	x	
Poland	x	x		
Portugal	x	x	s	s
Romania	x	s	x	s
Russia	x		s	s
San Marino	x		s	s
Slovakia	x	x	s	s
Slovenia	x	s	x	s
Spain	x	x	s	

Table III.5.2. (*cont.*)

State	European Convention on Human Rights	European Social Charter	European Social Charter (Revised)	Protocol 12 to the European Convention (the Protocol against discrimination)
Sweden	x	x	x	
Switzerland	x	s		
The Former Yugoslav Rep. of Macedonia	x	s		s
Turkey	x	x		s
Ukraine	x	s	s	s
United Kingdom	x	x	s	
TOTAL NO. OF RATIFICATIONS	43	25	12	2

Notes: x = ratification, accession, notification of succession, acceptance, or definitive signature; s = signature not yet followed by ratification.

To check the current ratification status of European human rights documents, see conventions.coe.int/treaty/EN/cadreprincipal.htm.

Table III.5.3. States Parties to the Inter-American treaties, updated as of 30 June 2001

State	American Convention on Human Rights 'Pact of San Jose, Costa Rica'	Additional Protocol to the American Convention on Human Rights in the Area of Economic, Social and Cultural Rights 'Protocol of San Salvador'	Inter-American Convention on the Prevention, Punishment and Eradication of Violence against Women
Antigua & Barbuda			x
Argentina	x	s	x
Bahamas			x
Barbados	x		x
Belize			x
Bolivia	x	s	x
Brazil	x	x	x
Canada			
Chile	x	s	x
Colombia	x	x	x
Costa Rica	x	x	x
Cuba			
Dominica	x		x
Dominican Republic	x	s	x
Ecuador	x	x	x
El Salvador	x	x	x
Grenada	x		x
Guatemala	x	x	x
Guyana			x
Haiti	x	s	x
Honduras	x		x
Jamaica	x		
Mexico	x	x	x
Nicaragua	x	s	x
Panama	x	x	x
Paraguay	x	x	x
Peru	x	x	x
St Kitts & Nevis			x
St Lucia			x
St Vincent & the Grenadines			x
Suriname	x	x	
Trinidad & Tobago	x		x
United States	s		
Uruguay	x	x	x
Venezuela	x	s	x
TOTAL NO. OF RATIFICATIONS	25	12	30

Notes: x = ratification, accession, notification of succession, acceptance, or definitive signature; s = signature not yet followed by ratification.

To check the current ratification of Inter-American human rights conventions, see www.cidh.oas.org basic.htm, last accessed 9 May 2002.

Table III.5.4. States Parties to the African charters, updated as of 2002

State	African Charter on Human and Peoples' Rights	African Charter on the Rights and Welfare of the Child
Algeria	x	s
Angola	x	x
Benin	x	x
Botswana	x	
Burkina Faso	x	x
Burundi	x	
Cameroon	x	x
Cape Verde	x	x
Central African Republic	x	
Chad	x	x
Comoros	x	
Congo	x	s
Côte d'Ivoire	x	
Dem. Rep. of Congo	x	
Djibouti	x	s
Egypt	x	s
Equatorial Guinea	x	
Eritrea	x	x
Ethiopia	x	
Gabon	x	s
Gambia	x	
Ghana	x	s
Guinea	x	x
Guinea-Bissau	x	
Kenya	x	x
Lesotho	x	x
Liberia	x	s
Libya	x	s
Madagascar	x	s
Malawi	x	x
Mali	x	x
Mauritania	x	
Mauritius	x	x
Mozambique	x	x
Namibia	x	s
Niger	x	x
Nigeria	x	
Rwanda	x	s
Sahrawi Arab Dem. Rep.	x	s
Sao Tome & Principe	x	
Senegal	x	x

Table III.5.4. (*cont.*)

State	African Charter on Human and Peoples' Rights	African Charter on the Rights and Welfare of the Child
Seychelles	x	x
Sierra Leone	x	s
Somalia	x	s
South Africa	x	x
Sudan	x	
Swaziland	x	s
Tanzania	x	s
Togo	x	x
Tunisia	x	s
Uganda	x	x
Zambia	x	s
Zimbabwe	x	x
TOTAL NO. OF RATIFICATIONS	53	21

Notes: x = ratification, accession, notification of succession, acceptance, or definitive signature; s = signature not yet followed by ratification.

Status of African Charter on Human and People's Rights, updated as of 1 Jan. 2002, and African Charter on the Rights and Welfare of the Child, updated as of 10 Aug. 2000, taken from the University of Minnesota Human Rights Library at www.umn.edu/humanrts/instree/afrinst.htm, last accessed 9 May 2002.

Table III.5.5. Arab Charter on Human Rights

Member States of the League of Arab States

Algeria	Morocco
Bahrain	Oman
Comoros	Palestine
Djibouti	Qatar
Egypt	Saudi Arabia
Iraq	Somalia
Jordan	Sudan
Kuwait	Syrian Arab Republic
Lebanon	Tunisia
Libyan Arab Jamahiriya	United Arab Emirates
Mauritania	Yemen

Note: The Arab Charter on Human Rights was adopted by the Council of the League of Arab States by its resolution 5437 (102nd regular session) on 15 September 1994.

6

Human Rights Treaty Committees:
General Recommendations/Comments

1. *Committee on the Elimination of Discrimination against Women, General Recommendation 19: Violence against Women*

CEDAW, *General Recommendation 19*, UN GAOR 1992, UN Doc. A/47/38.

1. Gender-based violence is a form of discrimination that seriously inhibits women's ability to enjoy rights and freedoms on a basis of equality with men.

2. In 1989, the Committee recommended that States should include in their reports information on violence and on measures introduced to deal with it (General recommendation 12, eighth session).

3. At its tenth session in 1991, it was decided to allocate part of the eleventh session to a discussion and study on Article 6 and other Articles of the Convention relating to violence towards women and the sexual harassment and exploitation of women. That subject was chosen in anticipation of the 1993 World Conference on Human Rights, convened by the General Assembly by its resolution 45/155 of 18 December 1990.

4. The Committee concluded that not all the reports of States parties adequately reflected the close connection between discrimination against women, gender-based violence, and violations of human rights and fundamental freedoms. The full implementation of the Convention required States to take positive measures to eliminate all forms of violence against women.

5. The Committee suggested to States parties that in reviewing their laws and policies, and in reporting under the Convention, they should have regard to the following comments of the Committee concerning gender-based violence.

6. The Convention in Article 1 defines discrimination against women. The definition of discrimination includes gender-based violence, that is, violence that is directed against a woman because she is a woman or that affects women disproportionately. It includes acts that inflict physical, mental or sexual harm or suffering, threats of such acts, coercion and other deprivations of liberty. Gender-based violence may breach specific provisions of the Convention, regardless of whether those provisions expressly mention violence.

7. Gender-based violence, which impairs or nullifies the enjoyment by women of human rights and fundamental freedoms under general international law or under human rights conventions, is discrimination within the meaning of Article 1 of the Convention. These rights and freedoms include:

(a) The right to life;

(b) The right not to be subject to torture or to cruel, inhuman or degrading treatment or punishment;

(c) The right to equal protection according to humanitarian norms in time of international or internal armed conflict;

(d) The right to liberty and security of person;

(e) The right to equal protection under the law;

(f) The right to equality in the family;

(g) The right to the highest standard attainable of physical and mental health;

(h) The right to just and favourable conditions of work.

8. The Convention applies to violence perpetrated by public authorities. Such acts of violence may breach that State's obligations under general international human rights law and under other conventions, in addition to breaching this Convention.

9. It is emphasized, however, that discrimination under the Convention is not restricted to action by or on behalf of Governments (see Articles 2(e), 2 (f) and 5). For example, under Article 2(e) the Convention calls on States parties to take all appropriate measures to eliminate discrimination against women by any person, organization or enterprise. Under general international law and specific human rights covenants, States may also be responsible for private acts if they fail to act with due diligence to prevent violations of rights or to investigate and punish acts of violence, and for providing compensation.

Comments on Specific Articles of the Convention

Articles 2 and 3

10. Articles 2 and 3 establish a comprehensive obligation to eliminate discrimination in all its forms in addition to the specific obligations under Articles 5–16.

Articles 2(f), 5 and 10(c)

11. Traditional attitudes by which women are regarded as subordinate to men or as having stereotyped roles perpetuate widespread practices involving violence or coercion, such as family violence and abuse, forced marriage, dowry deaths, acid attacks and female circumcision. Such prejudices and practices may justify gender-based violence as a form of protection or control of

women. The effect of such violence on the physical and mental integrity of women is to deprive them of the equal enjoyment, exercise and knowledge of human rights and fundamental freedoms. While this comment addresses mainly actual or threatened violence the underlying consequences of these forms of gender-based violence help to maintain women in subordinate roles and contribute to their low level of political participation and to their lower level of education, skills and work opportunities.

12. These attitudes also contribute to the propagation of pornography and the depiction and other commercial exploitation of women as sexual objects, rather than as individuals. This in turn contributes to gender-based violence.

Article 6

13. States parties are required by Article 6 to take measures to suppress all forms of traffic in women and exploitation of the prostitution of women.

14. Poverty and unemployment increase opportunities for trafficking in women. In addition to established forms of trafficking there are new forms of sexual exploitation, such as sex tourism, the recruitment of domestic labour from developing countries to work in developed countries, and organized marriages between women from developing countries and foreign nationals. These practices are incompatible with the equal enjoyment of rights by women and with respect for their rights and dignity. They put women at special risk of violence and abuse.

15. Poverty and unemployment force many women, including young girls, into prostitution. Prostitutes are especially vulnerable to violence because their status, which may be unlawful, tends to marginalize them. They need the equal protection of laws against rape and other forms of violence.

16. Wars, armed conflicts and the occupation of territories often lead to increased prostitution, trafficking in women and sexual assault of women, which require specific protective and punitive measures.

Article 11

17. Equality in employment can be seriously impaired when women are subjected to gender-specific violence, such as sexual harassment in the workplace.

18. Sexual harassment includes such unwelcome sexually determined behaviour as physical contact and advances, sexually coloured remarks, showing pornography and sexual demands, whether by words or actions. Such conduct can be humiliating and may constitute a health and safety problem; it is discriminatory when the woman has reasonable ground to believe that her objection would disadvantage her in connection with her employment, including recruitment or promotion, or when it creates a hostile working environment.

Article 12

19. States parties are required by Article 12 to take measures to ensure equal access to health care. Violence against women puts their health and lives at risk.

20. In some States there are traditional practices perpetuated by culture and tradition that are harmful to the health of women and children. These practices include dietary restrictions for pregnant women, preference for male children and female circumcision or genital mutilation.

Article 14

21. Rural women are at risk of gender-based violence because of traditional attitudes regarding the subordinate role of women that persist in many rural communities. Girls from rural communities are at special risk of violence and sexual exploitation when they leave the rural community to seek employment in towns.

Article 16 (and Article 5)

22. Compulsory sterilization or abortion adversely affects women's physical and mental health, and infringes the right of women to decide on the number and spacing of their children.

23. Family violence is one of the most insidious forms of violence against women. It is prevalent in all societies. Within family relationships women of all ages are subjected to violence of all kinds, including battering, rape, other forms of sexual assault, mental and other forms of violence, which are perpetuated by traditional attitudes. Lack of economic independence forces many women to stay in violent relationships. The abrogation of their family responsibilities by men can be a form of violence, and coercion. These forms of violence put women's health at risk and impair their ability to participate in family life and public life on a basis of equality.

Specific recommendations

24. In light of these comments, the Committee on the Elimination of Discrimination against Women recommends:

  (a) States parties should take appropriate and effective measures to overcome all forms of gender-based violence, whether by public or private act;

  (b) States parties should ensure that laws against family violence and abuse, rape, sexual assault and other gender-based violence give adequate protection to all women, and respect their integrity and dignity. Appropriate protective and support services should be provided for victims. Gender-sensitive training of judicial and law enforcement officers and other public officials is essential for the effective implementation of the Convention;

(*c*) States parties should encourage the compilation of statistics and research on the extent, causes and effects of violence, and on the effectiveness of measures to prevent and deal with violence;

(*d*) Effective measures should be taken to ensure that the media respect and promote respect for women;

(*e*) States parties in their report should identify the nature and extent of attitudes, customs and practices that perpetuate violence against women, and the kinds of violence that result. They should report the measures that they have undertaken to overcome violence, and the effect of those measures;

(*f*) Effective measures should be taken to overcome these attitudes and practices. States should introduce education and public information programmes to help eliminate prejudices which hinder women's equality (recommendation No. 3, 1987);

(*g*) Specific preventive and punitive measures are necessary to overcome trafficking and sexual exploitation;

(*h*) States parties in their reports should describe the extent of all these problems and the measures, including penal provisions, preventive and rehabilitation measures, that have been taken to protect women engaged in prostitution or subject to trafficking and other forms of sexual exploitation. The effectiveness of these measures should also be described;

(*i*) Effective complaints procedures and remedies, including compensation, should be provided;

(*j*) States parties should include in their reports information on sexual harassment, and on measures to protect women from sexual harassment and other forms of violence or coercion in the workplace;

(*k*) States parties should establish or support services for victims of family violence, rape, sex assault and other forms of gender-based violence, including refuges, specially trained health workers, rehabilitation and counselling;

(*l*) States parties should take measures to overcome such practices and should take account of the Committee's recommendation on female circumcision (recommendation No. 14) in reporting on health issues;

(*m*) States parties should ensure that measures are taken to prevent coercion in regard to fertility and reproduction, and to ensure that women are not forced to seek unsafe medical procedures such as illegal abortion because of lack of appropriate services in regard to fertility control;

(*n*) States parties in their reports should state the extent of these problems and should indicate the measures that have been taken and their effect;

(*o*)   States parties should ensure that services for victims of violence are accessible to rural women and that where necessary special services are provided to isolated communities;

(*p*)   Measures to protect them from violence should include training and employment opportunities and the monitoring of the employment conditions of domestic workers;

(*q*)   States parties should report on the risks to rural women, the extent and nature of violence and abuse to which they are subject, their need for and access to support and other services and the effectiveness of measures to overcome violence;

(*r*)   Measures that are necessary to overcome family violence should include:

   (i)   Criminal penalties where necessary and civil remedies in case of domestic violence;

   (ii)   Legislation to remove the defence of honour in regard to the assault or murder of a female family member;

   (iii)   Services to ensure the safety and security of victims of family violence, including refuges, counselling and rehabilitation programmes;

   (iv)   Rehabilitation programmes for perpetrators of domestic violence;

   (v)   Support services for families where incest or sexual abuse has occurred;

(*s*)   States parties should report on the extent of domestic violence and sexual abuse, and on the preventive, punitive and remedial measures that have been taken;

(*t*)   That States parties should take all legal and other measures that are necessary to provide effective protection of women against gender-based violence, including, inter alia:

   (i)   Effective legal measures, including penal sanctions, civil remedies and compensatory provisions to protect women against all kinds of violence, including, inter alia, violence and abuse in the family, sexual assault and sexual harassment in the workplace;

   (ii)   Preventive measures, including public information and education programmes to change attitudes concerning the roles and status of men and women;

   (iii)   Protective measures, including refuges, counselling, rehabilitation and support services for women who are the victims of violence or who are at risk of violence;

(*u*)   That States parties should report on all forms of gender-based violence, and that such reports should include all available data on the incidence of each form of violence, and on the effects of such violence on the women who are victims;

(v) That the reports of States parties should include information on the legal, preventive and protective measures that have been taken to overcome violence against women, and on the effectiveness of such measures.

2. *Committee on the Elimination of Discrimination against Women, General Recommendation 24: Women and Health (Article 12)*

CEDAW, *General Recommendation 24*, UN GAOR 1999, UN Doc. A/54/38/ Rev.1, pp. 3–7.

Introduction

1. The Committee on the Elimination of Discrimination against Women, affirming that access to health care, including reproductive health is a basic right under the Convention on the Elimination of All Forms of Discrimination against Women, determined at its 20th session, pursuant to article 21, to elaborate a general recommendation on article 12 of the Convention.

Background

2. States parties' compliance with article 12 of the Convention is central to the health and well-being of women. It requires States to eliminate discrimination against women in their access to health care services, throughout the life cycle, particularly in the areas of family planning, pregnancy, confinement and during the post-natal period. The examination of reports submitted by States parties pursuant to article 18 of the Convention demonstrates that women's health is an issue that is recognized as a central concern in promoting the health and well-being of women. For the benefit of States parties and those who have a particular interest in and concern with the issues surrounding women's health, the present general recommendation seeks to elaborate the Committee's understanding of article 12 and to address measures to eliminate discrimination in order to realize the right of women to the highest attainable standard of health.

3. Recent United Nations world conferences have also considered these objectives. In preparing this general recommendation, the Committee has taken into account relevant programmes of action adopted at United Nations world conferences and, in particular, those of the 1993 World Conference on Human Rights, the 1994 International Conference on Population and

Development and the 1995 Fourth World Conference on Women. The Committee has also noted the work of the World Health Organization (WHO), the United Nations Population Fund (UNFPA) and other United Nations bodies. It has also collaborated with a large number of non-governmental organizations with a special expertise in women's health in preparing this general recommendation.

4. The Committee notes the emphasis which other United Nations instruments place on the right to health and to the conditions which enable good health to be achieved. Among such instruments are the Universal Declaration of Human Rights, the International Covenant on Economic, Social and Cultural Rights, the International Covenant on Civil and Political Rights, the Convention on the Rights of the Child and the Convention on the Elimination of All Forms of Racial Discrimination.

5. The Committee refers also to its earlier general recommendations on female circumcision, human immunodeficiency virus/acquired immunodeficiency syndrome (HIV/AIDS), disabled women, violence against women and equality in family relations, all of which refer to issues which are integral to full compliance with article 12 of the Convention.

6. While biological differences between women and men may lead to differences in health status, there are societal factors which are determinative of the health status of women and men and which can vary among women themselves. For that reason, special attention should be given to the health needs and rights of women belonging to vulnerable and disadvantaged groups, such as migrant women, refugee and internally displaced women, the girl child and older women, women in prostitution, indigenous women and women with physical or mental disabilities.

7. The Committee notes that the full realization of women's right to health can be achieved only when States parties fulfil their obligation to respect, protect and promote women's fundamental human right to nutritional well-being throughout their life span by means of a food supply that is safe, nutritious and adapted to local conditions. Towards this end, States parties should take steps to facilitate physical and economic access to productive resources especially for rural women, and to otherwise ensure that the special nutritional needs of all women within their jurisdiction are met.

Article 12

1. States Parties shall take all appropriate measures to eliminate discrimination against women in the field of health care in order to ensure, on a basis of equality of men and women, access to health care services, including those related to family planning.
2. Notwithstanding the provisions of paragraph 1 of this article, States Parties shall ensure to women appropriate services in connection with

pregnancy, confinement and the post-natal period, granting free services where necessary, as well as adequate nutrition during pregnancy and lactation.

8. States parties are encouraged to address the issue of women's health throughout the woman's lifespan. For the purposes of this general recommendation, therefore, women includes girls and adolescents. This general recommendation will set out the Committee's analysis of the key elements of article 12.

Key elements

Article 12(1)

9. States parties are in the best position to report on the most critical health issues affecting women in that country. Therefore, in order to enable the Committee to evaluate whether measures to eliminate discrimination against women in the field of health care are appropriate, States parties must report on their health legislation, plans and policies for women with reliable data disaggregated by sex on the incidence and severity of diseases and conditions hazardous to women's health and nutrition and on the availability and cost-effectiveness of preventive and curative measures. Reports to the Committee must demonstrate that health legislation, plans and policies are based on scientific and ethical research and assessment of the health status and needs of women in that country and take into account any ethnic, regional or community variations or practices based on religion, tradition or culture.

10. States parties are encouraged to include in their reports information on diseases, health conditions and conditions hazardous to health that affect women or certain groups of women differently from men, as well as information on possible intervention in this regard.

11. Measures to eliminate discrimination against women are considered to be inappropriate if a health care system lacks services to prevent, detect and treat illnesses specific to women. It is discriminatory for a State party to refuse to legally provide for the performance of certain reproductive health services for women. For instance, if health service providers refuse to perform such services based on conscientious objection, measures should be introduced to ensure that women are referred to alternative health providers.

12. States parties should report on their understanding of how policies and measures on health care address the health rights of women from the perspective of women's needs and interests and how it addresses distinctive features and factors which differ for women in comparison to men, such as:

(*a*) Biological factors which differ for women in comparison with men, such as their menstrual cycle and their reproductive function and menopause. Another example is the higher risk of exposure to sexually transmitted diseases which women face;

(*b*) Socio-economic factors that vary for women in general and some groups of women in particular. For example, unequal power relationships between women and men in the home and workplace may negatively affect women's nutrition and health. They may also be exposed to different forms of violence which can affect their health. Girl children and adolescent girls are often vulnerable to sexual abuse by older men and family members, placing them at risk of physical and psychological harm and unwanted and early pregnancy. Some cultural or traditional practices such as female genital mutilation also carry a high risk of death and disability;

(*c*) Psychosocial factors which vary between women and men include depression in general and post-partum depression in particular as well as other psychological conditions, such as those that lead to eating disorders such as anorexia and bulimia;

(*d*) While lack of respect for the confidentiality of patients will affect both men and women, it may deter women from seeking advice and treatment and thereby adversely affect their health and well-being. Women will be less willing , for that reason, to seek medical care for diseases of the genital tract, for contraception or for incomplete abortion and in cases where they have suffered sexual or physical violence.

13. The duty of States parties to ensure, on a basis of equality between men and women, access to health care services, information and education implies an obligation to respect, protect and fulfil women's rights to health care. States parties have the responsibility to ensure that legislation and executive action and policy comply with these three obligations. They must also put in place a system which ensures effective judicial action. Failure to do so will constitute a violation of article 12.

14. The obligation to respect rights requires States parties to refrain from obstructing action taken by women in pursuit of their health goals. States parties should report on how public and private health care providers meet their duties to respect women's rights to have access to health care. For example, States parties should not restrict women's access to health services or to the clinics that provide those services on the ground that women do not have the authorization of husbands, partners, parents or health authorities, because they are unmarried[1] or because they are women. Other barriers to women's access to appropriate health care include laws that criminalize medical procedures only needed by women and that punish women who undergo those procedures.

[1] General Recommendation 21, para. 29.

15. The obligation to protect rights relating to women's health requires States parties, their agents and officials to take action to prevent and impose sanctions for violations of rights by private persons and organizations. Since gender-based violence is a critical health issue for women, States parties should ensure:

(*a*) The enactment and effective enforcement of laws and the formulation of policies, including health care protocols and hospital procedures to address violence against women and abuse of girl children and the provision of appropriate health services;

(*b*) Gender-sensitive training to enable health care workers to detect and manage the health consequences of gender-based violence;

(*c*) Fair and protective procedures for hearing complaints and imposing appropriate sanctions on health care professionals guilty of sexual abuse of women patients;

(*d*) The enactment and effective enforcement of laws that prohibit female genital mutilation and marriage of girl children.

16. States parties should ensure that adequate protection and health services, including trauma treatment and counselling, are provided for women in especially difficult circumstances, such as those trapped in situations of armed conflict and women refugees.

17. The duty to fulfil rights places an obligation on States parties to take appropriate legislative, judicial, administrative, budgetary, economic and other measures to the maximum extent of their available resources to ensure that women realize their rights to health care. Studies such as those which emphasize the high maternal mortality and morbidity rates worldwide and the large numbers of couples who would like to limit their family size but lack access to or do not use any form of contraception provide an important indication for States parties of possible breaches of their duties to ensure women's access to health care. The Committee asks States parties to report on what they have done to address the magnitude of women's ill-health, in particular when it arises from preventable conditions, such as tuberculosis and HIV/AIDS. The Committee is concerned at the growing evidence that States are relinquishing these obligations as they transfer State health functions to private agencies. States parties cannot absolve themselves of responsibility in these areas by delegating or transferring these powers to private sector agencies. States parties should therefore report on what they have done to organize governmental processes and all structures through which public power is exercised to promote and protect women's health. They should include information on positive measures taken to curb violations of women's rights by third parties, to protect their health and the measures they have taken to ensure the provision of such services.

18. The issues of HIV/AIDS and other sexually transmitted disease are central to the rights of women and adolescent girls to sexual health. Adolescent girls and women in many countries lack adequate access to information and services necessary to ensure sexual health. As a consequence of unequal power relations based on gender, women and adolescent girls are often unable to refuse sex or insist on safe and responsible sex practices. Harmful traditional practices, such as female genital mutilation, polygamy, as well as marital rape, may also expose girls and women to the risk of contracting HIV/AIDS and other sexually transmitted diseases. Women in prostitution are also particularly vulnerable to these diseases. States parties should ensure, without prejudice and discrimination, the right to sexual health information, education and services for all women and girls, including those who have been trafficked, including those who have been trafficked, even if they are not legally resident in the country. In particular, States parties should ensure the rights of female and male adolescents to sexual and reproductive health education by properly trained personnel in specially designed programmes that respect their rights to privacy and confidentiality.

19. In their reports States parties should identify the test by which they assess whether women have access to health care on a basis of equality of men and women in order to demonstrate compliance with article 12. In applying these tests, States parties should bear in mind the provisions of article 1 of the Convention. Reports should therefore include comments on the impact that health policies, procedures, laws and protocols have on women when compared with men.

20. Women have the right to be fully informed, by properly trained personnel, of their options in agreeing to treatment or research, including likely benefits and potential adverse effects of proposed procedures and available alternatives.

21. States parties should report on measures taken to eliminate barriers that women face in gaining access to health care services and what measures they have taken to ensure women timely and affordable access to such services. Barriers include requirements or conditions that prejudice women's access such as high fees for health care services, the requirement for preliminary authorization by spouse, parent or hospital authorities, distance from health facilities and absence of convenient and affordable public transport.

22. States parties should also report on measures taken to ensure access to quality health care services, for example, by making them acceptable to women. Acceptable services are those which are delivered in a way that ensures that a woman gives her fully informed consent, respects her dignity, guarantees her confidentiality and is sensitive to her needs and perspectives. States parties should not permit forms of coercion, such as non-consensual sterilization, mandatory testing for sexually transmitted diseases or mandatory pregnancy

testing as a condition of employment that violate women's rights to informed consent and dignity.

23. In their reports, States parties should state what measures they have taken to ensure timely access to the range of services which are related to family planning, in particular, and to sexual and reproductive health in general. Particular attention should be paid to the health education of adolescents, including information and counselling on all methods of family planning.[2]

24. The Committee is concerned about the conditions of health care services for older women, not only because women often live longer than men and are more likely than men to suffer from disabling and degenerative chronic diseases, such as osteoporosis and dementia, but because they often have the responsibility for their aging spouses. Therefore, States parties should take appropriate measures to ensure the access of older women to health services that address the handicaps and disabilities associated with aging.

25. Women with disabilities, of all ages, often have difficulty with physical access to health services. Women with mental disabilities are particularly vulnerable, while there is limited understanding, in general, of the broad range of risks to mental health to which women are disproportionately susceptible as a result of gender discrimination, violence, poverty, armed conflict, dislocation and other forms of social deprivation. States parties should take appropriate measures to ensure that health services are sensitive to the needs of women with disabilities and are respectful of their human rights and dignity.

Article 12(2)

26. Reports should also include what measures States parties have taken to ensure women appropriate services in connection with pregnancy, confinement and the post-natal period. Information on the rates at which these measures have reduced maternal mortality and morbidity in their countries, in general, and in vulnerable groups, regions and communities, in particular, should also be included.[3]

27. States parties should include in their reports how they supply free services where necessary to ensure safe pregnancies, childbirth and post-partum periods for women. Many women are at risk of death or disability from pregnancy-related causes because they lack the funds to obtain or access the necessary services, which include ante-natal, maternity and post-natal services. The Committee notes that it is the duty of States parties to ensure women's right to safe motherhood and emergency obstetric services and they should allocate to these services the maximum extent of available resources.

---

[2] Health education for adolescents should further address, *inter alia*, gender equality, violence, prevention of sexually transmitted diseases and reproductive and sexual health rights.

[3] Reference to resolutions in which the Committee adopted the Cairo and Beijing recommendations to reduce maternal mortality and morbidity.

Other relevant articles in the Convention

28. When reporting on measures taken to comply with article 12, States parties are urged to recognize its interconnection with other articles in the Convention that have a bearing on women's health. Those articles include article 5(*b*), which requires States parties to ensure that family education includes a proper understanding of maternity as a social function; article 10, which requires States parties to ensure equal access to education, thus enabling women to access health care more readily and reducing female students' dropout rates, which are often due to premature pregnancy; article 10(*h*) which provides that States parties provide to women and girls specific educational information to help ensure the well-being of families, including information and advice on family planning; article 11, which is concerned, in part, with the protection of women's health and safety in working conditions, including the safeguarding of the reproductive function, special protection from harmful types of work during pregnancy and with the provision of paid maternity leave; article 14(2)(*b*), which requires States parties to ensure access for rural women to adequate health care facilities, including information, counselling and services in family planning, and (*h*), which obliges States parties to take all appropriate measures to ensure adequate living conditions, particularly housing, sanitation, electricity and water supply, transport and communications, all of which are critical for the prevention of disease and the promotion of good health care; and article 16(1)(*e*), which requires States parties to ensure that women have the same rights as men to decide freely and responsibly on the number and spacing of their children and to have access to information, education and means to enable them to exercise these rights. Article 16(2) also proscribes the betrothal and marriage of children, an important factor in preventing the physical and emotional harm which arise from early childbirth.

Recommendations for government action

29. States parties should implement a comprehensive national strategy to promote women's health throughout their lifespan. This will include interventions aimed at both the prevention and treatment of diseases and conditions affecting women, as well as responding to violence against women, and will ensure universal access for all women to a full range of high-quality and affordable health care, including sexual and reproductive health services.

30. States parties should allocate adequate budgetary, human and administrative resources to ensure that women's health receives a share of the overall health budget comparable with that for men's health, taking into account their different health needs.

31. States parties should also, in particular:

(a) Place a gender perspective at the centre of all policies and programmes affecting women's s health and should involve women in the planning, implementation and monitoring of such policies and programmes and in the provision of health services to women;

(b) Ensure the removal of all barriers to women's access to health services, education and information, including in the area of sexual and reproductive health, and, in particular, allocate resources for programmes directed at adolescents for the prevention and treatment of sexually transmitted diseases, including HIV/AIDS;

(c) Prioritize the prevention of unwanted pregnancy through family planning and sex education and reduce maternal mortality rates through safe motherhood services and prenatal assistance. When possible, legislation criminalizing abortion could be amended to remove punitive provisions imposed on women who undergo abortion;

(d) Monitor the provision of health services to women by public, non-governmental and private organizations, to ensure equal access and quality of care;

(e) Require all health services to be consistent with the human rights of women, including the rights to autonomy, privacy, confidentiality, informed consent and choice;

(f) Ensure that the training curricula of health workers includes comprehensive, mandatory, gender-sensitive courses on women's health and human rights, in particular gender-based violence.

3. Committee on Economic, Social and Cultural Rights, General Comment 14: The Right to the Highest Attainable Standard of Health (Article 12)

CESCR, *General Comment 14*, UN ESCOR 2000, UN Doc. E/C.12/2000/4, 11 August 2000.

1. Health is a fundamental human right indispensable for the exercise of other human rights. Every human being is entitled to the enjoyment of the highest attainable standard of health conducive to living a life in dignity. The realization of the right to health may be pursued through numerous, complementary approaches, such as the formulation of health policies, or the implementation of health programmes developed by the World Health Organization (WHO), or the adoption of specific legal instruments. Moreover, the right to health includes certain components which are legally enforceable.[4]

---

[4] e.g. the principle of non-discrimination in relation to health facilities, goods, and services is legally enforceable in numerous national jurisdictions.

2. The human right to health is recognized in numerous international instruments. Article 25.1 of the Universal Declaration of Human Rights affirms: 'Everyone has the right to a standard of living adequate for the health of himself and of his family, including food, clothing, housing and medical care and necessary social services'. The International Covenant on Economic, Social and Cultural Rights provides the most comprehensive article on the right to health in international human rights law. In accordance with article 12.1 of the Covenant, States parties recognize 'the right of everyone to the enjoyment of the highest attainable standard of physical and mental health', while article 12.2 enumerates, by way of illustration, a number of 'steps to be taken by the States parties . . . to achieve the full realization of this right'. Additionally, the right to health is recognized, *inter alia*, in article 5(*e*)(iv) of the International Convention on the Elimination of All Forms of Racial Discrimination of 1965, in articles 11.1(*f*) and 12 of the Convention on the Elimination of All Forms of Discrimination against Women of 1979 and in article 24 of the Convention on the Rights of the Child of 1989. Several regional human rights instruments also recognize the right to health, such as the European Social Charter of 1961 as revised (art. 11), the African Charter on Human and Peoples' Rights of 1981 (art. 16) and the Additional Protocol to the American Convention on Human Rights in the Area of Economic, Social and Cultural Rights of 1988 (art. 10). Similarly, the right to health has been proclaimed by the Commission on Human Rights,[5] as well as in the Vienna Declaration and Programme of Action of 1993 and other international instruments.[6]

3. The right to health is closely related to and dependent upon the realization of other human rights, as contained in the International Bill of Rights, including the rights to food, housing, work, education, human dignity, life, non-discrimination, equality, the prohibition against torture, privacy, access to information, and the freedoms of association, assembly and movement. These and other rights and freedoms address integral components of the right to health.

4. In drafting article 12 of the Covenant, the Third Committee of the United Nations General Assembly did not adopt the definition of health contained in the preamble to the Constitution of WHO, which conceptualizes health as

---

[5] In its resolution 1989/11.

[6] The Principles for the Protection of Persons with Mental Illness and for the Improvement of Mental Health Care adopted by the United Nations General Assembly in 1991 (resolution 46/119) and the Committee's General Comment No. 5 on persons with disabilities apply to persons with mental illness; the Programme of Action of the International Conference on Population and Development held at Cairo in 1994, as well as the Declaration and Programme for Action of the Fourth World Conference on Women held in Beijing in 1995 contain definitions of reproductive health and women's health, respectively.

'a state of complete physical, mental and social well-being and not merely the absence of disease or infirmity'. However, the reference in article 12.1 of the Covenant to 'the highest attainable standard of physical and mental health' is not confined to the right to health care. On the contrary, the drafting history and the express wording of article 12.2 acknowledge that the right to health embraces a wide range of socio-economic factors that promote conditions in which people can lead a healthy life, and extends to the underlying determinants of health, such as food and nutrition, housing, access to safe and potable water and adequate sanitation, safe and healthy working conditions, and a healthy environment.

5. The Committee is aware that, for millions of people throughout the world, the full enjoyment of the right to health still remains a distant goal. Moreover, in many cases, especially for those living in poverty, this goal is becoming increasingly remote. The Committee recognizes the formidable structural and other obstacles resulting from international and other factors beyond the control of States that impede the full realization of article 12 in many States parties.

6. With a view to assisting States parties' implementation of the Covenant and the fulfilment of their reporting obligations, this General Comment focuses on the normative content of article 12 (Part I), States parties' obligations (Part II), violations (Part III) and implementation at the national level (Part IV), while the obligations of actors other than States parties are addressed in Part V. The General Comment is based on the Committee's experience in examining States parties' reports over many years.

I. Normative Content of Article 12

7. Article 12.1 provides a definition of the right to health, while article 12.2 enumerates illustrative, non-exhaustive examples of States parties' obligations.

8. The right to health is not to be understood as a right to be *healthy*. The right to health contains both freedoms and entitlements. The freedoms include the right to control one's health and body, including sexual and reproductive freedom, and the right to be free from interference, such as the right to be free from torture, non-consensual medical treatment and experimentation. By contrast, the entitlements include the right to a system of health protection which provides equality of opportunity for people to enjoy the highest attainable level of health.

9. The notion of 'the highest attainable standard of health' in article 12.1 takes into account both the individual's biological and socio-economic preconditions and a State's available resources. There are a number of aspects which cannot be addressed solely within the relationship between States and

individuals; in particular, good health cannot be ensured by a State, nor can States provide protection against every possible cause of human ill health. Thus, genetic factors, individual susceptibility to ill health and the adoption of unhealthy or risky lifestyles may play an important role with respect to an individual's health. Consequently, the right to health must be understood as a right to the enjoyment of a variety of facilities, goods, services and conditions necessary for the realization of the highest attainable standard of health.

10. Since the adoption of the two International Covenants in 1966 the world health situation has changed dramatically and the notion of health has undergone substantial changes and has also widened in scope. More determinants of health are being taken into consideration, such as resource distribution and gender differences. A wider definition of health also takes into account such socially-related concerns as violence and armed conflict.[7] Moreover, formerly unknown diseases, such as Human Immunodeficiency Virus and Acquired Immunodeficiency Syndrome (HIV/AIDS), and others that have become more widespread, such as cancer, as well as the rapid growth of the world population, have created new obstacles for the realization of the right to health which need to be taken into account when interpreting article 12.

11. The Committee interprets the right to health, as defined in article 12.1, as an inclusive right extending not only to timely and appropriate health care but also to the underlying determinants of health, such as access to safe and potable water and adequate sanitation, an adequate supply of safe food, nutrition and housing, healthy occupational and environmental conditions, and access to health-related education and information, including on sexual and reproductive health. A further important aspect is the participation of the population in all health-related decision-making at the community, national and international levels.

12. The right to health in all its forms and at all levels contains the following interrelated and essential elements, the precise application of which will depend on the conditions prevailing in a particular State party:

(a) *Availability.* Functioning public health and health care facilities, goods and services, as well as programmes, have to be available in sufficient quantity within the State party. The precise nature of the facilities, goods and services will vary depending on numerous factors, including the State party's developmental level. They will include, however, the underlying determinants of health, such as safe and potable drinking

---

[7] Common Article 3 of the Geneva Conventions for the protection of war victims (1949); Additional Protocol I (1977) relating to the Protection of Victims of International Armed Conflicts, Art. 75(2)(*a*); Additional Protocol II (1977) relating to the Protection of Victims of Non-International Armed Conflicts, Art. 4(*a*).

water and adequate sanitation facilities, hospitals, clinics and other health-related buildings, trained medical and professional personnel receiving domestically competitive salaries, and essential drugs, as defined by the WHO Action Programme on Essential Drugs.[8]

(b) *Accessibility*. Health facilities, goods and services[9] have to be accessible to everyone without discrimination, within the jurisdiction of the State party. Accessibility has four overlapping dimensions:

Non-discrimination: health facilities, goods and services must be accessible to all, especially the most vulnerable or marginalized sections of the population, in law and in fact, without discrimination on any of the prohibited grounds.[10]

Physical accessibility: health facilities, goods and services must be within safe physical reach for all sections of the population, especially vulnerable or marginalized groups, such as ethnic minorities and indigenous populations, women, children, adolescents, older persons, persons with disabilities and persons with HIV/AIDS. Accessibility also implies that medical services and underlying determinants of health, such as safe and potable water and adequate sanitation facilities, are within safe physical reach, including in rural areas. Accessibility further includes adequate access to buildings for persons with disabilities.

Economic accessibility (affordability): health facilities, goods and services must be affordable for all. Payment for health-care services, as well as services related to the underlying determinants of health, has to be based on the principle of equity, ensuring that these services, whether privately or publicly provided, are affordable for all, including socially disadvantaged groups. Equity demands that poorer households should not be disproportionately burdened with health expenses as compared to richer households.

Information accessibility: accessibility includes the right to seek, receive and impart information and ideas[11] concerning health issues. However, accessibility of information should not impair the right to have personal health data treated with confidentiality.

(c) *Acceptability*. All health facilities, goods and services must be respectful of medical ethics and culturally appropriate, i.e. respectful of the culture

---

[8] See WHO Model List of Essential Drugs, revised December 1999, *WHO Drug Information*, 13/4 (1999).

[9] Unless expressly provided otherwise, any reference in this General Comment to health facilities, goods, and services includes the underlying determinants of health outlined in paras. 11 and 12(a) of this General Comment.

[10] See paras. 18 and 19 of this General Comment.

[11] See Article 19.2 of the International Covenant on Civil and Political Rights. This General Comment gives particular emphasis to access to information because of the special importance of this issue in relation to health.

of individuals, minorities, peoples and communities, sensitive to gender and life-cycle requirements, as well as being designed to respect confidentiality and improve the health status of those concerned.

(*d*) *Quality*. As well as being culturally acceptable, health facilities, goods and services must also be scientifically and medically appropriate and of good quality. This requires, *inter alia*, skilled medical personnel, scientifically approved and unexpired drugs and hospital equipment, safe and potable water, and adequate sanitation.

13. The non-exhaustive catalogue of examples in article 12.2 provides guidance in defining the action to be taken by States. It gives specific generic examples of measures arising from the broad definition of the right to health contained in article 12.1, thereby illustrating the content of that right, as exemplified in the following paragraphs.[12]

Article 12.2(a). The right to maternal, child and reproductive health

14. 'The provision for the reduction of the stillbirth rate and of infant mortality and for the healthy development of the child' (art. 12.2(*a*))[13] may be understood as requiring measures to improve child and maternal health, sexual and reproductive health services, including access to family planning, pre- and post-natal care,[14] emergency obstetric services and access to information, as well as to resources necessary to act on that information.[15]

---

[12] In the literature and practice concerning the right to health, three levels of health care are frequently referred to: *primary health care* typically deals with common and relatively minor illnesses and is provided by health professionals and/or generally trained doctors working within the community at relatively low cost; *secondary health care* is provided in centres, usually hospitals, and typically deals with relatively common minor or serious illnesses that cannot be managed at community level, using specialty-trained health professionals and doctors, special equipment and sometimes in-patient care at comparatively higher cost; *tertiary health care* is provided in relatively few centres, typically deals with small numbers of minor or serious illnesses requiring specialty-trained health professionals and doctors and special equipment, and is often relatively expensive. Since forms of primary, secondary, and tertiary health care frequently overlap and often interact, the use of this typology does not always provide sufficient distinguishing criteria to be helpful for assessing which levels of health care States parties must provide, and is therefore of limited assistance in relation to the normative understanding of Article 12.

[13] According to WHO, the stillbirth rate is no longer commonly used, infant and under-5 mortality rates being measured instead.

[14] *Prenatal* denotes existing or occurring before birth; *perinatal* refers to the period shortly before and after birth (in medical statistics the period begins with the completion of 28 weeks of gestation and is variously defined as ending one to four weeks after birth); *neonatal*, by contrast, covers the period pertaining to the first four weeks after birth; while *post-natal* denotes occurrence after birth. In this General Comment, the more generic terms pre- and post-natal are exclusively employed.

[15] Reproductive health means that women and men have the freedom to decide if and when to reproduce and the right to be informed and to have access to safe, effective, affordable, and acceptable methods of family planning of their choice as well as the right of access to appropriate health care services that will, for example, enable women to go safely through pregnancy and childbirth.

Article 12.2(b). The right to healthy natural and workplace environments

15. 'The improvement of all aspects of environmental and industrial hygiene' (art. 12.2(*b*)) comprises, *inter alia*, preventive measures in respect of occupational accidents and diseases; the requirement to ensure an adequate supply of safe and potable water and basic sanitation; the prevention and reduction of the population's exposure to harmful substances such as radiation and harmful chemicals or other detrimental environmental conditions that directly or indirectly impact upon human health.[16] Furthermore, industrial hygiene refers to the minimization, so far as is reasonably practicable, of the causes of health hazards inherent in the working environment.[17] Article 12.2(*b*) also embraces adequate housing and safe and hygienic working conditions, an adequate supply of food and proper nutrition, and discourages the abuse of alcohol, and the use of tobacco, drugs and other harmful substances.

Article 12.2(c). The right to prevention, treatment and control of diseases

16. 'The prevention, treatment and control of epidemic, endemic, occupational and other diseases' (art. 12.2(*c*)) requires the establishment of prevention and education programmes for behaviour-related health concerns such as sexually transmitted diseases, in particular HIV/AIDS, and those adversely affecting sexual and reproductive health, and the promotion of social determinants of good health, such as environmental safety, education, economic development and gender equity. The right to treatment includes the creation of a system of urgent medical care in cases of accidents, epidemics and similar health hazards, and the provision of disaster relief and humanitarian assistance in emergency situations. The control of diseases refers to States' individual and joint efforts to, *inter alia*, make available relevant technologies, using and improving epidemiological surveillance and data collection on a disaggregated basis, the implementation or enhancement of immunization programmes and other strategies of infectious disease control.

Article 12.2(d). The right to health facilities, goods and services[18]

17. 'The creation of conditions which would assure to all medical service and medical attention in the event of sickness' (art. 12.2(*d*)), both physical and

---

[16] The Committee takes note, in this regard, of Principle 1 of the Stockholm Declaration of 1972 which states: 'Man has the fundamental right to freedom, equality and adequate conditions of life, in an environment of a quality that permits a life of dignity and well-being', as well as of recent developments in international law, including General Assembly resolution 45/94 on the need to ensure a healthy environment for the well-being of individuals; Principle 1 of the Rio Declaration; and regional human rights instruments such as article 10 of the San Salvador Protocol to the American Convention on Human Rights.

[17] ILO Convention No. 155, Art. 4.2.   [18] See para. 12(*b*) and n. 8 above.

mental, includes the provision of equal and timely access to basic preventive, curative, rehabilitative health services and health education; regular screening programmes; appropriate treatment of prevalent diseases, illnesses, injuries and disabilities, preferably at community level; the provision of essential drugs; and appropriate mental health treatment and care. A further important aspect is the improvement and furtherance of participation of the population in the provision of preventive and curative health services, such as the organization of the health sector, the insurance system and, in particular, participation in political decisions relating to the right to health taken at both the community and national levels.

Article 12. Special topics of broad application

Non-discrimination and equal treatment

18. By virtue of article 2.2 and article 3, the Covenant proscribes any discrimination in access to health care and underlying determinants of health, as well as to means and entitlements for their procurement, on the grounds of race, colour, sex, language, religion, political or other opinion, national or social origin, property, birth, physical or mental disability, health status (including HIV/AIDS), sexual orientation and civil, political, social or other status, which has the intention or effect of nullifying or impairing the equal enjoyment or exercise of the right to health. The Committee stresses that many measures, such as most strategies and programmes designed to eliminate health-related discrimination, can be pursued with minimum resource implications through the adoption, modification or abrogation of legislation or the dissemination of information. The Committee recalls General Comment No. 3, paragraph 12, which states that even in times of severe resource constraints, the vulnerable members of society must be protected by the adoption of relatively low-cost targeted programmes.

19. With respect to the right to health, equality of access to health care and health services has to be emphasized. States have a special obligation to provide those who do not have sufficient means with the necessary health insurance and health-care facilities, and to prevent any discrimination on internationally prohibited grounds in the provision of health care and health services, especially with respect to the core obligations of the right to health.[19] Inappropriate health resource allocation can lead to discrimination that may not be overt. For example, investments should not disproportionately favour expensive curative health services which are often accessible only to a small, privileged fraction of the population, rather than primary and preventive health care benefiting a far larger part of the population.

---

[19] For the core obligations, see paras. 43 and 44 of the present General Comments.

Gender perspective

20. The Committee recommends that States integrate a gender perspective in their health-related policies, planning, programmes and research in order to promote better health for both women and men. A gender-based approach recognizes that biological and socio-cultural factors play a significant role in influencing the health of men and women. The disaggregation of health and socio-economic data according to sex is essential for identifying and remedying inequalities in health.

Women and the right to health

21. To eliminate discrimination against women, there is a need to develop and implement a comprehensive national strategy for promoting women's right to health throughout their life span. Such a strategy should include interventions aimed at the prevention and treatment of diseases affecting women, as well as policies to provide access to a full range of high quality and affordable health care, including sexual and reproductive services. A major goal should be reducing women's health risks, particularly lowering rates of maternal mortality and protecting women from domestic violence. The realization of women's right to health requires the removal of all barriers interfering with access to health services, education and information, including in the area of sexual and reproductive health. It is also important to undertake preventive, promotive and remedial action to shield women from the impact of harmful traditional cultural practices and norms that deny them their full reproductive rights.

Children and adolescents

22. Article 12.2(*a*) outlines the need to take measures to reduce infant mortality and promote the healthy development of infants and children. Subsequent international human rights instruments recognize that children and adolescents have the right to the enjoyment of the highest standard of health and access to facilities for the treatment of illness.[20]

The Convention on the Rights of the Child directs States to ensure access to essential health services for the child and his or her family, including pre- and post-natal care for mothers. The Convention links these goals with ensuring access to child-friendly information about preventive and health-promoting behaviour and support to families and communities in implementing these practices. Implementation of the principle of non-discrimination requires that girls, as well as boys, have equal access to adequate nutrition, safe environments, and physical as well as mental health services. There is a need to adopt effective and appropriate measures to abolish harmful traditional practices

---

[20] Article 24.1 of the Convention on the Rights of the Child.

affecting the health of children, particularly girls, including early marriage, female genital mutilation, preferential feeding and care of male children.[21] Children with disabilities should be given the opportunity to enjoy a fulfilling and decent life and to participate within their community.

23. States parties should provide a safe and supportive environment for adolescents, that ensures the opportunity to participate in decisions affecting their health, to build life-skills, to acquire appropriate information, to receive counselling and to negotiate the health-behaviour choices they make. The realization of the right to health of adolescents is dependent on the development of youth-friendly health care, which respects confidentiality and privacy and includes appropriate sexual and reproductive health services.

24. In all policies and programmes aimed at guaranteeing the right to health of children and adolescents their best interests shall be a primary consideration.

Older persons

25. With regard to the realization of the right to health of older persons, the Committee, in accordance with paragraphs 34 and 35 of General Comment No. 6 (1995), reaffirms the importance of an integrated approach, combining elements of preventive, curative and rehabilitative health treatment. Such measures should be based on periodical check-ups for both sexes; physical as well as psychological rehabilitative measures aimed at maintaining the functionality and autonomy of older persons; and attention and care for chronically and terminally ill persons, sparing them avoidable pain and enabling them to die with dignity.

Persons with disabilities

26. The Committee reaffirms paragraph 34 of its General Comment No. 5, which addresses the issue of persons with disabilities in the context of the right to physical and mental health. Moreover, the Committee stresses the need to ensure that not only the public health sector but also private providers of health services and facilities comply with the principle of non-discrimination in relation to persons with disabilities.

Indigenous peoples

27. In the light of emerging international law and practice and the recent measures taken by States in relation to indigenous peoples,[22] the Committee deems it useful to identify elements that would help to define indigenous

---

[21] See World Health Assembly resolution WHA47.10, 1994, entitled 'Maternal and child health and family planning: traditional practices harmful to the health of women and children'.

[22] Recent emerging international norms relevant to indigenous peoples include the ILO Convention No. 169 concerning Indigenous and Tribal Peoples in Independent Countries (1989); Articles 29 (c) and (d) and 30 of the Convention on the Rights of the Child (1989); Article 8 (j) of the Convention on Biological Diversity (1992), recommending that States respect, preserve and

peoples' right to health in order better to enable States with indigenous peoples to implement the provisions contained in article 12 of the Covenant. The Committee considers that indigenous peoples have the right to specific measures to improve their access to health services and care. These health services should be culturally appropriate, taking into account traditional preventive care, healing practices and medicines. States should provide resources for indigenous peoples to design, deliver and control such services so that they may enjoy the highest attainable standard of physical and mental health. The vital medicinal plants, animals and minerals necessary to the full enjoyment of health of indigenous peoples should also be protected. The Committee notes that, in indigenous communities, the health of the individual is often linked to the health of the society as a whole and has a collective dimension. In this respect, the Committee considers that development-related activities that lead to the displacement of indigenous peoples against their will from their traditional territories and environment, denying them their sources of nutrition and breaking their symbiotic relationship with their lands, has a deleterious effect on their health.

Limitations

28. Issues of public health are sometimes used by States as grounds for limiting the exercise of other fundamental rights. The Committee wishes to emphasize that the Covenant's limitation clause, article 4, is primarily intended to protect the rights of individuals rather than to permit the imposition of limitations by States. Consequently a State party which, for example, restricts the movement of, or incarcerates, persons with transmissible diseases such as HIV/AIDS, refuses to allow doctors to treat persons believed to be opposed to a government, or fails to provide immunization against the community's major infectious diseases, on grounds such as national security or the preservation of public order, has the burden of justifying such serious measures in relation to each of the elements identified in article 4. Such restrictions must be in accordance with the law, including international human rights standards, compatible with the nature of the rights protected by the Covenant, in the interest of legitimate aims pursued, and strictly necessary for the promotion of the general welfare in a democratic society.

maintain knowledge, innovation and practices of indigenous communities; Agenda 21 of the United Nations Conference on Environment and Development (1992), in particular ch. 26; and Part I, para. 20, of the Vienna Declaration and Programme of Action (1993), stating that States should take concerted positive steps to ensure respect for all human rights of indigenous people, on the basis of non-discrimination. See also the preamble and Article 3 of the United Nations Framework Convention on Climate Change (1992); and Article 10(2)(e) of the United Nations Convention to Combat Desertification in Countries Experiencing Serious Drought and/or Desertification, Particularly in Africa (1994). During recent years an increasing number of States have changed their constitutions and introduced legislation recognizing specific rights of indigenous peoples.

29. In line with article 5.1, such limitations must be proportional, i.e. the least restrictive alternative must be adopted where several types of limitations are available. Even where such limitations on grounds of protecting public health are basically permitted, they should be of limited duration and subject to review.

II. States Parties' Obligations

General legal obligations

30. While the Covenant provides for progressive realization and acknowledges the constraints due to the limits of available resources, it also imposes on States parties various obligations which are of immediate effect. States parties have immediate obligations in relation to the right to health, such as the guarantee that the right will be exercised without discrimination of any kind (art. 2.2) and the obligation to take steps (art. 2.1) towards the full realization of article 12. Such steps must be deliberate, concrete and targeted towards the full realization of the right to health.[23]

31. The progressive realization of the right to health over a period of time should not be interpreted as depriving States parties' obligations of all meaningful content. Rather, progressive realization means that States parties have a specific and continuing obligation to move as expeditiously and effectively as possible towards the full realization of article 12.[24]

32. As with all other rights in the Covenant, there is a strong presumption that retrogressive measures taken in relation to the right to health are not permissible. If any deliberately retrogressive measures are taken, the State party has the burden of proving that they have been introduced after the most careful consideration of all alternatives and that they are duly justified by reference to the totality of the rights provided for in the Covenant in the context of the full use of the State party's maximum available resources.[25]

33. The right to health, like all human rights, imposes three types or levels of obligations on States parties: the obligations to *respect*, *protect* and *fulfil*. In turn, the obligation to fulfil contains obligations to facilitate, provide and promote.[26] The obligation to *respect* requires States to refrain from interfering directly or indirectly with the enjoyment of the right to health. The obligation to *protect* requires States to take measures that prevent third parties from interfering with article 12 guarantees. Finally, the obligation to *fulfil* requires

---

[23] See General Comment No. 13, para. 43.

[24] See General Comment No. 3, para. 9; General Comment No. 13, para. 44.

[25] See General Comment No. 3, para. 9; General Comment No. 13, para. 45.

[26] According to General Comments Nos. 12 and 13, the obligation to fulfil incorporates an obligation to *facilitate* and an obligation to *provide*. In the present General Comment, the obligation to fulfil also incorporates an obligation to *promote* because of the critical importance of health promotion in the work of WHO and elsewhere.

States to adopt appropriate legislative, administrative, budgetary, judicial, promotional and other measures towards the full realization of the right to health.

Specific legal obligations

34. In particular, States are under the obligation to *respect* the right to health by, *inter alia*, refraining from denying or limiting equal access for all persons, including prisoners or detainees, minorities, asylum seekers and illegal immigrants, to preventive, curative and palliative health services; abstaining from enforcing discriminatory practices as a State policy; and abstaining from imposing discriminatory practices relating to women's health status and needs. Furthermore, obligations to respect include a State's obligation to refrain from prohibiting or impeding traditional preventive care, healing practices and medicines, from marketing unsafe drugs and from applying coercive medical treatments, unless on an exceptional basis for the treatment of mental illness or the prevention and control of communicable diseases. Such exceptional cases should be subject to specific and restrictive conditions, respecting best practices and applicable international standards, including the Principles for the Protection of Persons with Mental Illness and the Improvement of Mental Health Care.[27]

In addition, States should refrain from limiting access to contraceptives and other means of maintaining sexual and reproductive health, from censoring, withholding or intentionally misrepresenting health-related information, including sexual education and information, as well as from preventing people's participation in health-related matters. States should also refrain from unlawfully polluting air, water and soil, e.g. through industrial waste from State-owned facilities, from using or testing nuclear, biological or chemical weapons if such testing results in the release of substances harmful to human health, and from limiting access to health services as a punitive measure, e.g. during armed conflicts in violation of international humanitarian law.

35. Obligations to *protect* include, *inter alia*, the duties of States to adopt legislation or to take other measures ensuring equal access to health care and health-related services provided by third parties; to ensure that privatization of the health sector does not constitute a threat to the availability, accessibility, acceptability and quality of health facilities, goods and services; to control the marketing of medical equipment and medicines by third parties; and to ensure that medical practitioners and other health professionals meet appropriate standards of education, skill and ethical codes of conduct. States are also obliged to ensure that harmful social or traditional practices do not interfere with access to pre- and post-natal care and family-planning; to prevent third parties from coercing women to undergo traditional practices, e.g. female genital mutilation; and to take measures to protect all vulnerable or marginalized

---

[27] General Assembly resolution 46/119 (1991).

groups of society, in particular women, children, adolescents and older persons, in the light of gender-based expressions of violence. States should also ensure that third parties do not limit people's access to health-related information and services.

36. The obligation to *fulfil* requires States parties, *inter alia*, to give sufficient recognition to the right to health in the national political and legal systems, preferably by way of legislative implementation, and to adopt a national health policy with a detailed plan for realizing the right to health. States must ensure provision of health care, including immunization programmes against the major infectious diseases, and ensure equal access for all to the underlying determinants of health, such as nutritiously safe food and potable drinking water, basic sanitation and adequate housing and living conditions. Public health infrastructures should provide for sexual and reproductive health services, including safe motherhood, particularly in rural areas. States have to ensure the appropriate training of doctors and other medical personnel, the provision of a sufficient number of hospitals, clinics and other health-related facilities, and the promotion and support of the establishment of institutions providing counselling and mental health services, with due regard to equitable distribution throughout the country. Further obligations include the provision of a public, private or mixed health insurance system which is affordable for all, the promotion of medical research and health education, as well as information campaigns, in particular with respect to HIV/AIDS, sexual and reproductive health, traditional practices, domestic violence, the abuse of alcohol and the use of cigarettes, drugs and other harmful substances. States are also required to adopt measures against environmental and occupational health hazards and against any other threat as demonstrated by epidemiological data. For this purpose they should formulate and implement national policies aimed at reducing and eliminating pollution of air, water and soil, including pollution by heavy metals such as lead from gasoline. Furthermore, States parties are required to formulate, implement and periodically review a coherent national policy to minimize the risk of occupational accidents and diseases, as well as to provide a coherent national policy on occupational safety and health services.[28]

---

[28] Elements of such a policy are the identification, determination, authorization, and control of dangerous materials, equipment, substances, agents, and work processes; the provision of health information to workers and the provision, if needed, of adequate protective clothing and equipment; the enforcement of laws and regulations through adequate inspection; the requirement of notification of occupational accidents and diseases, the conduct of inquiries into serious accidents and diseases, and the production of annual statistics; the protection of workers and their representatives from disciplinary measures for actions properly taken by them in conformity with such a policy; and the provision of occupational health services with essentially preventive functions. See ILO Occupational Safety and Health Convention, 1981 (No. 155) and Occupational Health Services Convention, 1985 (No. 161).

37. The obligation to *fulfil (facilitate)* requires States *inter alia* to take positive measures that enable and assist individuals and communities to enjoy the right to health. States parties are also obliged to *fulfil (provide)* a specific right contained in the Covenant when individuals or a group are unable, for reasons beyond their control, to realize that right themselves by the means at their disposal. The obligation to *fulfil (promote)* the right to health requires States to undertake actions that create, maintain and restore the health of the population. Such obligations include: (i) fostering recognition of factors favouring positive health results, e.g. research and provision of information; (ii) ensuring that health services are culturally appropriate and that health care staff are trained to recognize and respond to the specific needs of vulnerable or marginalized groups; (iii) ensuring that the State meets its obligations in the dissemination of appropriate information relating to healthy lifestyles and nutrition, harmful traditional practices and the availability of services; (iv) supporting people in making informed choices about their health.

International obligations

38. In its General Comment No. 3, the Committee drew attention to the obligation of all States parties to take steps, individually and through international assistance and cooperation, especially economic and technical, towards the full realization of the rights recognized in the Covenant, such as the right to health. In the spirit of article 56 of the Charter of the United Nations, the specific provisions of the Covenant (articles 12, 2.1, 22 and 23) and the Alma-Ata Declaration on primary health care, States parties should recognize the essential role of international cooperation and comply with their commitment to take joint and separate action to achieve the full realization of the right to health. In this regard, States parties are referred to the Alma-Ata Declaration which proclaims that the existing gross inequality in the health status of the people, particularly between developed and developing countries, as well as within countries, is politically, socially and economically unacceptable and is, therefore, of common concern to all countries.[29]

39. To comply with their international obligations in relation to article 12, States parties have to respect the enjoyment of the right to health in other countries, and to prevent third parties from violating the right in other countries, if they are able to influence these third parties by way of legal or political means, in accordance with the Charter of the United Nations and applicable international law. Depending on the availability of resources, States should facilitate access to essential health facilities, goods and services in other countries, wherever possible and provide the necessary aid when

[29] Article II, Alma-Ata Declaration, Report of the International Conference on Primary Health Care, Alma-Ata, 6–12 September 1978, in WHO, 'Health for All' Series, No. 1, Geneva: WHO, 1978.

required.[30] States parties should ensure that the right to health is given due attention in international agreements and, to that end, should consider the development of further legal instruments. In relation to the conclusion of other international agreements, States parties should take steps to ensure that these instruments do not adversely impact upon the right to health. Similarly, States parties have an obligation to ensure that their actions as members of international organizations take due account of the right to health. Accordingly, States parties which are members of international financial institutions, notably the International Monetary Fund, the World Bank, and regional development banks, should pay greater attention to the protection of the right to health in influencing the lending policies, credit agreements and international measures of these institutions.

40. States parties have a joint and individual responsibility, in accordance with the Charter of the United Nations and relevant resolutions of the United Nations General Assembly and of the World Health Assembly, to cooperate in providing disaster relief and humanitarian assistance in times of emergency, including assistance to refugees and internally displaced persons. Each State should contribute to this task to the maximum of its capacities. Priority in the provision of international medical aid, distribution and management of resources, such as safe and potable water, food and medical supplies, and financial aid should be given to the most vulnerable or marginalized groups of the population. Moreover, given that some diseases are easily transmissible beyond the frontiers of a State, the international community has a collective responsibility to address this problem. The economically developed States parties have a special responsibility and interest to assist the poorer developing States in this regard.

41. States parties should refrain at all times from imposing embargoes or similar measures restricting the supply of another State with adequate medicines and medical equipment. Restrictions on such goods should never be used as an instrument of political and economic pressure. In this regard, the Committee recalls its position, stated in General Comment No. 8, on the relationship between economic sanctions and respect for economic, social and cultural rights.

42. While only States are parties to the Covenant and thus ultimately accountable for compliance with it, all members of society—individuals, including health professionals, families, local communities, intergovernmental and non-governmental organizations, civil society organizations, as well as the private business sector—have responsibilities regarding the realization of the right to health. State parties should therefore provide an environment which facilitates the discharge of these responsibilities.

---

[30] See para. 45 of this General Comment.

Core obligations

43. In General Comment No. 3, the Committee confirms that States parties have a core obligation to ensure the satisfaction of, at the very least, minimum essential levels of each of the rights enunciated in the Covenant, including essential primary health care. Read in conjunction with more contemporary instruments, such as the Programme of Action of the International Conference on Population and Development,[31] the Alma-Ata Declaration provides compelling guidance on the core obligations arising from article 12. Accordingly, in the Committee's view, these core obligations include at least the following obligations:

(a) To ensure the right of access to health facilities, goods and services on a non-discriminatory basis, especially for vulnerable or marginalized groups;

(b) To ensure access to the minimum essential food which is nutritionally adequate and safe, to ensure freedom from hunger to everyone;

(c) To ensure access to basic shelter, housing and sanitation, and an adequate supply of safe and potable water;

(d) To provide essential drugs, as from time to time defined under the WHO Action Programme on Essential Drugs;

(e) To ensure equitable distribution of all health facilities, goods and services;

(f) To adopt and implement a national public health strategy and plan of action, on the basis of epidemiological evidence, addressing the health concerns of the whole population; the strategy and plan of action shall be devised, and periodically reviewed, on the basis of a participatory and transparent process; they shall include methods, such as right to health indicators and benchmarks, by which progress can be closely monitored; the process by which the strategy and plan of action are devised, as well as their content, shall give particular attention to all vulnerable or marginalized groups.

44. The Committee also confirms that the following are obligations of comparable priority:

(a) To ensure reproductive, maternal (pre-natal as well as post-natal) and child health care;

(b) To provide immunization against the major infectious diseases occurring in the community;

(c) To take measures to prevent, treat and control epidemic and endemic diseases;

---

[31] *Report of the International Conference on Population and Development, Cairo, 5–13 September 1994* (United Nations publication, Sales No. E.95.XIII.18), ch. I, resolution 1, annex, chaps. VII and VIII.

(*d*) To provide education and access to information concerning the main health problems in the community, including methods of preventing and controlling them;

(*e*) To provide appropriate training for health personnel, including education on health and human rights.

45. For the avoidance of any doubt, the Committee wishes to emphasize that it is particularly incumbent on States parties and other actors in a position to assist, to provide 'international assistance and cooperation, especially economic and technical'[32] which enable developing countries to fulfil their core and other obligations indicated in paragraphs 43 and 44 above.

III. Violations

46. When the normative content of article 12 (Part I) is applied to the obligations of States parties (Part II), a dynamic process is set in motion which facilitates identification of violations of the right to health. The following paragraphs provide illustrations of violations of article 12.

47. In determining which actions or omissions amount to a violation of the right to health, it is important to distinguish the inability from the unwillingness of a State party to comply with its obligations under article 12. This follows from article 12.1, which speaks of the highest attainable standard of health, as well as from article 2.1 of the Covenant, which obliges each State party to take the necessary steps to the maximum of its available resources. A State which is unwilling to use the maximum of its available resources for the realization of the right to health is in violation of its obligations under article 12. If resource constraints render it impossible for a State to comply fully with its Covenant obligations, it has the burden of justifying that every effort has nevertheless been made to use all available resources at its disposal in order to satisfy, as a matter of priority, the obligations outlined above. It should be stressed, however, that a State party cannot, under any circumstances whatsoever, justify its non-compliance with the core obligations set out in paragraph 43 above, which are non-derogable.

48. Violations of the right to health can occur through the direct action of States or other entities insufficiently regulated by States. The adoption of any retrogressive measures incompatible with the core obligations under the right to health, outlined in paragraph 43 above, constitutes a violation of the right to health. Violations through *acts of commission* include the formal repeal or suspension of legislation necessary for the continued enjoyment of the right to health or the adoption of legislation or policies which are manifestly

---

[32] Covenant, Art. 2.1.

incompatible with pre-existing domestic or international legal obligations in relation to the right to health.

49. Violations of the right to health can also occur through the omission or failure of States to take necessary measures arising from legal obligations. Violations through *acts of omission* include the failure to take appropriate steps towards the full realization of everyone's right to the enjoyment of the highest attainable standard of physical and mental health, the failure to have a national policy on occupational safety and health as well as occupational health services, and the failure to enforce relevant laws.

Violations of the obligation to respect

50. Violations of the obligation to respect are those State actions, policies or laws that contravene the standards set out in article 12 of the Covenant and are likely to result in bodily harm, unnecessary morbidity and preventable mortality. Examples include the denial of access to health facilities, goods and services to particular individuals or groups as a result of de jure or de facto discrimination; the deliberate withholding or misrepresentation of information vital to health protection or treatment; the suspension of legislation or the adoption of laws or policies that interfere with the enjoyment of any of the components of the right to health; and the failure of the State to take into account its legal obligations regarding the right to health when entering into bilateral or multilateral agreements with other States, international organizations and other entities, such as multinational corporations.

Violations of the obligation to protect

51. Violations of the obligation to protect follow from the failure of a State to take all necessary measures to safeguard persons within their jurisdiction from infringements of the right to health by third parties. This category includes such omissions as the failure to regulate the activities of individuals, groups or corporations so as to prevent them from violating the right to health of others; the failure to protect consumers and workers from practices detrimental to health, e.g. by employers and manufacturers of medicines or food; the failure to discourage production, marketing and consumption of tobacco, narcotics and other harmful substances; the failure to protect women against violence or to prosecute perpetrators; the failure to discourage the continued observance of harmful traditional medical or cultural practices; and the failure to enact or enforce laws to prevent the pollution of water, air and soil by extractive and manufacturing industries.

Violations of the obligation to fulfil

52. Violations of the obligation to fulfil occur through the failure of States parties to take all necessary steps to ensure the realization of the right to health. Examples include the failure to adopt or implement a national health policy

designed to ensure the right to health for everyone; insufficient expenditure or misallocation of public resources which results in the non-enjoyment of the right to health by individuals or groups, particularly the vulnerable or marginalized; the failure to monitor the realization of the right to health at the national level, for example by identifying right to health indicators and benchmarks; the failure to take measures to reduce the inequitable distribution of health facilities, goods and services; the failure to adopt a gender-sensitive approach to health; and the failure to reduce infant and maternal mortality rates.

IV. Implementation at the National Level

Framework legislation

53. The most appropriate feasible measures to implement the right to health will vary significantly from one State to another. Every State has a margin of discretion in assessing which measures are most suitable to meet its specific circumstances. The Covenant, however, clearly imposes a duty on each State to take whatever steps are necessary to ensure that everyone has access to health facilities, goods and services so that they can enjoy, as soon as possible, the highest attainable standard of physical and mental health. This requires the adoption of a national strategy to ensure to all the enjoyment of the right to health, based on human rights principles which define the objectives of that strategy, and the formulation of policies and corresponding right to health indicators and benchmarks. The national health strategy should also identify the resources available to attain defined objectives, as well as the most cost-effective way of using those resources.

54. The formulation and implementation of national health strategies and plans of action should respect, *inter alia*, the principles of non-discrimination and people's participation. In particular, the right of individuals and groups to participate in decision-making processes, which may affect their development, must be an integral component of any policy, programme or strategy developed to discharge governmental obligations under article 12. Promoting health must involve effective community action in setting priorities, making decisions, planning, implementing and evaluating strategies to achieve better health. Effective provision of health services can only be assured if people's participation is secured by States.

55. The national health strategy and plan of action should also be based on the principles of accountability, transparency and independence of the judiciary, since good governance is essential to the effective implementation of all human rights, including the realization of the right to health. In order to create a favourable climate for the realization of the right, States parties should take appropriate steps to ensure that the private business sector and civil society are aware of, and consider the importance of, the right to health in pursuing their activities.

56. States should consider adopting a framework law to operationalize their right to health national strategy. The framework law should establish national mechanisms for monitoring the implementation of national health strategies and plans of action. It should include provisions on the targets to be achieved and the time-frame for their achievement; the means by which right to health benchmarks could be achieved; the intended collaboration with civil society, including health experts, the private sector and international organizations; institutional responsibility for the implementation of the right to health national strategy and plan of action; and possible recourse procedures. In monitoring progress towards the realization of the right to health, States parties should identify the factors and difficulties affecting implementation of their obligations.

Right to health indicators and benchmarks

57. National health strategies should identify appropriate right to health indicators and benchmarks. The indicators should be designed to monitor, at the national and international levels, the State party's obligations under article 12. States may obtain guidance on appropriate right to health indicators, which should address different aspects of the right to health, from the ongoing work of WHO and the United Nations Children's Fund (UNICEF) in this field. Right to health indicators require disaggregation on the prohibited grounds of discrimination.

58. Having identified appropriate right to health indicators, States parties are invited to set appropriate national benchmarks in relation to each indicator. During the periodic reporting procedure the Committee will engage in a process of scoping with the State party. Scoping involves the joint consideration by the State party and the Committee of the indicators and national benchmarks which will then provide the targets to be achieved during the next reporting period. In the following five years, the State party will use these national benchmarks to help monitor its implementation of article 12. Thereafter, in the subsequent reporting process, the State party and the Committee will consider whether or not the benchmarks have been achieved, and the reasons for any difficulties that may have been encountered.

Remedies and accountability

59. Any person or group victim of a violation of the right to health should have access to effective judicial or other appropriate remedies at both national and international levels.[33] All victims of such violations should be entitled to

---

[33] Regardless of whether groups as such can seek remedies as distinct holders of rights, States parties are bound by both the collective and individual dimensions of Article 12. Collective rights are critical in the field of health; modern public health policy relies heavily on prevention and promotion which are approaches directed primarily to groups.

adequate reparation, which may take the form of restitution, compensation, satisfaction or guarantees of non-repetition. National ombudsmen, human rights commissions, consumer forums, patients' rights associations or similar institutions should address violations of the right to health.

60. The incorporation in the domestic legal order of international instruments recognizing the right to health can significantly enhance the scope and effectiveness of remedial measures and should be encouraged in all cases.[34] Incorporation enables courts to adjudicate violations of the right to health, or at least its core obligations, by direct reference to the Covenant.

61. Judges and members of the legal profession should be encouraged by States parties to pay greater attention to violations of the right to health in the exercise of their functions.

62. States parties should respect, protect, facilitate and promote the work of human rights advocates and other members of civil society with a view to assisting vulnerable or marginalized groups in the realization of their right to health.

V. Obligations of Actors Other than States Parties

63. The role of the United Nations agencies and programmes, and in particular the key function assigned to WHO in realizing the right to health at the international, regional and country levels, is of particular importance, as is the function of UNICEF in relation to the right to health of children. When formulating and implementing their right to health national strategies, States parties should avail themselves of technical assistance and cooperation of WHO. Further, when preparing their reports, States parties should utilize the extensive information and advisory services of WHO with regard to data collection, disaggregation, and the development of right to health indicators and benchmarks.

64. Moreover, coordinated efforts for the realization of the right to health should be maintained to enhance the interaction among all the actors concerned, including the various components of civil society. In conformity with articles 22 and 23 of the Covenant, WHO, the International Labour Organization, the United Nations Development Programme, UNICEF, the United Nations Population Fund, the World Bank, regional development banks, the International Monetary Fund, the World Trade Organization and other relevant bodies within the United Nations system, should cooperate effectively with States parties, building on their respective expertise, in relation to the implementation of the right to health at the national level, with due respect to their individual mandates. In particular, the international financial institutions, notably the World Bank and the International Monetary Fund,

[34] See General Comment No. 2, para. 9.

should pay greater attention to the protection of the right to health in their lending policies, credit agreements and structural adjustment programmes. When examining the reports of States parties and their ability to meet the obligations under article 12, the Committee will consider the effects of the assistance provided by all other actors. The adoption of a human rights-based approach by United Nations specialized agencies, programmes and bodies will greatly facilitate implementation of the right to health. In the course of its examination of States parties' reports, the Committee will also consider the role of health professional associations and other non-governmental organizations in relation to the States' obligations under article 12.

65. The role of WHO, the Office of the United Nations High Commissioner for Refugees, the International Committee of the Red Cross/Red Crescent and UNICEF, as well as non-governmental organizations and national medical associations, is of particular importance in relation to disaster relief and humanitarian assistance in times of emergencies, including assistance to refugees and internally displaced persons. Priority in the provision of international medical aid, distribution and management of resources, such as safe and potable water, food and medical supplies, and financial aid should be given to the most vulnerable or marginalized groups of the population.

4. *Human Rights Committee, General Comment 28: Equality of Rights between Men and Women (Article 3)*

HRC, *General Comment 28*, UN GAOR 2000, UN Doc. A/55/40, Annex VI, p. 133.

1. The Committee has decided to update its General Comment on Article 3 of this Covenant[35] and to replace General Comment 4 (thirteenth session 1981), in the light of the experience it has gathered in its activities over the last 20 years. This revision seeks to take account of the important impact of this article on the enjoyment by women of the human rights protected under the Covenant.

2. Article 3 implies that all human beings should enjoy the rights provided for in the Covenant, on an equal basis and in their totality. The full effect of this provision is impaired whenever any person is denied the full and equal enjoyment of any right. Consequently, States should ensure to men and women equally the enjoyment of all rights provided for in the Covenant.

3. The obligation to ensure to all individuals the rights recognized in the Covenant, established in articles 2 and 3 of the Covenant, requires that State parties take all necessary steps to enable every person to enjoy those rights. These steps include the removal of obstacles to the equal enjoyment [of] each

---

[35] The International Covenant on Civil and Political Rights.

of such rights, the education of the population and of state officials in human rights and the adjustment of domestic legislation so as to give effect to the undertakings set forth in the Covenant. The State party must not only adopt measures of protection but also positive measures in all areas so as to achieve the effective and equal empowerment of women. States parties must provide information regarding the actual role of women in society so that the Committee may ascertain what measures, in addition to legislative provisions, have been or should be taken to give effect to these obligations, what progress has been made, what difficulties are encountered and what steps are being taken to overcome them.

4. State parties are responsible for ensuring the equal enjoyment of rights without any discrimination. Articles 2 and 3 mandate States parties to take all steps necessary, including the prohibition of discrimination on the ground of sex, to put an end to discriminatory actions both in the public and the private sector which impair the equal enjoyment of rights.

5. Inequality in the enjoyment of rights by women throughout the world is deeply embedded in tradition, history and culture, including religious attitudes. The subordinate role of women in some countries is illustrated by the high incidence of pre-natal sex selection and abortion of female fetuses. States parties should ensure that traditional, historical, religious or cultural attitudes are not used to justify violations of women's right to equality before the law and to equal enjoyment of all Covenant rights. States parties should furnish appropriate information on those aspects of tradition, history, cultural practices and religious attitudes which jeopardise, or may jeopardise, compliance with article 3, and indicate what measures they have taken or intend to take to overcome such factors.

6. In order to fulfil the obligation set forth in article 3 States parties should take account of the factors which impede the equal enjoyment by women and men of each right specified in the Covenant. To enable the Committee to obtain a complete picture of the situation of women in each State party as regards the implementation of the rights in the Covenant, this general comment identifies some of the factors affecting the equal enjoyment by women of the rights under the Covenant, and spells out the type of information that is required with regard to these various rights.

7. The equal enjoyment of human rights by women must be protected during a state of emergency (article 4). States parties which take measures derogating from their obligations under the Covenant in time of public emergency, as provided in article 4, should provide information to the Committee with respect to the impact on the situation of women of such measures and should demonstrate that they are non-discriminatory.

8. Women are particularly vulnerable in times of internal or international armed conflicts. States parties should inform the Committee of all measures

taken during these situations to protect women from rape, abduction and other forms of gender based violence.

9. In becoming parties to the Covenant, States undertake, in accordance with article 3, to ensure the equal right of men and women to the enjoyment of all civil and political rights set forth in the Covenant, and in accordance with article 5, nothing in the Covenant may be interpreted as implying for any State, group or person any right to engage in any activity or perform any act aimed at the destruction of any of the rights provided for in article 3, or at limitations not covered by the Covenant. Moreover, there shall be no restriction upon or derogation from the equal enjoyment by women of all fundamental human rights recognized or existing pursuant to law, conventions, regulations or customs, on the pretext that the Covenant does not recognize such rights or that it recognizes them to a lesser extent.

10. When reporting on the right to life protected by article 6, States parties should provide data on birth rates and on pregnancy and childbirth-related deaths of women. Gender-disaggregated data should be provided on infant mortality rates. States parties should give information on any measures taken by the State to help women prevent unwanted pregnancies, and to ensure that they do not have to undertake life-threatening clandestine abortions. States parties should also report on measures to protect women from practices that violate their right to life, such as female infanticide, the burning of widows and dowry killings. The Committee also wishes to have information on the particular impact on women of poverty and deprivation that may pose a threat to their lives.

11. To assess compliance with article 7 of the Covenant, as well as with article 24, which mandates special protection for children, the Committee needs to be provided information on national laws and practice with regard to domestic and other types of violence against women, including rape. It also needs to know whether the State party gives access to safe abortion to women who have become pregnant as a result of rape. The States parties should also provide the Committee information on measures to prevent forced abortion or forced sterilization. In States parties where the practice of genital mutilation exists information on its extent and on measures to eliminate it should be provided. The information provided by States parties on all these issues should include measures of protection, including legal remedies, for women whose rights under article 7 have been violated.

12. Having regard to their obligations under article 8, States parties should inform the Committee of measures taken to eliminate trafficking of women and children, within the country or across borders, and forced prostitution. They must also provide information on measures taken to protect women and children, including foreign women and children, from slavery, disguised inter alia as domestic or other kinds of personal service. States parties where women

and children are recruited, and from which they are taken, and States parties where they are received should provide information on measures, national or international, which have been taken in order to prevent the violation of women's and children's rights.

13. States parties should provide information on any specific regulation of clothing to be worn by women in public. The Committee stresses that such regulations may involve a violation of a number of rights guaranteed by the Covenant, such as:

- article 26, on non-discrimination;
- article 7, if corporal punishment is imposed in order to enforce such a regulation;
- article 9, when failure to comply with the regulation is punished by arrest;
- article 12, if liberty of movement is subject to such a constraint;
- article 17, which guarantees all persons the right to privacy without arbitrary or unlawful interference;
- articles 18 and 19, when women are subjected to clothing requirements that are not in keeping with their religion or their right of self-expression; and, lastly,
- article 27, when the clothing requirements conflict with the culture to which the woman can lay a claim.

14. With regards to article 9 States parties should provide information on any laws or practices which may deprive women of their liberty on an arbitrary or unequal basis, such as by confinement within the house. (See General Comment No. 8 paragraph 1.)

15. As regards articles 7 and 10, States parties must provide all information relevant to ensuring that the right of persons deprived of their liberty are protected on equal terms for men and women. In particular, States parties should report on whether men and women are separated in prisons and whether women are guarded only by female guards. States parties should also report about compliance with the rule that accused juvenile females shall be separated from adults and on any difference in treatment between male and female persons deprived of liberty, such as, for example, access to rehabilitation and education programmes and to conjugal and family visits. Pregnant women who are deprived of their liberty should receive humane treatment and respect for their inherent dignity at all times surrounding the birth and while caring for their newly-born children; States parties should report on facilities to ensure this and on medical and health care for such mothers and their babies.

16. As regards article 12, States parties should provide information on any legal provision or any practice which restricts women's right to freedom of movement as, for example, the exercise of marital powers over the wife or parental powers over adult daughters, legal or de facto requirements which

prevent women from travelling such as the requirement of consent of a third party to the issuance of a passport or other type of travel documents to an adult woman. States parties should also report on measures taken to eliminate such laws and practices and to protect women against them, including reference to available domestic remedies. (See General Comment No 27 paragraphs 6 and 18.)

17. States parties should ensure that alien women are accorded on an equal basis the right to submit reasons against their expulsion, and to have their case reviewed as provided in article 13. In this regard, they should be entitled to submit reasons based on gender specific violations of the Covenant such as those mentioned in paragraphs [10 and 11] above.

18. State parties should provide information to enable the Committee to ascertain whether access to justice and the right to a fair trial, provided for in article 14, are enjoyed by women on equal terms to men. In particular States parties should inform the Committee whether there are legal provisions preventing women from direct and autonomous access to the courts (Case 202/1986, Ato del Avellanal v. Peru (views of 28 October 1988); whether women may give evidence as witnesses on the same terms as men; and whether measures are taken to ensure women equal access to legal aid, in particular in family matters. States parties should report on whether certain categories of women are denied the enjoyment of the presumption of innocence under article 14, paragraph 2, and on the measures which have been taken to put an end to this situation.

19. The right of everyone under article 16 to be recognized everywhere as a person before the law is particularly pertinent for women, who often see it curtailed by reason of sex or marital status. This right implies that the capacity of women to own property, to enter into a contract or to exercise other civil rights may not be restricted on the basis of marital status or any other discriminatory ground. It also implies that women may not be treated as objects to be given together with the property of the deceased husband to his family. States must provide information on laws or practices that prevent women from being treated or from functioning as full legal persons and the measures taken to eradicate laws or practices that allow such treatment.

20. States parties must provide information to enable the Committee to assess the effect of any laws and practices that may interfere with women's right to enjoy privacy and other rights protected by article 17 on the basis of equality with men. An example of such interference arises where the sexual life of a woman is taken into consideration to decide the extent of her legal rights and protections, including protection against rape. Another area where States may fail to respect women's privacy relates to their reproductive functions, for example, where there is a requirement for the husband's authorization to make a decision in regard to sterilization, where general requirements are imposed

for the sterilization of women, such as having a certain number of children or being of a certain age, or where States impose a legal duty upon doctors and other health personnel to report cases of women who have undergone abortion. In these instances, other rights in the Covenant, such as those of articles 6 and 7, might also be at stake. Women's privacy may also be interfered with by private actors, such as employers who request a pregnancy test before hiring a woman. States parties should report on any laws and public or private actions that interfere with the equal enjoyment by women of the rights under article 17, and on the measures taken to eliminate such interference and to afford women protection from any such interference.

21. States parties must take measures to ensure that freedom of thought, conscience and religion, and the freedom to adopt the religion or belief of one's choice—including the freedom to change religion or belief and to express one's religion or belief—will be guaranteed and protected in law and in practice for both men and women, on the same terms and without discrimination. These freedoms protected by article 18, must not be subject to restrictions other than those authorized by the Covenant, and must not be constrained by, inter alia, rules requiring permission from third parties, or by interference from fathers, husbands, brothers or others. Article 18 may not be relied upon to justify discrimination against women by reference to freedom of thought, conscience and religion; States parties should therefore provide information on the status of women as regards their freedom of thought, conscience and religion, and indicate what steps they have taken or intend to take both to eliminate and prevent infringements of these freedoms in respect of women and to protect their rights against any discrimination.

22. In relation to article 19 States parties should inform the Committee of any laws or other factors which may impede women from exercising the rights protected under this provision on an equal basis. As the publication and dissemination of obscene and pornographic material which portrays women and girls as objects of violence or degrading or inhuman treatment is likely to promote these kinds of treatment of women and girls, States parties should provide information about legal measures to restrict the publication or dissemination of such material.

23. States are required to treat men and women equally in regard to marriage in accordance with article 23, which has been elaborated further by General Comment 19 (1990). Men and women have the right to enter into marriage only with their free and full consent, and States have an obligation to protect the enjoyment of this right on an equal basis. Many factors may prevent women from being able to make the decision to marry freely. One factor relates to the minimum age for marriage. That age should be set by the State on the basis of equal criteria for men and women. These criteria should ensure women's capacity to make an informed and uncoerced decision. A second factor

in some States may be that either by statutory or customary law a guardian, who is generally male, consents to the marriage instead of the woman herself, thereby preventing women from exercising a free choice.

24. A different factor that may affect women's right to marry only when they have given free and full consent is the existence of social attitudes which tend to marginalize women victims of rape and put pressure on them to agree to marriage. A woman's free and full consent to marriage may also be undermined by laws which allow the rapist to have his criminal responsibility extinguished or mitigated if he marries the victim. States parties should indicate whether marrying the victim extinguishes or mitigates criminal responsibility and in the case in which the victim is a minor whether the rape reduces the marriageable age of the victim, particularly in societies where rape victims have to endure marginalization from society. A different aspect of the right to marry may be affected when States impose restrictions on remarriage by women as compared to men. Also the right to choose one's spouse may be restricted by laws or practices that prevent the marriage of a woman of a particular religion with a man who professes no religion or a different religion. States should provide information on these laws and practices and on the measures taken to abolish the laws and eradicate the practices which undermine the right of women to marry only when they have given free and full consent. It should also be noted that equality of treatment with regard to the right to marry implies that polygamy is incompatible with this principle. Polygamy violates the dignity of women. It is an inadmissible discrimination against women. Consequently, it should be definitely abolished wherever it continues to exist.

25. To fulfill their obligations under article 23, paragraph 4, States must ensure that the matrimonial regime contains equal rights and obligations for both spouses, with regard to the custody and care of children, the children's religious and moral education, the capacity to transmit to children the parent's nationality, and the ownership or administration of property, whether common property or property in the sole ownership of either spouse. States should review their legislation to ensure that married women have equal rights in regard to the ownership and administration of such property, where necessary. Also, States should ensure that no sex-based discrimination occurs in respect of the acquisition or loss of nationality by reason of marriage, of residence rights and of the right of each spouse to retain the use of his or her original family name or to participate on an equal basis in the choice of a new family name. Equality during marriage implies that husband and wife should participate equally in responsibility and authority within the family.

26. States must also ensure equality in regard to the dissolution of marriage, which excludes the possibility of repudiation. The grounds for divorce and annulment should be the same for men and women, as well as decisions with regard to property distribution, alimony and the custody of children. The need

to maintain contact between children and the non-custodian parent, should be based on equal considerations. Women should also have equal inheritance rights to those of men when the dissolution of marriage is caused by the death of one of the spouses.

27. In giving effect to recognition of the family in the context of article 23, it is important to accept the concept of the various forms of family, including unmarried couples and their children and single parents and their children and to ensure the equal treatment of women in these contexts (General Comment 19 paragraph 2 last sentence). Single parent families frequently consist of a single woman caring for one or more children, and States parties should describe what measures of support are in place to enable her to discharge her parental functions on the basis of equality with a man in a similar position.

28. The obligation of states to protect children (article 24) should be carried out equally for boys and girls. States should report on measures taken to ensure that girls are treated equally to boys in education, in feeding and in health care, and provide the Committee with disaggregated data in this respect. States should eradicate, both through legislation and any other appropriate measures, all cultural or religious practices which jeopardize the freedom and well-being of female children.

29. The right to participate in the conduct of public affairs is not fully implemented everywhere on an equal basis. States must ensure that the law guarantees to women article 25 rights on equal terms with men and take effective and positive measures to promote and ensure women's participation in the conduct of public affairs and in public office, including appropriate affirmative action. Effective measures taken by States parties to ensure that all persons entitled to vote are able to exercise that right should not be discriminatory on the grounds of sex. The Committee requires States parties to provide statistical information on the percentage of women in publicly elected offices including the legislature as well as in high-ranking civil service positions and the judiciary.

30. Discrimination against women is often intertwined with discrimination on other grounds such as race, colour, language, religion, political or other opinion, national or social origin, property, birth or other status. States parties should address the ways in which any instances of discrimination on other grounds affect women in a particular way, and include information on the measures taken to counter these effects.

31. The right to equality before the laws and freedom from discrimination, protected by article 26, requires States to act against discrimination by public and private agencies in all fields. Discrimination against women in areas such as social security laws—Case 172/84, Broeks v. Netherlands (views of 9 April 1987); case 182/84, Zwaan de Vries v. The Netherlands (views of 9 April 1987); case 218/1986, Vos v. The Netherlands (views of 29 March 1989)—, as well as

in the area of citizenship or rights of non-citizens in a country—Case 035/1978, Aumeeruddy-Cziffra et al. v. Mauritius (views adopted 9 April 1981)—, violates article 26. The commission of so called 'honour crimes' which remain unpunished, constitutes a serious violation of the Covenant and in particular of articles 6, 14 and 26. Laws which impose more severe penalties on women than on men for adultery or other offences also violate the requirement of equal treatment. The Committee has also often observed in reviewing States reports that a large proportion of women are employed in areas which are not protected by labor laws, that prevailing customs and traditions discriminate against women, particularly with regard to access to better paid employment and to equal pay for work of equal value. States should review their legislation and practices and take the lead in implementing all measures necessary in order to eliminate discrimination against women, in all fields, for example by prohibiting discrimination by private actors in areas such as employment, education, political activities and the provision of accommodation, goods and services. States parties should report on all these measures and provide information on the remedies available to victims of such discrimination.

32. The rights which persons belonging to minorities enjoy under article 27 of the Covenant in respect of their language, culture and religion do not authorize any State, group or person to violate the right to equal enjoyment by women of any Covenant rights, including the right to equal protection of the law. States should report on any legislation or administrative practices related to membership in a minority community that might constitute an infringement of the equal rights of women under the Covenant—Case 24/1977 Lovelace v. Canada (views adopted July 1981)—and on measures taken or envisaged to ensure the equal right of men and women to enjoy all civil and political rights in the Covenant. Likewise, States should report on measures taken to discharge their responsibilities in relation to cultural or religious practices within minority communities that affect the rights of women. In their reports, States parties should pay attention to the contribution made by women to the cultural life of their communities.

5. Committee on the Elimination of Racial Discrimination, General Recommendation 25: Gender Related Dimensions of Racial Discrimination

CERD, *General Recommendation 25*, UN GAOR 2000, UN Doc. A/55/18, Annex V, p. 152.

1. The Committee notes that racial discrimination does not always affect women and men equally or in the same way. There are circumstances in which

racial discrimination only or primarily affects women, or affects women in a different way, or to a different degree than men. Such racial discrimination will often escape detection if there is no explicit recognition or acknowledgement of the different life experiences of women and men, in areas of both public and private life.

2. Certain forms of racial discrimination may be directed towards women specifically because of their gender, such as sexual violence committed against women members of particular racial or ethnic groups in detention or during armed conflict; the coerced sterilization of indigenous women; abuse of women workers in the informal sector or domestic workers employed abroad by their employers. Racial discrimination may have consequences that affect primarily or only women, such as pregnancy resulting from racial bias-motivated rape; in some societies women victims of such rape may also be ostracized. Women may also be further hindered by a lack of access to remedies and complaint mechanisms for racial discrimination because of gender-related impediments, such as gender bias in the legal system and discrimination against women in private spheres of life.

3. Recognizing that some forms of racial discrimination have a unique and specific impact on women, the Committee will endeavour in its work to take into account gender factors or issues which may be interlinked with racial discrimination. The Committee believes that its practices in this regard would benefit from developing, in conjunction with the States parties, a more systematic and consistent approach to evaluating and monitoring racial discrimination against women, as well as the disadvantages, obstacles and difficulties women face in the full exercise and enjoyment of their civil, political, economic, social and cultural rights on grounds of race, colour, descent, or national or ethnic origin.

4. Accordingly, the Committee, when examining forms of racial discrimination, intends to enhance its efforts to integrate gender perspectives, incorporate gender analysis, and encourage the use of gender-inclusive language in its sessional working methods, including its review of reports submitted by States parties, concluding observations, early warning mechanisms and urgent action procedures, and general recommendations.

5. As part of the methodology for fully taking into account the gender-related dimensions of racial discrimination, the Committee will include in its sessional working methods an analysis of the relationship between gender and racial discrimination, by giving particular consideration to:

(*a*) the form and manifestation of racial discrimination;
(*b*) the circumstances in which racial discrimination occurs;
(*c*) the consequences of racial discrimination; and
(*d*) the availability and accessibility of remedies and complaint mechanisms for racial discrimination.

6. Noting that reports submitted by States parties often do not contain specific or sufficient information on the implementation of the Convention with respect to women, States parties are requested to describe, as far as possible in quantitative and qualitative terms, factors affecting and difficulties experienced in ensuring the equal enjoyment by women, free from racial discrimination, of rights under the Convention. Data which have been categorized by race or ethnic origin, and which are then disaggregated by gender within those racial or ethnic groups, will allow the States parties and the Committee to identify, compare and take steps to remedy forms of racial discrimination against women that may otherwise go unnoticed and unaddressed.

7

Summary of the International Guidelines on HIV/AIDS and Human Rights (1996)

HIV/AIDS continues to spread throughout the world at an alarming rate. The widespread abuse of human rights and fundamental freedoms associated with HIV/AIDS has emerged in all parts of the world in the wake of the epidemic. In response to this situation the experts at the Second International Consultation on HIV/AIDS and Human Rights concluded the following:

(*a*) The protection of human rights is essential to safeguard human dignity in the context of HIV/AIDS and to ensure an effective, rights-based response to HIV/AIDS. An effective response requires the implementation of all human rights, civil and political, economic, social and cultural, and fundamental freedoms of all people, in accordance with existing international human rights standards;

(*b*) Public health interests do not conflict with human rights. On the contrary, it has been recognized that when human rights are protected, fewer people become infected and those living with HIV/AIDS and their families can better cope with HIV/AIDS;

(*c*) A rights-based, effective response to the HIV/AIDS epidemic involves establishing appropriate governmental institutional responsibilities, implementing law reform and support services and promoting a supportive environment for groups vulnerable to HIV/AIDS and for those living with HIV/AIDS;

(*d*) In the context of HIV/AIDS, international human rights norms and pragmatic public health goals require States to consider measures that may be considered controversial, particularly regarding the status of women and children, sex workers, injecting drug users and men having sex with men. It is, however, the responsibility of all States to identify how they can best meet their human rights obligations and protect public health within their specific political, cultural and religious contexts;

International Guidelines on HIV/AIDS and Human Rights (Geneva: Office of the UN High Commissioner for Human Rights and UNAIDS, 1996); annotated international guidelines are available in UNAIDS and Inter-Parliamentary Union, *Handbook for Legislators on HIV/AIDS, Law and Human Rights* (Geneva: UNAIDS, 1999).

(*e*) Although States have primary responsibility for implementing strategies that protect human rights and public health, United Nations bodies, agencies and programmes, regional intergovernmental bodies and non-governmental organizations, including networks of people living with HIV/AIDS, play critical roles in this regard.

The Consultation adopted Guidelines on HIV/AIDS and Human Rights, the purpose of which is to translate international human rights norms into practical observance in the context of HIV/AIDS. To this end, the Guidelines consist of two parts: first, the human rights principles underlying a positive response to HIV/AIDS and second, action-oriented measures to be employed by Governments in the areas of law, administrative policy and practice that will protect human rights and achieve HIV-related public health goals.

There are many steps that States can take to protect HIV-related human rights and to achieve public health goals. The 12 Guidelines elaborated by the Consultation for States to implement an effective, rights-based response are summarized below.

Guideline 1: States should establish an effective national framework for their response to HIV/AIDS which ensures a coordinated, participatory, transparent and accountable approach, integrating HIV/AIDS policy and programme responsibilities across all branches of government.

Guideline 2: States should ensure, through political and financial support, that community consultation occurs in all phases of HIV/AIDS policy design, programme implementation and evaluation and that community organizations are enabled to carry out their activities, including in the field of ethics, law and human rights, effectively.

Guideline 3: States should review and reform public policy laws to ensure that they adequately address public health issues raised by HIV/AIDS, that their provisions applicable to casually transmitted diseases are not inappropriately applied to HIV/AIDS and that they are consistent with international human rights obligations.

Guideline 4: States should review and reform criminal laws and correctional systems to ensure that they are consistent with international human rights obligations and are not misused in the context of HIV/AIDS or targeted against vulnerable groups.

Guideline 5: States should enact or strengthen anti-discrimination and other protective laws that protect vulnerable groups, people living with HIV/ AIDS and people with disabilities from discrimination in both the public and private sectors, ensure privacy and confidentiality and ethics in research involving human subjects, emphasize education and conciliation, and provide for speedy and effective administrative and civil remedies.

Guideline 6: States should enact legislation to provide for the regulation of HIV-related goods, services and information, so as to ensure widespread availability of qualitative prevention measures and services, adequate HIV prevention and care information and safe and effective medication at an affordable price. (Revised 10 September 2002, available at www.unaids.org.)

Guideline 7: States should implement and support legal support services that will educate people affected by HIV/AIDS about their rights, provide free legal services to enforce those rights, develop expertise on HIV-related legal issues and utilize means of protection in addition to the courts, such as offices of ministries of justice, ombudspersons, health complaint units and human rights commissions.

Guideline 8: States, in collaboration with and through the community, should promote a supportive and enabling environment for women, children and other vulnerable groups by addressing underlying prejudices and inequalities through community dialogue, specially designed social and health services and support to community groups.

Guideline 9: States should promote the wide and ongoing distribution of creative education, training and media programmes explicitly designed to change attitudes of discrimination and stigmatization associated with HIV/AIDS to understanding and acceptance.

Guideline 10: States should ensure that government and the private sector develop codes of conduct regarding HIV/AIDS issues that translate human rights principles into codes of professional responsibility and practice, with accompanying mechanisms to implement and enforce these codes.

Guideline 11: States should ensure monitoring and enforcement mechanisms to guarantee the protection of HIV-related human rights, including those of people living with HIV/AIDS, their families and communities.

Guideline 12: States should cooperate through all relevant programmes and agencies of the United Nations system, including UNAIDS, to share knowledge and experience concerning HIV-related human rights issues and should ensure effective mechanisms to protect human rights in the context of HIV/AIDS at international level.

8

Sample Application to Petition
a Human Rights Treaty Body

Various treaty-based bodies of the United Nations Human Rights System offer avenues of communication through which individuals or groups of individuals, who claim to be victims of human rights violations, may lodge a complaint against their state. Specifically, the available communications are as follows:

1. The *Optional Protocol to the International Covenant on Civil and Political Rights* outlines, in Articles 1 through 5, a complaints procedure to the Human Rights Committee for individuals or groups of individuals whose state is a party to both the *Political Covenant* and the *Optional Protocol*.

2. The *Optional Protocol to the Convention on the Elimination of All Forms of Discrimination against Women* provides, in Articles 2 through 7, a Communications Procedure to *the Committee on the Elimination of Discrimination Against Women* (CEDAW) for individuals or groups of individuals whose state is a party to both the *Women's Convention* and the *Optional Protocol*, and for an Inquiry Procedure in Articles 8 and 9 for examination of grave or systemic violations in States that are Party to the *Women's Convention*, its *Optional Protocol* and that accept the competence of CEDAW to conduct such Inquiries.

3. *Article 14 of the International Convention on the Elimination of All Forms of Racial Discrimination* establishes a procedure which makes it possible for an individual or a group of persons who claim to be victims of racial discrimination to lodge a complaint with the *Committee on the Elimination of Racial Discrimination* (CERD) against their state. This may only be done if the state concerned is a party to the Convention and has declared that it recognizes the competence of CERD to receive such complaints.

Each procedure referred to above should be examined carefully to ensure that a communication or complaint meets the technical and substantive requirements imposed by that particular system. For communications to the Human Rights Committee, for instance, a sample form is available,[1] although its use is not required.

---

[1] See www.unhchr.ch/html/menu2/complain.htm.

The following sample form can by utilized as a model for any of the communications procedures to the treaty-based bodies discussed, with the caveat that careful attention must be paid to the specific scope of each. For example, some procedures permit any person or NGO to raise questions of human rights violations; others permit only the alleged victim or a direct representative to file a complaint. The requirement to exhaust domestic remedies is common to nearly every procedure, but its interpretation varies considerably.[2]

Model Communication to UN-Based Treaty Bodies

Date

Communication to:

[Type address here]

Note: Communications to the Human Rights Committee and Committee on the Elimination of Racial Discrimination should be addressed as follows (indicate Committee for which communication is intended):

Office of the High Commission for Human Rights
United Nations
CH-1211 Geneva 10
Switzerland
Tel.: (41) (22) 917-9000; fax: (41) (22) 917-9022

Communications to the Committee on the Elimination of Discrimination Against Women should be addressed to:

Division for Advancement of Women
United Nations
2 UN Plaza, DC2-12th Floor
New York, NY 10017
USA
Tel.: (1) (212) 963-3177; fax: (1) (212) 963-3463

submitted for consideration under the [add relevant Convention]

I. Information Concerning the Author of the Communication

Name: First Name(s):
Nationality: Profession:
Date and Place of Birth:
Present address or whereabouts:

---

[2] H. Hannum (ed.), *Guide to International Human Rights Practice* (Ardsley, NY: Transnational Publishers, Inc. and The Procedural Aspects of International Law Institute, 3rd edn., 1999).

Address for exchange of confidential correspondence (if other than present address):

Submitting the communication as:

(*a*) Victim of the violation or violations set forth below

(*b*) Appointed representative/legal counsel of the alleged victim(s)

(*c*) Other

If box (*c*) is marked, the author should explain:

  (i) In what capacity s/he is acting on behalf of the victim(s) (e.g. family rela-
       tionship or other personal links with the alleged victim(s)):
  (ii) Why the victim(s) is (are) unable to submit the communication him/her
       self (themselves):

*An unrelated third party having no link to the victim(s) cannot submit a com-
munication on their behalf.*

II. Information Concerning the Alleged Victim(s) (if Other than Author)

Name: First Name:
Nationality: Profession:
Date and place of birth:
Present address or whereabouts:

III. State Concerned/Articles Violated/Domestic Remedies

Name of the State party (country) against which the communication is
directed:

Articles allegedly violated:

Steps taken by or on behalf of the alleged victim(s) to exhaust domestic remedies—recourse to the courts or other public authorities, when and with what results (if possible, enclose copies of all relevant judicial or administrative decisions):

If domestic remedies have not been exhausted, explain why:

IV. Other International Procedures

Has the same matter been submitted for examination under another procedure of international investigation or settlement (e.g. the Inter-American Commission of Human Rights, the European Court of Human Rights)? If so, when and with what results?

V. Facts of the Claim

Detailed description of the facts of the alleged violation or violations (including relevant dates):[3]

Author's signature

[3] Add as many pages as needed for this description.

Annotated Table of Cases

Select Bibliography by Chapter

Although not exhaustive, the following select bibliography of books is intended as a guide to additional readings to Chapters 2–7 in Part I of this book.

Chapter 2. Reproductive and Sexual Health

Berer, M., and T. K. S. Ravindran (eds.), *Safe Motherhood Initiatives: Critical Issues, Special Edition* (London: Reproductive Health Matters, 1999).

Fathalla, M. F., *From Obstetrics and Gynecology to Women's Health: The Road Ahead* (New York and London: Parthenon, 1997).

—— A. Rosenfield, and C. Indriso (eds.), *FIGO Manual of Human Reproduction*, iii. *Global Issues in Reproductive Health* (New York and London: Parthenon, 1998)

Maine, D., *et al.*, *Guidelines for Monitoring the Availability and Use of Obstetric Services* (New York: UNICEF, 2nd edn., 1997).

Murray, C., and A. Lopez (eds.), *Health Dimensions of Sex and Reproduction* (Boston, Mass.: Harvard School of Public Health on Behalf of the World Health Organization and the World Bank, 1998).

Starrs, A., *The Safe Motherhood Action Agenda: Priorities for the Next Decade, Report on the Safe Motherhood Technical Consultation, 18–23 October 1997, Colombo, Sri Lanka* (New York: Family Care International, 1998).

World Health Organization, Department of Reproductive Health and Research, *The WHO Reproductive Health Library* (Geneva: WHO, 2001, CD-Rom format).

Chapter 3. Health Care Systems

Alan Guttmacher Institute, *Sharing Responsibility: Women, Society and Abortion Worldwide* (New York and Washington: AGI, 1999).

Ford Foundation, *Globalization, Health Sector Reform, Gender and Reproductive Health* (New York: Ford Foundation, 2002).

United Nations, *Women and Health: Mainstreaming the Gender Perspective into the Health Sector. Report of the Expert Group Meeting 28 September–2 October 1998, Tunis* (New York: United Nations, Publication Sales No. 99.IV.4, 1999).

United Nations, *Population and Development*, i. *Programme of Action Adopted at the International Conference on Population and Development, Cairo, 5–13 September 1994* (New York: United Nations, Department for Economic and Social Information and Policy Analysis, ST/ESA/SER.A/149, 1994).

—— Department of Public Information, *Platform for Action and Beijing Declaration. Fourth World Conference on Women, Beijing, China, 4–15 September 1995* (New York: United Nations, 1995).

—— General Assembly, *Report of the Ad Hoc Committee of the Whole of the Twenty-First Special Session of the General Assembly: Overall Review and Appraisal of the Implementation of the Programme of Action of the International Conference on Population and Development*, A/S-21/5/Add.1 (New York: United Nations, 1999).

—— —— *Report of the Ad Hoc Committee of the Whole of the Twenty-Third Special Session of the General Assembly: Further Actions and Initiatives to Implement the Beijing Declaration and the Platform for Action*, A/S-23/10/Rev.1 (New York: United Nations, 2000).

World Bank, *World Development Report: Investing in Health* (New York: Oxford University Press, 1993).

World Health Organization, *The World Health Report 2000. Health Systems: Improving Performance* (Geneva: WHO, 2000).

—— *Reproductive Health Indicators for Global Monitoring: Report of the Second Interagency Meeting* (Geneva: WHO, 2001).

—— *Transforming Health Systems: Gender and Rights in Reproductive Health* (Geneva: WHO, 2001).

Chapter 4. Ethics

American College of Obstetricians and Gynecologists, *Ethics in Obstetrics and Gynecology* (Washington, DC: ACOG, 2002).

Beauchamp, T. L., and J. F. Childress, *Principles of Biomedical Ethics* (New York: Oxford University Press, 5th edn., 2001).

British Medical Association, *Medical Ethics Today: Its Practice and Philosophy* (London: BMA, 1993).

Gillon, R. (ed.), *Principles of Health Care Ethics* (Chichester: John Wiley & Sons, 1994).

Harris, J. (ed.), *Bioethics* (Oxford: Oxford University Press, 2001).

—— and S. Holm (eds.), *The Future of Human Reproduction* (Oxford: Clarendon Press, 1998).

International Federation of Gynecology and Obstetrics, *FIGO Committee for the Ethical Aspects of Human Reproduction and Women's Health, Recommendations on Ethical Issues in Obstetrics and Gynecology* (London: FIGO, 2000).

Jonsen, A. R., M. Siegler, and W. J. Winslade, *Clinical Ethics* (New York: McGraw Hill, 4th edn., 1998).

Kerridge, J., M. Lowe, and J. McPhee, *Ethics and Law for the Health Professions* (Katoomba, NSW: Social Science Press, 1998).

Macklin, R., *Against Relativism: Cultural Diversity and the Search for Ethical Universals in Medicine* (New York: Oxford University Press 1997).

Snyder, L. (ed.), *Ethical Choices: Case Studies for Medical Practice* (Philadelphia: American College of Physicians, 1996).

Chapter 5. Legal Origins and Principles

Center for Reproductive Law and Policy (CRLP), *Women of the World: Laws and Policies Affecting their Reproductive Lives: Anglophone Africa—2001 Progress Report* (New York: CRLP, 2001).

—— *Women of the World: Laws and Policies Affecting their Reproductive Lives: East Central Europe* (New York: CRLP, 2000).

—— and Demus, Estudio para la Defensa de los Derechos de la Mujer, *Women of the World: Laws and Policies Affecting their Reproductive Lives—Latin America and the Caribbean* (New York: CRLP, 1997).

———— *Mujeres del Mundo: Leyes y Politicas que afectan sus vidas reproductivas, America Latina y el Caribe, Suplemento 2000* (New York: CRLP, 2001).

—— and Groupe de recherche femmes et lois au Sénégal, *Women of the World: Laws and Policies Affecting their Reproductive Lives: Francophone Africa* (New York: CRLP, 1999).

—— and International Federation of Women Lawyers; Kenya Chapter; *Women of the World: Laws and Policies Affecting their Reproductive Lives: Anglophone Africa* (New York: CRLP, 1997).

Cook, R. J., and B. M. Dickens, *Considerations for Formulating Reproductive Health Laws* (Geneva: WHO, 2nd edn., 2000).

Gostin, L. O., *Public Health Law: Power, Duty and Restraint* (Berkeley, Calif.: University of California Press, 2000).

Jayasuriya, D. C. (ed.), *HIV Law, Ethics and Human Rights* (New Delhi: United Nations Development Programme, 1995).

Jost, T. S., *Readings in Comparative Health Law and Bioethics* (Durham, NC: Carolina Academic Press, 2001).

Kennedy, I., and A. Grubb (eds.), *Principles of Medical Law* (Oxford: Oxford University Press, 1998).

Mason, J. K., *Medico-Legal Aspects of Reproduction and Parenthood* (Aldershot: Ashgate Dartmouth, 2nd edn., 1998).

Robertson, J. A., *Children of Choice: Freedom and the New Reproductive Technologies* (Princeton: Princeton University Press, 1994).

Spece, R. G., D. S. Shimm, and A. E. Buchanan (eds.), *Conflicts of Interest in Clinical Practice and Research* (New York: Oxford University Press, 1996).

United Nations, *Abortion Policies: A Global Review*, 3 vols. (New York: United Nations, 1995).

Chapter 6. Human Rights Principles

Alfredsson, G., and K. Tomasevski (eds.), *A Thematic Guide to Documents on Health and Human Rights* (The Hague: Martinus Nijhoff Publishers, 1998).

American University Law Review, 44/4 (symposium edition on reproductive and sexual rights) (1995).

British Medical Association, *The Medical Profession and Human Rights: Handbook for a Changing Agenda* (London: Zed Books, 2001).

Brownlie, I., and G. S. Goodwin-Gill (eds.), *Basic Instruments on Human Rights* (Oxford: Oxford University Press, 4th edn., 2002).

Buergenthal, T., R. Norris, and D. Shelton, *Protecting Human Rights in the Americas: Selected Problems* (Arlington, Va.: N. P. Engel, 3rd edn., 1990).

Coliver, S. (ed.), *The Right to Know: Human Rights and Access to Reproductive Health Information* (London and Philadelphia: Article 19 and University of Pennsylvania Press, 1995).

Cook, R. J., *Women's Health and Human Rights: The Promotion and Protection of Women's Health through International Human Rights Law* (Geneva: WHO, 1994).

—— B. M. Dickens, O. A. Wilson, and S. E. Scarrow, *Advancing Safe Motherhood through Human Rights* (Geneva: WHO, 2001).

Eriksson, M. K., *Reproductive Freedom in the Context of International Human Rights and Humanitarian Law* (The Hague: Martinus Nijhoff, 2000).

Garling, M., and C. Anselm Odinkalu, *Building Bridges for Rights: Inter-African Initiatives in the Field of Human Rights* (London: Interights, 2001).

Gostin, L. O., and Z. Lazzarini, *Human Rights and Public Health in the AIDS Pandemic* (New York: Oxford University Press, 1997).

Health and Human Rights, 1/4 (symposium edition on women's health and human rights) (1995).

Health and Human Rights, 4/2 (symposium edition on reproductive and sexual rights) (2000).

Hodgkin, R., and P. Newhall, *Implementation Handbook for the Convention on the Rights of the Child* (New York: UNICEF, 1998).

International Planned Parenthood Federation, *Charter on Sexual and Reproductive Rights* (London: IPPF, 1996).

Joseph, S., J. Schulz, and M. Castan, *The International Covenant on Civil and Political Rights: Cases, Materials and Commentary* (Oxford: Oxford University Press, 2000).

Mann, J. M., S. Gruskin, M. A. Grodin, and G. J. Annas (eds.), *Health and Human Rights* (New York: Routledge, 1999).

Medicine and the Law, 18/2–3 (symposium edition on reproductive and sexual rights) (1999).

Nordic Journal of International Law, 67/1 (symposium edition on reproductive and sexual rights) (1998).

Packer, C. A. A., *The Right to Reproductive Choice* (Turku, Finland: Åabo Akademi University, Institute for Human Rights, 1996).

Petchesky, R. P., and K. Judd (eds.), *Negotiating Reproductive Rights: Women's Perspectives Across Countries and Cultures* (London: Zed Books, 1998).

Rahman, A., and N. Toubia, *Female Genital Mutilation: A Guide to Laws and Policies Worldwide* (London: Zed Books, 2000).

Stanchieri, J., I. Merali, and R. J. Cook, *The Application of Human Rights to Reproductive and Sexual Health: A Compilation of the Work of UN Treaty Bodies* (Ottawa: Action Canada for Population and Development, 2001).

Toebes, B. C. A., *The Right to Health as a Human Right in International Law* (Antwerp: Intersentia-Hart, 1999).

UNAIDS, Inter-Parliamentary Union, *Handbook for Legislators on HIV/AIDS, Law and Human Rights* (Geneva: UNAIDS, 1999).

United Nations, *HIV/AIDS and Human Rights —International Guidelines: The Results of the Second International Consultation on HIV/AIDS and Human Rights, 23–25 Sept. 1999* (Geneva: United Nations, HR/PUB/98/1, 1998).

United Nations Division for the Advancement of Women, United Nations Population Fund, and United Nations High Commissioner for Human Rights, *Round Table of Human Rights Treaty Bodies on Human Rights Approaches to Women's Health, with a Focus on Sexual and Reproductive Health and Rights: Summary of the Proceedings and Recommendations* (New York: UNFPA, 1998).

United Nations Population Fund, *The State of World Population: 1997—The Right to Choose: Reproductive Rights and Reproductive Health* (New York: UNFPA, 1997).

Chapter 7. Implementation of Legal and Human Rights Principles

Ahmed An-Na'im, A. (ed.), *Universal Rights, Local Remedies: Implementing Human Rights in the Legal Systems of Africa* (London: Interights, 1999).

Alston, P., and J. Crawford (eds.), *The Future of UN Human Rights Treaty Monitoring* (Cambridge: Cambridge University Press, 2000).

Blaustein, A. P., and G. H. Flanz, *Constitutions of the Countries of the World* (Dobbs Ferry, NY: Oceana Publications, 1999).

Byrnes, A., J. Connors, and L. Bik (eds.), *Advancing the Human Rights of Women: Using International Human Rights Standards in Domestic Litigation* (London: Commonwealth Secretariat, 1997).

Carbert, A., J. Stanchieri, and R. J. Cook, *Advocating for Reproductive and Sexual Health Rights in the African Regional Human Rights System* (Chapel Hill, NC: Ipas, 2002).

Cook, R. J. (ed.), *Human Rights of Women: National and International Perspectives* (Philadelphia: University of Pennsylvania Press, 1994).

Hannum, H. (ed.), *Guide to International Human Rights Practice* (Ardsley, NY: Transnational Publishers and Procedural Aspects of International Law Institute, 3rd edn., 1999).

International Human Rights Internship Program and Asia Forum for Human Rights and Development, *Circle of Rights: Economic, Social and Cultural Rights Activism. A Training Resource* (Washington, DC: International Human Rights Internship Program, Institute of International Education, 2000).

Lockwood, C. E., D. B. Magraw, M. F. Spring, and S. I. Strong (eds.), *The International Human Rights of Women: Instruments of Change* (Chicago: American Bar Association Section of International Law and Practice, 1998).

McChesney, A., *Promoting and Defending Economic, Social and Cultural Rights: A Handbook* (Washington, DC: American Association for the Advancement of Science, 2000).

Mertus, J., N. Flowers, and M. Dutt, *Local Action Global Change: Learning about the Human Rights of Women and Girls* (New York: UNIFEM and the Center for Women's Global Leadership, 1999).

Murray, R., *The African Commission on Human and Peoples' Rights and International Law* (Oxford: Hart Publishing, 2000).

Profamilia Servicio Juridico and International Programme on Reproductive and Sexual Health Law, University of Toronto, *El Sistema Interamericano de Derechos Humanos: Derechos Sexuales y Reproductivos en Acción* (The Inter-American Human Rights System: Sexual and Reproductive Rights in Action) (Bogotá: Profamilia Servicio Juridico, 4 vols., 2001).

Schuler, M. A., and D. Q. Thomas (eds.), *Women's Human Rights Step by Step* (Washington, DC: Women, Law and Development International and Human Rights Watch, 1999).

Stanchieri, J., I. Merali, and R. J. Cook, *The Application of Human Rights to Reproductive and Sexual Health: A Compilation of the Work of International Human Rights Treaty Bodies* (Ottawa: Action Canada for Population and Development, 2001).

—— —— N. Rasmussen, D. Bogecho, and R. J. Cook, *The Application of Human Rights to Reproductive and Sexual Health: A Compilation of the Work of the European*

Human Rights System (Warsaw: Federation for Women and Family Planning and ASTRA—Central and Eastern European Women's Network for Sexual and Reproductive Rights; Toronto: International Programme of Reproductive and Sexual Health Law, Faculty of Law, University of Toronto; Copenhagen: Danish Centre for Human Rights, 2002).

United Nations, *Assessing the Status of Women: A Guide to Reporting under the Convention on the Elimination of All Forms of Discrimination against Women* (New York: United Nations, 2000).

—— *Manual on Human Rights Reporting* (New York: United Nations, 1997).

Zajkowski, J., Martinez, K. H., and Cook, R. J., *Bringing Rights to Bear on Reproductive and Sexual Rights: An Analysis of the Work of UN Treaty Monitoring Bodies* (New York: Center for Reproductive Law and Policy, 2003).

Annotated Listing of Relevant Websites

Although not exhaustive, the following is an annotated listing of relevant websites. Those included below are functional as of April 2002.

Action Canada for Population and Development

www.acpd.ca

This website, maintained by Action Canada for Population and Development, contains online resources and links relating to reproductive and sexual rights. In addition, this site contains an online version of *The Application of Human Rights to Reproductive and Sexual Health: A Compilation of the Work of International Human Rights Treaty Bodies.*

African Commission on Human Rights

www1.umn.edu/humanrts/africa/comision.html

This website provides links to documents issued by the African Commission including final communiqués and examinations of state reports. There are also links to the African (Banjul) Charter on Human and Peoples' Rights, and information regarding the Commission's upcoming sessions.

Alan Guttmacher Institute (AGI)

www.agi-usa.org/index.html

The AGI website contains information on reproductive and sexual health issues, such as sexual behaviour, pregnancy and birth, contraception, abortion, sexually transmitted infections, youth, law, and policy.

American College of Obstetrics and Gynecology (ACOG)

http://www.acog.org

The website, maintained by ACOG, provides a list of books on women's health, news releases, US government's legislation and regulation activities relating to women's health.

Annual Review of Population Law, Harvard Law Library

www.law.harvard.edu/Programs/annual_review/

This website contains excerpts of recent legislation, constitutions, and court decisions on reproductive and sexual health from most countries in the world. The website is a source of texts of national laws on reproductive and sexual health, including texts of abortion laws of a number of countries.

Center for Reproductive Law and Policy (CRLP)

www.crlp.org

This website contains information on CRLP projects pertaining to reproductive and sexual health in the United States and worldwide. It also provides online access to newsletters and some publications of the CRLP.

CLADEM

http://www.eurosur.org/CLADEM/

This website contains various resources relating to women's rights with specific emphasis on Latin America and the Caribbean countries. Besides the information in the website, it links to national legislation, public policies, and resources of other organizations.

Coalition against Trafficking in Women—Asia Pacific (CATWAP)

http://www.catw-ap.org/

This website is maintained by the Coalition Against Trafficking in Women—Asia Pacific which is an international network of feminist groups, organizations and individuals fighting the sexual exploitation of women globally. The website contains statistics and other relevant facts regarding the topic of trafficking in women. It also contains speeches, papers, and publications on this topic, including, the Asia-Pacific Coalition report.

Commonwealth Medical Association Trust (ComMAT)

http://www.commat.org

This website contains an overview of upcoming sessions of UN Treaty Bodies, including, CEDAW, CRC, HRC, CESCR, CERD and CAT. It also provides the schedules for States Parties' reports to these human rights treaty bodies. In addition, ComMAT posts the portions of States Parties' reports pertaining to health of Commonwealth countries.

Consortium for Health and Human Rights

http://www.healthandhumanrights.org

The activities of the consortium of health and human rights organizations are posted on this website. They include conferences, curriculum development, and support for student organizing.

Constitution Finder

http://confinder.richmond.edu/

This website is an index of constitutions, charters, amendments and other related documents. Nations of the world are listed alphabetically, and each is linked to its constitutional text posted somewhere on the internet.

Demographic and Health Survey (DHS)

http://www.measuredhs.com

The website, maintained by the Measure project of DHS, assists developing countries in the collection and use of data to evaluate population, health, and nutrition programmes. It also provides information on family planning, maternal and child health, and reproductive health. The website contains various data on surveys conducted worldwide, analysis on secondary data, publications, and links to relevant resources.

Emergency Contraception for Diverse Communities Project

http://www.path.org/index.htm

The website, maintained by Program for Appropriate Technology in Health (PATH), provides information on health with special emphasis on that of women and children. The website provides resources on emergency contraception for clinical and non-clinical providers prepared by Program Appropriate Technology in Health, including the Emergency Contraception Tools Notebook.

EngenderHealth

www.engenderhealth.org

This website contains information about various reproductive and sexual health issues, including family planning, maternal/child health, male reproductive health, post-abortion care, infections (STI/HIV), and sexuality and gender. Online courses on reproductive health and infection prevention are also available on this site to provide training for health care staff who work in low-resource settings.

European Court of Human Rights

www.echr.coe.int

This website contains a list of recent judgments and press releases on those judgments. There is also a link to the searchable database of the Court's previous judgments.

European NGOs for Sexual and Reproductive Health and Rights, Population and Development

http://www.eurongos.org

This website links to a number of European-based NGOs working in reproductive health and rights, population, and development. It provides information concerning donors, various manuals, and a link to international organizations.

Family Care International (FCI)

www.familycareintl.org

This website contains information about FCI initiatives in different regions of the world, as well as a list and summary of FCI publications that can be ordered online. FCI aims to improve women's sexual and reproductive health and rights in developing countries, with a special emphasis on making pregnancy and childbirth safer.

Family Health International (FHI)

www.fhi.org

This website contains information on the projects and initiatives undertaken by FHI, an organization that works to improve reproductive and family health around the world through biomedical and social science research, health service delivery interventions, training, and information programmes. More than 1,500 full-text materials are available on this site, including books, reports, case studies, research summaries, periodicals, and training materials, which provide information on family planning, reproductive health, maternal health, gender issues, sexually transmitted diseases, reproductive tract infections, and HIV/AIDS prevention and care.

Global Reproductive Health Forum

www.hsph.harvard.edu/organizations/healthnet

This website provides interactive electronic forums and global discussion groups, and links to a variety of full-text reproductive health and rights materials through an extensive online research library.

Harvard AIDS Institute

http://www.hsph.harvard.edu/hai/lab_research/bhp.html

This website contains information regarding upcoming conferences, forums, workshops, and other training opportunities relating to AIDS and a link to the AIDS enhancing care initiative website, which focuses on methods of improvement of care for people living with AIDS. There are also links to scientific resources for researchers, and an online version of the Harvard AIDS Review from 1995 to present.

Human Rights Internet

www.hri.ca

This website is maintained by Human Rights Internet which is dedicated to empowering human rights activists worldwide, governmental and non-governmental, through dissemination of information and education. The website is dedicated to international NGOs, with a database of human rights websites, including those pertaining to reproductive and sexual health, a documentation centre, and publishing house. It also provides a world calendar of human rights events occurring each month around the globe on which visitors can post information on events in their regions.

Human Rights Library

www.umn.edu/humanrts

This database, maintained by the University of Minnesota, contains direct links to more than 6,900 documents relating to human rights around the world, including educational materials, annotated bibliographies, UN documents, regional documents, and numerous treaties and conventions. This site is particularly useful for documents and information relating to the African human rights system.

Human Rights Watch

www.hrw.org

This website provides a list of publications, current events, and the Human Rights Watch World Report, focused on protecting the human rights of people around the world by bringing offenders to justice, preventing discrimination, upholding political freedom and protecting people from inhuman conduct. A section on Women's Rights includes information pertaining to reproductive and sexual health.

Inter-American Commission on Human Rights

http://www.cidh.oas.org/DefaultE.htm (English)
http://www.cidh.oas.org/french.htm (French)
http://www.cidh.oas.org/Default.htm (Spanish)
http://www.cidh.oas.org/comissao.htm (Portuguese)

This multilingual website contains basic documents used by the Inter-American Commission on Human Rights, as well as annual reports, press releases, and information on how to present a petition to the Commission.

Inter-American Court of Human Rights

www.corteidh.or.cr/ (Spanish)
http://www.oas.org/default.htm (English)
http://www.oas.org/default_fr.htm (French)
http://www.oas.org/defaultpt.htm (Portuguese)

This website contains general information about the Court's composition and functions. The site also contains jurisprudence of the Court, press releases, and links to international courts and related institutions.

Interights

www.interights.org

The website is maintained by the International Centre for the Legal Protection of Human Rights, an international human rights law centre dedicated to support and promote the development of legal protection for human rights and freedoms worldwide. The website contains databases for Commonwealth and International human rights case law. Both databases may be searched by subject-matter or by keywords. Case titles, dates, and summaries are provided.

International Center for Research on Women

http://www.icrw.org

The website provides recent research on poverty reduction, HIV/AIDS, reproductive health, social change, and adolescence, amongst others.

International Council of AIDS Services Organizations (ICASO)

http://www.icaso.org/icaso.htm

This website contains online documents relating to AIDS, including information about vaccines. There are links to ICASO's five regional offices, and descriptions of human rights violations that NGOs often encounter. In addition, the site contains information about forthcoming AIDS conferences.

International Federation of Gynecology and Obstetrics (FIGO)

www.figo.org

This site contains information on FIGO projects, activities, and conferences, and provides links to some FIGO publications, including guidelines on the ethical aspects of issues that impact obstetrics, gynaecology, and women's health.

International HIV/AIDS Alliance

www.aidsalliance.org
www.aidsmap.com

This website contains online publications and resources, as well as numerous links which are divided into the following categories: general HIV/AIDS, People Living with HIV/AIDS, prevention, care and support, organizational development, impact mitigation, and regional websites.

International Lesbian and Gay Association

http://www.ilga.org

The website provides information and news from around the globe relating to gays and lesbians. It includes comprehensive data on laws affecting lesbians and gays around the world on a country-by-country basis.

International Planned Parenthood Federation (IPPF)

www.ippf.org/index.htm

This website contains online documents and reports relating to reproductive and sexual health, as well as links to IPPF regional offices and other organizations concerned with reproductive health issues.

International Women's Health Coalition

http://www.iwhc.org/

This website contains information on international programmes relating to reproductive and sexual health, and online publications and reports. Highlights include updates on follow-up measures taken by the international community and non-governmental organizations to ensure women's health and rights. The site features initiatives on adolescent health and rights, sexual rights, and access to safe abortion. Most sections now appear in Spanish, French, and Portuguese as well as English.

International Women's Rights Action Watch (IWRAW)

www.igc.org/iwraw/

This website provides online access to the IWRAW newsletter, their publication list and updates on the work of the Committee on the Elimination of Discrimination Against Women. This Committee reviews what states have done to bring their laws, policies, and practices into compliance with the Convention on the Elimination of All Forms of Discrimination against Women.

IPAS

www.ipas.org

This website provides information on IPAS's strategies and projects to improve the reproductive health of women, with a focus on preventing unsafe abortion, improving treatment of its complications, and reducing its consequences. It also makes available a number of full-text IPAS documents and publications.

Measure Communication

http://www.prb.org/MeasureTemplate.cfm

The website consists of resources to foster better dissemination and use of data and information to support improved population, health, and nutrition policies in developing countries.

Pan American Health Organization (PAHO)—Program on Women, Health and Development

http://www.paho.org/default.htm (English)
http://www.paho.org/default_spa.htm (Spanish)

The website consists of extensive resources of PAHO, which is the inter-American regional office of the World Health Organization. The website contains health-related data, periodic publications, databases, and other technical documents.

Partners for Health Reform-plus (PHRplus)

http://www.phrproject.com/globali/mrh.htm

The website is maintained by PHRplus, a US Agency for International Development flagship project in health policy and systems. The website offers extensive resources of health policy reform, management, financing, and strengthening.

PopNet

http://www.prb.org/PopTemplate.cfm

The website, maintained by the Population Reference Bureau, presents information on population topics such as demographic statistics, economics, education, environment, gender, policy, and reproductive health. It provides a comprehensive directory of population-related websites available by organization, by region or country, and by topic within countries.

Population Council

www.popcouncil.org

This website includes extensive information on the Council's efforts on a range of reproductive health and family planning issues, as well as numerous full-text documents published by the Council.

Q Web: A Women's Empowerment Base

http://www.qweb.kvinnoforum.se/main.html

This website is run by Kvinnoforum, an independent organization working to enhance women's empowerment in their personal life, their working life, and at a societal level around the globe. The site contains online articles, references and discussion forums in the areas of gender equality, society and women's health, sexuality and reproduction, violence and abuse, adolescents and trafficking.

Reproductive Health Gateway

http://www.rhgateway.org

This website is maintained by Population and Health Materials Working Group (PHWMG), to encourage cooperation among organizations, eliminate duplication of materials, and promote the dissemination and utilization of each organization's materials. The website offers a quick access to relevant, accurate information about reproductive health on the web. It links to a number of websites carefully selected for accuracy, authority, and relevance.

Reproductive Health Outlook

http://www.rho.org

The website, maintained by Program for Appropriate Technology in Health (PATH), provides up-to-date summaries of research findings, programme experience, and clinical guidelines related to key reproductive health topics, as well as analyses of policy and programme implications.

Rising Daughters Aware

http://www.fgm.org

This website is maintained by Rising Daughters Aware/FGM Network. It consists of extensive information on female genital mutilation practices including medical articles and protocols, legal texts, information, and links. It also provides useful links to various international organizations and NGOs.

Safe Motherhood

www.safemotherhood.org

This website contains information about initiatives developed by the Inter-Agency group for Safe Motherhood, created in 1987 by the United Nations Population Fund (UNFPA), the United Nations Children's Fund (UNICEF), the World Health Organization (WHO), the World Bank, the International Planned Parenthood

Federation (IPPF), and the Population Council. The agency aims to assess the problem of maternal deaths and disability and to recommend solutions. Links to a number of full-text fact sheets, pamphlets, and compilations of data are provided.

UNAIDS

www.unaids.org

This site includes information on the projects, research, and conferences sponsored by UNAIDS and aimed at strengthening and supporting an expanded worldwide response to the HIV/AIDS epidemic. The site contains an extensive collection of full-text documents and publications, including country-by-country data on HIV/AIDS prevalence and prevention indicators, and the most recent *Global Reports* published by the organization.

United Nations Children's Emergency Fund (UNICEF)

www.unicef.org/safe

This site provides information on all UNICEF programmes and research. The site also makes available UNICEF's annual *Progress of Nations and State of the World's Children* reports. There are sections within the site that summarize UNICEF research into children's and women's health, and in particular the organization's research into promoting safe motherhood and preventing mother-to-child transmission of HIV/AIDS. The statistical section of the website (www.unicef.org/statis/) allows users to click on a map to obtain statistics for specific countries or a given region. The information includes statistics on reproductive health (Total Fertility Rate, Contraceptive Prevalence, and Maternal Mortality Ratio), education rates, and other health and welfare indicators.

United Nations High Commissioner for Human Rights (UNHCHR)

www.unhchr.ch

This website offers image and text versions of the organizational structure for the United Nations system in the field of human rights. From this site, one can access the United Nations Treaty Bodies State Party Reports and Concluding Observations for the following: the Economic Covenant, the Political Covenant, the Women's Convention, the Race Conventions and the Children's Convention, among others. 'Status of Ratification' information is also listed by country and by treaty.

Committee against Torture
www.unhchr.ch/html/menu2/6/cat.htm

Committee on Economic, Social and Cultural Rights
www.unhchr.ch/html/menu2/6/cescr.htm

Committee on the Elimination of Discrimination against Women
www.un.org/womenwatch/daw/cedaw/

Committee on the Elimination of Racial Discrimination
www.unhchr.ch/html/menu2/6/cerd.htm

Committee on the Rights of the Child

www.unhchr.ch/html/menu2/6/crc.htm

Human Rights Committee

www.unhchr.ch/html/menu2/6/crc.htm

United Nations, Population Division

http://www.unpopulation.org/htm

A United Nation website maintained by the Population Division, Department of Economic and Social Affairs whose responsibility is monitoring and appraisal of the broad range of areas in the field of population. The website provides first-hand information such as up-to-date statistics, publications, and various reports prepared by the UN bodies.

United Nations Population Fund (UNFPA)

www.unfpa.org

This website provides an overview of UNFPA's work in the programme area of reproductive health, including family planning and sexual health. The site also provides links to a number of full-text UNFPA publications, including its advocacy series collection, technical publications for health service providers, and its annual *State of World Population* report.

Women's Human Rights Resources (WHRR)

www.law-lib.utoronto.ca/Diana/mainpage.htm

This site is maintained by the Women's Human Rights Resources group of the Bora Laskin Law Library at the Faculty of Law, University of Toronto, in collaboration with law librarians, lawyers, students, researchers, activists, and human rights experts around the world. The section on reproductive rights and sexual health contains annotated lists of articles, documents, cases, and other resources on the subject, many of which are linked to full-text online versions. In addition, the site provides many specific topics that contain information related to reproductive and sexual health, including, but not limited to: age of marriage, marriage and family life, health and well-being, and violence against women. There are also research guides available online which describe briefly some strategies for researching in the areas of international human rights, and international women's rights.

Women Link Worldwide

http://www.womenslinkworldwide.org

This website functions as an information clearinghouse on judicial precedent affecting women's rights from various regions. It consists of national case-laws and case-laws decided by international courts such as Inter-American and European courts of human rights.

Women Watch

http://www.un.org/womenwatch

A UN website consisting of materials on different activities of the UN bodies working on advancement and empowerment of women. It also provides a link to a number of relevant UN agencies.

World Bank

www.worldbank.org

This website provides information on World Bank projects and initiatives to alleviate poverty around the world. It contains sections which focus on the economic aspects of reproductive health, including safe motherhood and HIV/AIDS.

World Health Organization, Department of Reproductive Health and Research

www.who.int/reproductive-health

This section of the WHO website contains information on WHO research projects on family and reproductive health, as well as links to a number of online versions of WHO documents, including guidelines for health care providers, WHO fact sheets, and training manuals.

World Health Organization, Gender and Women's Health Department

http://www.who.int/frh-whd

This section of the WHO website provides various online papers addressing issues on women and health such as female genital cutting, women and HIV/AIDS, violence against women, and women and tobacco.

Index